Laboratory Medicine in Clinical Practice

Practical and Efficient Use of the Laboratory in Patient Management

Harvey N. Mandell
Editor

Margaret Johnson Bia
Associate Editor

John Wright • PSG Inc
Boston   Bristol   London
1983

Library of Congress Cataloging in Publication Data
Main entry under title:

Laboratory medicine in clinical practice.
  Bibliography: p.
  Includes index.
    1. Diagnosis, Laboratory.   I. Mandell, Harvey N.
II. Bia, Margaret Johnson.   [DNLM: 1. Diagnosis,
Laboratory.   2. Laboratories—Utilization.   QY 4 L1232]
RB37.L275   1983   616.07′5   83-1253
ISBN 0-7236-7051-X

Published simultaneously by:
John Wright • PSG Inc, 545 Great Road, Littleton,
Massachusetts 01460, U.S.A.
John Wright & Sons Ltd. 823–825 Bath Road,
Bristol BS4 5NU, England

Medicine is an ever-changing science. As new research and clinical experience broaden our knowledge, changes in treatment and drug therapy are
required. The authors and the publisher of this work have made every effort to ensure that the treatment and drug dosage schedules herein are
accurate and in accord with the standards accepted at the time of publication. Readers are advised, however, to check the product information
sheet included in the package of each drug they plan to administer to be
certain that changes have not been made in the recommended dose or in
the indications and contraindications for administration. This recommendation is of particular importance in regard to new or infrequently used
drugs.

Printed in the United States of America

International Standard Book Number: 0-7236-7051-X

Library of Congress Catalog Card Number: 83-1253

To Marjorie

Dr. Harvey N. Mandell is Medical Director of The William W. Backus Hosptial in Norwich, Connecticut, a post he assumed after 22 years of private practice in internal medicine. He is Associate Clinical Professor of Medicine at Yale University School of Medicine. An alumnus of Dartmouth College, Dr. Mandell attended Dartmouth Medical School before transferring to the College of Physicians and Surgeons, Columbia University in the City of New York, where he was graduated. He is a Diplomate of the American Board of Internal Medicine, a Fellow of the American College of Physicians, and a member of the Connecticut and American Societies of Internal Medicine. Other professional organizations in which Dr. Mandell holds member-ship are the American Medical Writers Association and the Medical Chess Club of America, where he meets with indifferent success.

About the Editor

P. W. Askenase, MD Professor of Medicine, Department of Medicine, Yale University School of Medicine, New Haven, Connecticut

Colin E. Atterbury, MD Associate Professor of Medicine, Liver Disease Unit, Department of Internal Medicine, Yale University School of Medicine

Chief, Intermediate Care Section, Veterans Administration Medical Center, West Haven, Connecticut

D. N. Baron, MD, DSc Professor of Chemical Pathology, Royal Free Hospital School of Medicine, London, United Kingdom

Frank J. Bia, MD, MPH Assistant Professor of Medicine and Laboratory Medicine, Infectious Disease Section, Department of Medicine and Department of Laboratory Medicine, Yale University School of Medicine

Veterans Administration Medical Center, West Haven, Connecticut

Margaret Johnson Bia, MD Assistant Professor of Medicine, Department of Internal Medicine, Section of Nephrology, Yale University School of Medicine, New Haven, Connecticut

John A. Bosso, PharmD Associate Professor of Clinical Pharmacy, Adjunct Associate Professor of Pediatrics, College of Pharmacy and School of Medicine, University of Utah, Salt Lake City, Utah

Yoram Bujanover, MD Lecturer in Pediatrics, Pediatric Gastroenterologist, Tel Aviv Medical Center and Sackler School of Medicine, Tel Aviv University, Tel Aviv, Israel

■ **John D. Clemens, MD** Assistant Professor of Medicine, Yale University School of Medicine, New Haven, Connecticut

Kenneth L. Cohen, MD Associate Professor of Medicine, Department of Internal Medicine, Yale University School of Medicine

Associate Chief of Staff for Ambulatory Care, Veterans Administration Medical Center, West Haven, Connecticut

Contributors

Donald R. Coustan, MD Associate Professor of Obstetrics and Gynecology, Brown University Program in Medicine

Director of Maternal-Fetal Medicine, Women and Infants Hospital of Rhode Island, Providence, Rhode Island

James Donaldson, MD Associate Professor of Neurology and Internal Medicine, University of Connecticut School of Medicine, Farmington, Connecticut

K. Erlendsson, MD Postdoctoral Fellow, Department of Medicine, Yale University School of Medicine, New Haven, Connecticut

Charles K. Francis, MD Associate Professor of Medicine (Cardiology), Yale University School of Medicine, New Haven, Connecticut

Eric P. Gall, MD Associate Professor, Internal Medicine (Clinical Immunology), Surgery (Orthopedics), University of Arizona College of Medicine, Tucson, Arizona

Tuvia Gilat, MD Professor of Medicine, Chief, Department of Gastroenterology, Tel Aviv Medical Center and Sackler School of Medicine, Tel Aviv University, Tel Aviv, Israel

Richard D. Kayne, MD Clinical Instructor of Medicine, Department of Internal Medicine, Yale University School of Medicine, New Haven, Connecticut

Gary T. Kinasewitz, MD Associate Professor of Medicine, Louisiana State University School of Medicine, Shreveport, Louisiana

Alan S. Kliger, MD Associate Clinical Professor of Medicine, Yale University School of Medicine,

Director, Dialysis Service, Yale-New Haven Hospital, New Haven, Connecticut

Harvey N. Mandell, MD Medical Director, The William W. Backus Hospital, Norwich, Connecticut

Associate Clinical Professor of Medicine, Yale University School of Medicine, New Haven, Connecticut

Peter McPhedran, MD Associate Professor of
Laboratory Medicine and Medicine, Yale University
School of Medicine

Director of Hematology Laboratory, Yale-New Haven
Hospital, New Haven, Connecticut

Jean M. Nappi, PharmD Assistant Professor of
Clinical Pharmacy, Adjunct Assistant Professor of
Medicine, College of Pharmacy and School of Medicine,
University of Utah, Salt Lake City, Utah

Yochanan Peled, PhD Lecturer in Pathological
Chemistry, Head, Gastrointestinal Laboratory, Tel Aviv
Medical Center and Sackler School of Medicine, Tel Aviv
University, Tel Aviv, Israel

Richard D. Plotz, MD Instructor in Pathology,
Brown University Program in Medicine

Attending Pathologist, Women and Infants Hospital of
Rhode Island, Providence, Rhode Island

David L. Rutlen, MD Assistant Professor of Medicine
(Cardiology), Yale University School of Medicine, New
Haven, Connecticut

Arthur P. Staddon, MD Assistant Professor of
Medicine (Hematology–Oncology), University of
Pennsylvania, Presbyterian–University of Pennsylvania
Medical Center, Philadelphia, Pennsylvania

T. J. Swartz, MD Postdoctoral Fellow, Department of
Medicine, Yale University School of Medicine, New
Haven, Connecticut

T. J. Tinghitella, PhD Assistant Director, Clinical
Immunology Laboratory, Lecturer in Laboratory
Medicine, Department of Laboratory Medicine, New
Haven, Connecticut

Contents

Preface xiii

Acknowledgments xv

Introduction xvii

1 "Normal" Results, Specificity, Sensitivity, Predictive Value 1
John D. Clemens

2 The International System of Units (SI) and Its Application to Laboratory Medicine 17
D. N. Baron

3 The Laboratory in Hematological Diseases 25
Peter McPhedran

4 Utilization of Drug Levels 61
Jean M. Nappi and John A. Bosso

5 Interpretation of Blood Gas and Electrolyte Values 77
Harvey N. Mandell and Margaret Johnson Bia

6 The Laboratory in Renal Diseases 91
Margaret Johnson Bia and Alan S. Kliger

7 The Laboratory in Cardiovascular Diseases 111
David L. Rutlen and Charles K. Francis

8 The Laboratory in Pulmonary Diseases .. 119
Gary T. Kinasewitz

9 Clinical Infectious Diseases and the Microbiology Laboratory 145
Frank J. Bia

10 Methods of Immunodiagnosis of Infectious Diseases 163
T. J. Tinghitella

11 Laboratory Tests in Clinical Immunology and Allergy 175
P. W. Askenase, T. J. Swartz, K. Erlendsson, and T. J. Tinghitella

12 The Laboratory in Rheumatic Diseases ..197
Eric P. Gall

13 The Laboratory in Diseases of the Gastrointestinal Tract 211
Tuvia Gilat, Yochanan Peled, and Yoram Bujanover

14 The Laboratory in Liver Diseases.............231
Colin E. Atterbury

15 The Laboratory in Neurological and Muscular Diseases..................................263
James Donaldson

16 The Laboratory in Diabetes Mellitus and Hypoglycemia 269
Kenneth L. Cohen and Richard D. Kayne

17 The Laboratory in Endocrinology.............281
Pituitary Disease, Thyroid Disease, Parathyroid Disease and Calcium Metabolism, Adrenal Gland, Gonadal Disease, The Multiple Endocrine Neoplasia Syndromes, Carcinoid Syndrome
Kenneth L. Cohen and Richard D. Kayne

18 The Laboratory in Oncology.....................347
Arthur P. Staddon

19 The Laboratory in Diseases Associated with Pregnancy..353
Donald R. Coustan and Richard D. Plotz

Index..387

Now, here, you see, it takes all the running you can do, to keep in the same place. If you want to get somewhere else, you must run at least twice as fast as that! **Lewis Carroll**
"Through the Looking Glass"

This view of life, through the looking glass, must seem painfully familiar to the practicing physician trying to keep up with the explosion in laboratory medicine. It is a paradox of modern medicine that, as the laboratory provides for greater precision in diagnosis and treatment, practicing physicians are becoming less critical and efficient in its use. The difficulties for the physician in practice are understandable. The last two to three decades have been historically unique in the rate at which new biomedical knowledge has been produced and applied. New insights into the basic mechanisms of disease have been translated into new diagnostic tests and therapeutic modalities. Both diagnosis and therapy have become more sophisticated and specialized. It is not surprising, then, that the busy clinician finds it difficult to keep abreast of the bewildering array of new laboratory tests. New tests are frequently introduced through journal articles, consultants' suggestions, conferences, postgraduate courses, and newsletters. Often there is inadequate perspective provided on the use of the test in a specific clinical circumstance, or in relation to other existing tests. The physician, understandably, continues to use the strategy of laboratory testing that has proven helpful in the past and merely adds new tests to established patterns. The result is proliferation of testing rather than substitution of newer and better approaches for outdated ones.

A laboratory medicine textbook should focus not only on what tests are available and what information they provide, but on a strategy of the use of tests in clinical circumstances. Unfortunately, many laboratory medicine textbooks are written more for the person performing the tests than for the person ordering them. In these kinds of textbooks, the test is primary and the clinical circumstance in which it is used is secondary. Textbooks of medicine tend to reverse the process, reporting appropriate laboratory diagnostic information under specific clinical diagnoses. The present text pulls together both kinds of information into a usable system-oriented approach. The practicing physician may pose questions about disorders of an organ system, approaches to the evaluation of a clinical or laboratory abnormality, or the usefulness of specific laboratory tests and find the answers easily in this book.

Physicians should order laboratory tests to answer specific diagnostic or therapeutic questions, not just to document well-established clinical–laboratory associations. When careful clinical assessment is followed by a clear formulation of questions, focused use of the laboratory permits more efficient, effective, and safer patient management. After formulating the correct clinical questions, physicians should be aware of the kinds of answers that can come from the laboratory. This requires knowledge of not only what is available, but also of the sensitivity, specificity, reproducibility, risk, and cost of the tests and their likelihood of answering the questions posed. All this information, along with a healthy respect for the biological variation and the potential for laboratory error, is necessary for proper use of the laboratory. This book permits easy access to this information in a well-written text, obviously intended for the practicing physician.

Samuel O. Thier, MD
Sterling Professor and Chairman
Department of Internal Medicine
Yale University School of Medicine
New Haven, Connecticut

I thank Tom Fleming, former editor of **Postgraduate Medicine** for publishing **Gases and 'Lytes Without Anguish,** which became the seed for this book. Thanks to Will Strauss of John Wright • PSG Inc for reading Gases and 'Lytes, inviting me to do this book, and guiding me through uncharted wilderness. An extraordinary thanks to Karen who did so many things so well with no more audible complaint than an occasional sigh. Thanks beyond words to Marjorie and to our three sons, Ross, Marc, and David, who have put up with so much.

Acknowledgments

Each of us physicians who has ever ordered a test from the laboratory has felt at least once the chagrin of not knowing what to do with the results when the report from the laboratory arrived. It did not mean necessarily that we were bad doctors or that we lacked intelligence. It did mean that we may have been, at such times, a little careless in thinking things through. It does not make sense to order a test if the ordering physician is not familiar with its significance unless it is something a consultant has asked for and whose results the consultant can use.

Yet, we all have done it. If anyone claims complete innocence from such an offense, let that physician wait. He or she will inevitably join the rest of us.

It is not entirely our fault. Like the rest of medicine and its sciences, the laboratory's activities have expanded rapidly, and no physician, whether generalist or specialist, can possibly know all that his or her laboratory can do. Clinical pathologists (chemical pathologists) who spend all day in their laboratories are surprised occasionally by the variety of procedures their own or referral laboratories can do.

When you first begin to use a clinical laboratory, it is a good idea to find out first what that laboratory can and cannot do for you. It is not helpful to find out at midnight that the laboratory will not do a stat serum amylase. The physician who uses a laboratory must either know or have ready access to all the normal ranges of tests in that laboratory. Methods differ, and the normal values you learned in medical school may not be sacred. Our English contributor suggests that the word normal should always be embraced by quotation marks when used to describe the "normal" range. No one can disagree, and we shall assume such limitations throughout the book.

The classical textbooks have, in general, handled explanations of laboratory tests admirably within sections of various disorders, but this type of material, by its nature, cannot be gathered in a single section of a textbook of internal medicine or surgery for quick referral by a searching physician. We have tried here to provide a single source where a doctor can find the clinical importance of the tests needed to help make a diagnosis, solve a problem, follow the course of a patient's progress, and help manage the patient.

We should not take the laboratory's excellence for granted. All laboratories are not excellent, as all of us physicians are not excellent. If your laboratory does not get the required financial backing or if the head of the laboratory does not demand high standards, you may get results which are inaccurate and possibly misleading. If you have any doubt, send samples of the same specimen to more than one laboratory and compare results.

Physicians should visit their laboratories and see what they are like. The clinician should find out who in the laboratory can answer questions and help with problem solving. Most of all, the practicing physician should use the clinical pathologist (chemical pathologist) as a consultant and not hesitate to discuss any questions he or she has about what the laboratory can offer in patient care.

To make the best use of laboratory results, you must have a firm understanding of the significance of false-positive and false-negative. This requires a knowledge of your patient. If you measure the alkaline phosphatase level of 1000 healthy, asymptomatic men and women, including those pregnant, a finding outside the normal range is more likely to be unimportant than the same result from a series of determinations of the same enzyme done on serum from 1000 men and women with known or suspected biliary, hepatic, and bone disease. Each chapter writer assumes that the tests requested are done in conjunction with a careful history and physical examination. No one has suggested that anything in this book should replace "Hx & Px."

I have asked each contributor to write his or her chapter solely for practicing physicians assuming that the reader's main goal in life is the diagnosis and treatment of patients who are or may be sick. Each contributor realizes that most practicing physicians are well trained in clinical medicine, but are not specialists in laboratory medicine and not superspecialists in narrow fields. The writers were asked to present their chapters in such a way that they could be read easily from beginning to end. Then the careful reader would finish with a good grasp of what the laboratory has to offer in that field, and the chapter could still be useful for quick reference when needed. Most owners of this book probably will not read from page one consecutively to the end. I hope that readers will first look at the chapters describing "normal" values, sensitivity and specificity, and the International System of Units, (SI). American readers need not panic at SI. The chapter is included for our education and to prepare us for the future. The book itself retains the old comfortable units of measurement, but if there should be another edition, SI may be accepted and required by then. The readers might then read the chapters in the fields best known to them that will either confirm their own knowledge or give them a clearer idea of what the laboratory can do when used wisely. From there, readers will probably be directed to the various chapters by the types of patients they serve that day or by innate curiosity leading them down new paths.

Failure to use a laboratory efficiently may delay proper diagnosis or lead to incorrect assumptions about a patient's course. Inevitably, increased and unnecessary costs to patients and expensive waste of laboratory personnel's time will follow. Optimal use of laboratories will, of course, be of inestimable aid in diagnosing and treating the ills of our patients.

Imaging techniques have, in general, been omitted because their inclusion would make a small book too big. The exception is the chapter on pulmonary medicine. Because imaging plays such an integral role in diagnosis there, no clinician could do without it.

Numbered references cited in a text can be distracting. For this reason, each contributor has concluded his or her chapter with a list of suggested readings. I hope readers will approve and be encouraged to read further.

Contributors were forbidden to use footnotes with the equal expectation of readers' approval.

Since the book will be published simultaneously in North America and the United Kingdom, contributors were asked to avoid jargon familiar to readers in one part of the world but mysterious to readers elsewhere. Whenever possible, the contributors have included British, American, Canadian, and Australian synonyms. If they have failed in any instance, I ask readers in the other countries not to feel slighted but to try to pick up each other's terminology. Perhaps the value of this book will overcome a bit of parochialism here and there.

Harvey N. Mandell, MD

All practicing physicians must interpret laboratory data. The manner in which they interpret such data depends a great deal upon the purposes for which the tests are obtained. Laboratory tests may be requested to establish diagnoses to estimate prognosis, to choose and regulate therapy, and to monitor the progression of disease. This chapter focuses on the evaluation of tests used for diagnostic purposes.

The diagnostic function of laboratory data is to identify the presence or absence of disease at the time the data are acquired. The results of some tests, often referred to as "gold standard tests," serve as the definitions of disease. For example, the result of liver biopsy obtained to diagnose hepatitis defines the presence or absence of the disease. Although one may be concerned about the expertise of the pathologists, or about observer variability among pathologists, one cannot resort to a more definitive procedure to confirm or deny the biopsy results. A different set of considerations applies to a second category of diagnostic tests, called "surrogate tests." Surrogate test results do not define a disease. Instead, such results correlate imperfectly with the results of suitable gold standard tests. Examples of surrogate tests include tuberculin tests for tuberculosis, serum transaminase levels for hepatitis, and exercise tolerance tests for ischemic heart disease.

Surrogate tests, often cheaper, less invasive, or more acceptable than definitive tests, are the predominant types of diagnostic tests ordered by clinicians. However, because surrogate test results correlate imperfectly with gold standard test results, the interpretation of surrogate test data frequently is not straightforward. Further confusing the situation is a bewildering array of terminology intended to guide surrogate test use and to evaluate surrogate test performance. These terms include "range of normal," "sensitivity," "specificity," "accuracy for positive prediction," and "accuracy for negative prediction." The following discussion explains these terms and describes their usefulness and limitations in clinical practice.

Range of Normal

Virtually all clinical laboratories provide a range of normal for test results reported on numerical scales. This range is intended to indicate a span of "normal" laboratory values attributable to the expected variation of test results among nondiseased persons. Values outside the range are designated "abnormal" because they cannot easily be attributed to variation in healthy persons. The determination of the normal range is accomplished by inspection of the distribution of test values in a selected healthy patient population (Figure 1-1). Typically, test values lying within the central 95% of this

"Normal" Results, Specificity, Sensitivity, Predictive Value

John D. Clemens

1

selected population (eg, excluding the 2.5% of the population with the lowest test values and the 2.5% of the population with the highest test values) is declared the "normal range." Values outside the central 95% of the population are termed "abnormal," despite their appearance in non-diseased subjects.

Although simple and intuitively appealing, the normal range has several problems. One major problem arises from the fact that the range of normal is derived from the distribution of test values for healthy persons, without consideration of the distribution of tests values for diseased patients. This "isolated" approach to constructing the limits of normal has at least two major adverse consequences. First, because the distribution of test values for diseased patients is not considered in the determination of the normal range, the normal range does not permit an assessment of the relative likelihood of disease and nondisease for any given test value. This problem is illustrated in Figure 1-2. Each of the three panels of this figure displays a different relationship between the distributions of laboratory values for diseased and nondiseased populations. The top panel depicts a test for which the distributions are entirely distinct and nonoverlapping. In this situation, 95% of nondiseased persons and 100% of diseased persons are correctly classified by the normal range. A normal test value always corresponds to a nondiseased individual, and an abnormal test value almost always corresponds to a

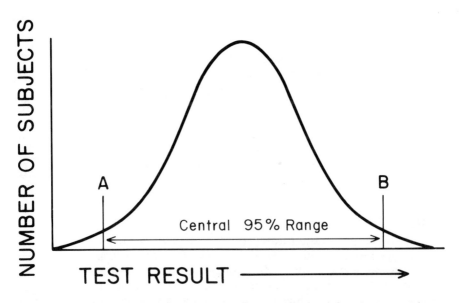

Figure 1-1 Range of normal for a hypothetical test whose results are expressed on a numerical scale. The abscissa notes the values for the test results, and the ordinate describes the number of persons in the population having each particular test result. The distribution of values in the population follows a smooth, symmetric, bell-shaped (Gaussian) configuration. The test result at A cuts off the 2.5% of the population with lowest values, and the result at B cuts off the 2.5% with highest values. The range between values A and B includes the central 95% of the population and commonly demarcates the limits of normal.

3

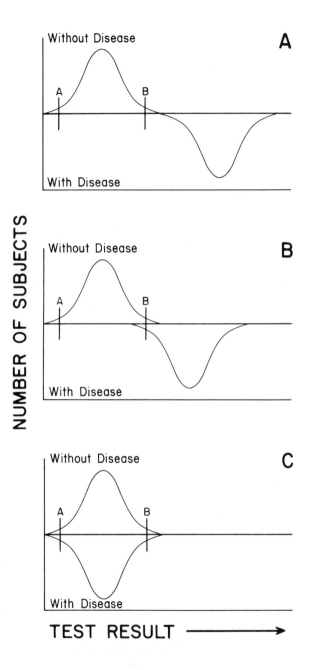

Figure 1-2 Relationship of test results for populations without disease (above the horizontal) and with disease (below the horizontal). The central 95% range of values for populations without disease defines the range of normal and is demarcated by lines A and B in each panel. The top panel **A** depicts the situation in which the distributions of test results for diseased and nondiseased populations are entirely distinct, the middle panel **B** depicts partial overlap of the distributions, and the bottom panel **C** shows identical distributions for the two populations.

diseased individual. The middle panel depicts a more typical clinical situation in which there is substantial overlap between the distributions of test results for nondiseased and diseased persons. Ninety-five percent of the nondiseased group is still correctly classified by the normal range, but a substantial fraction of the diseased is incorrectly classified as normal. As a result, a normal laboratory result no longer predicts that the person lacks disease with 100% confidence, and the ability of an abnormal test result to predict that a patient is diseased is less than in the situation where test value distributions do not overlap. In the bottom panel, the overlap between the two test value distributions has reached the extreme in which the two distributions entirely coincide. As a result, at each test value, both inside and outside of the normal range, patients have equal probabilities of being nondiseased and diseased. Thus, the confidence with which values within the normal range predict absence of disease and values outside of the normal range predict disease is dependent upon the relative distributions of test values for nondiseased and diseased populations. The range of normal concept ignores the distributions of test values for diseased populations.

Another problem arises from the practice of arbitrarily designating 5% of test values from healthy individuals as "abnormal." This convention creates a high likelihood of labeling a healthy individual "abnormal," especially when multiple tests are performed, as in multiphasic laboratory screening of patients.

If the results of tests are independent of one another (Table 1-1), there will be at least one abnormal result in 23% of completely healthy persons when five tests are performed. If 20 tests are performed, 65% of healthy persons will be falsely labeled as "abnormal" by at least one test result. To avoid this problem of falsely abnormal results, and the resulting problems of unnecessary further tests and therapies, it is desirable to determine the range of normal in a fashion that strikes a balance between mislabeling healthy persons "abnormal" and mislabeling diseased patients as "normal." These desiderata can only be accomplished by considering the joint distributions of test values for healthy and diseased populations when demarcating the limits of normal.

Several additional problems with the range of normal are epidemiologic in nature. Although the concept of the range of normal is based on the distribution of test values for healthy persons, in practice many such ranges are constructed from patient groups with variable admixtures of healthy and diseased subjects (eg, inpatient populations). Such admixtures often create wider normal ranges than would occur in a completely healthy population. Another defect is the frequent lack of attention given to several nondisease variables that have major effects on test results. Examples of these extraneous variables include age, gender, race, posture, level of activity, diet, drug intake, biorhythms, and unrelated illnesses. Inadequate consideration of the effects of these confounding variables may result in inapplicable and misleading normal ranges. For example, it is now appreciated that the upper limit of normal for blood glucose varies substantially with age, making it inappropriate to employ the same normal range for a 20 year old and an octogenarian. Another source of test variability often ignored in determining the range of normal is laboratory error, either in specimen collection or in laboratory analysis. Since laboratory error augments the variability of test

Table 1-1
Probability of Finding at Least One Falsely Abnormal
Test in a Completely Healthy Individual as Increasing Numbers
of Tests Are Performed

Number of Tests Performed	Probability that At Least One Test will be Abnormal in a Completely Healthy Individual
1	.05
5	.23
10	.40
15	.54
20	.64

results, it inevitably expands the width of the range of normal. If this expansion attributable to laboratory error is not considered, an excessive number of falsely abnormal results will fall outside of an inappropriately narrow normal range.

A final problem of the range of normal is statistical in nature. The actual distribution of test results in a population is rarely directly examined to demarcate the inner 95% range. Instead, a particular model distribution, often referred to as "Gaussian," is often assumed to describe the test values in the population. In a Gaussian distribution, test values assume a symmetric, bell-shaped configuration, such as the distribution displayed in Figure 1-1. Apart from its esthetic appeal, the Gaussian model affords tremendous computational convenience. To obtain the inner 95% range of values, one merely calculates the mean (or average) value as the center of the distribution and the span of test values corresponding to two standard deviations on either side of the mean as the desired central 95% range. The actual distribution of test values need not be plotted and directly examined. Unfortunately, the actual distribution of results for most tests is rarely symmetric or bell shaped. Therefore, calculations of the range of normal with Gaussian distributional assumptions frequently leads to aberrant limits of normal. For example, if most members of a population have low test values, but a few members have very high test values, the distribution of values will be skewed, not symmetric (Figure 1-3). If a mean is calculated, it will be affected by the high test values of a few members of the population and will lie to the right (at a higher value) of the values for most of the population. In addition, calculation of 2 standard deviations on either side of the mean creates an anomaly. Although the actual test results do not include negative values (eg, one never encounters negative values for serum sodium or potassium), the 95% range demarcated by the mean ± 2 standard deviations includes values extending far below zero. This aberrancy occurs because the distribution of values is not Gaussian. Only when the distribution of values is Gaussian does the mean ± 2 standard deviations demarcate the central 95% range of values for the population. Obviously, this defect, not an inherent flaw of the range of normal concept, can be remedied by examining the actual distribution of test values for the fulfillment of Gaussian assumptions. When these assumptions are not satisfied, normal ranges can be determined in a satisfactory fashion by directly inspecting the distribution of test values and demarcating the desired central range.

6

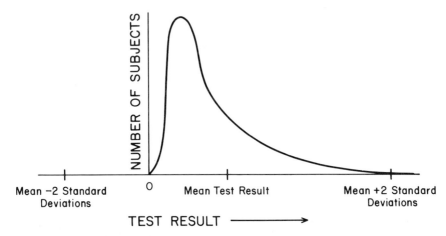

Figure 1-3 Skewed distribution of test values in a population without disease. Although all test values actually obtained in the population are positive, the use of the mean ± 2 standard deviations to demarcate the "normal" central 95% range in this non-Gaussian distribution causes the extension of the range to nonexistent negative test values.

The concept and the practice of the range of normal thus suffers from several flaws, creating substantial uncertainty in interpreting the meaning of normal and abnormal results. This uncertainty most frequently occurs when an unexpectedly abnormal result is obtained in an apparently healthy patient. This problem was addressed in a study performed by A. R. Bradwell and colleagues at the Queen Elizabeth Medical Centre in Birmingham, England. Among 174 patients with laboratory abnormalities that were not expected on the basis of the original clinical presentation, 71 (41%) had normal results on repeat testing. An additional 74 (42%) had abnormalities that were explainable on the basis of later-appreciated associations with illnesses known to be present at the time of testing, or on the basis of such factors as age, gender, and laboratory error that had not been accounted for in the original determination of the limits of normal. This study indicates that unexpectedly abnormal test results, particularly those that are marginally abnormal, are very likely falsely abnormal and should be repeated before initiating further diagnostic evaluation. Even remarkably abnormal results which are discrepant with clinical findings should be repeated to rule out laboratory error before extensive diagnostic evaluation or treatment is begun.

Indexes of Test Proficiency

The range of normal designates "normal" and "abnormal" test values without reference to the distribution of values for diseased persons. In contrast to this isolated approach to test results, the standard indexes of test proficiency consider the joint distributions of test values for diseased and nondiseased populations. These indexes, which are known as test sensitivity, test specificity, test accuracy for negative prediction, and test accuracy for positive prediction, are thus referred to as "correlated," rather than isolated, indexes.

The distributions of test values for diseased and nondiseased persons are considered jointly in Figure 1-4. The vertical line denotes the test cutoff: results to the right of the cutoff are considered "abnormal," whereas results to the left of the cutoff are deemed "normal." It can be seen that four groups of individuals are created by the conjunction of disease status and test status: a diseased group with abnormal, "true-positive," test results (region A); a diseased group with normal, "false-negative," test results (region C); a nondiseased group with normal, "true-negative," test results (region D); and a nondiseased group with abnormal, "false-positive," test results (region B). Since any population of tested individuals can be demarcated in this fashion, and since these demarcations denote the various ways that a test can correctly or incorrectly designate disease status, these four types of results comprise the basis for evaluating diagnostic test proficiency.

Sensitivity and Specificity

The most commonly used indexes of test proficiency are sensitivity and specificity. Sensitivity refers to the proportion of diseased patients who are correctly identified by abnormal test results. That is, test sensitivity is the

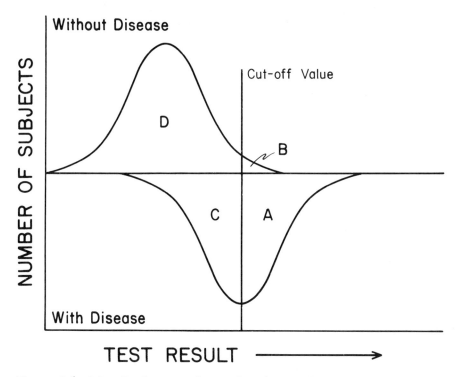

Figure 1-4 Joint distributions of test values for populations with and without a hypothetical disease. Test values to the right of the cutoff are "abnormal," and values to the left of the cutoff are "normal." Four groups of patients are demarcated by disease and test result status: patients with true-positive results (A), patients with false-negative results (C), patients with true-negative results (D), and patients with false-positive results (B).

proportion of the diseased persons with true-positive results. In contrast, specificity denotes the proportion of nondiseased persons who are correctly identified by normal test results. In other words, test specificity is the proportion of nondiseased persons who are correctly identified by true-negative test results. The calculation of sensitivity is illustrated by the results displayed in Table 1-2. The lowercase letters a, b, c, and d correspond to the number of persons in regions A, B, C, and D, respectively, in Figure 1-4. With this arrangement, sensitivity is $a/(a + c)$, and specificity is $d/(b + d)$. It can readily be seen that values for both sensitivity and specificity range from 0 (absent test proficiency) to 1 (perfect test proficiency).

The values for sensitivity and specificity for a given diagnostic test and a particular disease are often presented as if they are immutable. This is far from the truth. First, one can arbitrarily shift the cutoff between "normal" and "abnormal" test results. Thus, in Figure 1-4, by moving the cutoff to the right (eg, to a higher test value), regions D and C increase in size, whereas regions A and B decrease in size. The reverse occurs if the cutoff is moved to the left (eg, to a lower test value). With each change in the position of the test cutoff value, a different result for test sensitivity and test specificity emerges. A useful way of displaying the change of test sensitivity and test specificity with various test cutoff values is provided by the "receiver operator characteristic." The receiver operator characteristic of a given test is derived by plotting test sensitivity against $(1 - \text{test specificity})$ for each test cutoff value. In Figure 1-5, points A, B, C, D, and E denote sensitivity and $(1 - \text{specificity})$ values at five different test cutoff points for a single diagnostic test and a particular disease. As illustrated by the receiver operator characteristic in the figure, most tests cannot simultaneously attain both perfect sensitivity and perfect specificity, regardless of the test value chosen as the cutoff. Furthermore, increased test sensitivity is usually obtainable only at the expense of decreased test specificity, and increased test specificity is often attained at the expense of diminished test sensitivity.

Sensitivity and specificity may also vary as a function of the spectrum of disease represented in the tested patient population. Ransohoff and Feinstein have noted that the extent of disease may affect test sensitivity. Many tests give results revealing high sensitivity for anatomically or functionally extensive disease, but lower sensitivity for limited disease. For example, carcinoembryonic antigen (CEA) was initially regarded as a highly sensitive marker for colorectal carcinoma. Unfortunately, studies noting high sensitivity usually studied patients with widespread carcinoma. When CEA was subsequently evaluated for its sensitivity in detecting early colorectal carcinoma, the test was found to have an unacceptably low sensitivity for use as

Table 1-2
Results of Diagnostic Tests

Result of Test	Confirmed Disease Status		Total
	Present	*Absent*	
Positive	a	b	a + b
Negative	c	d	c + d
Total	a + c	b + d	a + b + c + d

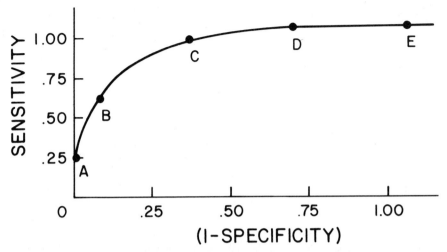

Figure 1-5 Receiver-operator characteristic for a hypothetical diagnostic test and disease. Points A, B, C, D, and E locate test sensitivity and (1 – specificity) at five different arbitrarily chosen test cutoff values.

a screening test. An additional phenomenon noted by Ransohoff and Feinstein is the variation of test specificity that occurs as a result of comorbid illnesses (eg, illnesses other than the disease of interest), demographic factors (eg, age and gender), and miscellaneous exogenous factors (eg, drug intake) which may generate false-positive test results in the nondiseased group chosen for testing. Depending on the prevalence of these factors in the nondiseased group, test specificity may be very high or very low. For example, many factors apart from colorectal carcinoma are known to elevate CEA. These factors include inflammatory bowel disease, pancreatitis, alcoholic cirrhosis, and a wide variety of other gastrointestinal and nongastrointestinal neoplasms. Several studies excluding such patients from the noncolorectal carcinoma group tested with CEA reported low numbers of false-positive test results and a high specificity of CEA for colorectal carcinoma. However, studies that included significant numbers of patients with these diseases reported substantial numbers of false-positive results and low test specificity.

Because test sensitivity often depends on the extensiveness of disease in the diseased population, and specificity depends on the prevalence of a variety of demographic and clinical factors in the nondiseased population, no single values for sensitivity and specificity are adequate to describe test performance. Consequently, the practicing clinician should carefully scrutinize reports evaluating test sensitivity and specificity to ascertain that the test was evaluated in populations of diseased and nondiseased individuals that are likely to be similar to the patients tested in clinical practice.

Accuracy for Positive and Negative Prediction

One impediment to applying values for sensitivity and specificity to clinical practice is that these values are constructed in a clinically backward fashion.

The calculation of test sensitivity answers the question, "Given that we know that the patient has the disease, what is the likelihood of an abnormal test result?," and the calculation of test specificity answers the question, "Given that we know the patient does not have the disease, what is the likelihood of a normal test result?" Unfortunately, at the time that a diagnostic test result is interpreted, the clinician does not know whether the patient is diseased. Indeed, if the clinician had this knowledge, there would be little reason to order the diagnostic test in the first place. In the usual circumstance, the clinician is confronted with abnormal and normal test results and must answer the questions, "Given that the patient has an abnormal test result, what is the likelihood that the patient has the disease?," and "Given that the patient has a normal test result, what is the likelihood that the patient lacks the disease?" The answer to the first question is called the accuracy for positive test prediction, and the answer to the second question is termed the accuracy for negative test prediction. Referring back to Table 1-2, the accuracy for positive prediction is calculated as $a/(a + b)$ (eg, the ratio of true-positive to total positive test results), and the accuracy for negative prediction is calculated as $d/(c + d)$ (eg, the ratio of true-negative to total negative test results).

Test sensitivity influences the number of true-positive results, and test specificity affects the number of false-positive results. Thus, the accuracy for positive test prediction is affected by both sensitivity and specificity. Similarly, since test specificity influences the number of true-negative results and test sensitivity affects the number of false-negative results, the accuracy for negative prediction is also modified by test sensitivity and specificity. In fact, perfect accuracy for positive test prediction, which requires zero false-positive results, can only be obtained with perfect specificity. Conversely, perfect accuracy for negative test prediction, which requires zero false-negative test results, demands perfect test sensitivity.

Another important determinant of the accuracy for positive and negative test prediction, apart from test sensitivity and specificity, is the proportion of the tested population having the disease of interest. The effect of this proportion, which is referred to as "disease prevalence," is illustrated in Table 1-3. In this table, a test with fixed levels of sensitivity (.9) and specificity (.9) is applied to two different patient populations. The first patient population, represented in the top panel of the table, has a high disease prevalence of .6. The second patient population, represented in the bottom panel, has a low disease prevalence of .01. In the high-prevalence population, the accuracy for both positive test prediction (.93) and negative test prediction (.86) is substantial. However, when the same test is applied to the population with low disease prevalence, test accuracy is dramatically altered. The accuracy for positive prediction declines to an extremely low level (.08), since true-positive results are "swamped" by the large number of false-positive results arising from the greatly increased number of nondiseased individuals in the population. In contrast, the accuracy for negative prediction rises to .99, since true-negative results, derived from the greatly increased group of non-diseased individuals, vastly outnumber false-negative results, arising from the reduced group of diseased individuals.

Thus, test sensitivity, test specificity, and disease prevalence must be incorporated into the calculation of the accuracy for positive and negative test

Table 1-3
Effect of Varying Disease Prevalence Upon Accuracy for Positive and Negative Prediction in a Test with Fixed Sensitivity (.9) and Specificity (.9)

Disease Prevalence = .6

Result of Test	Confirmed Disease Status		Total
	Present	*Absent*	
Positive	540	40	580
Negative	60	360	420
Total	600	400	1000

$$\text{Accuracy for Positive Prediction} = \frac{540}{540 + 40} = .93$$

$$\text{Accuracy for Negative Prediction} = \frac{360}{360 + 60} = .86$$

Disease Prevalence = .01

Result of Test	Confirmed Disease Status		Total
	Present	*Absent*	
Positive	9	99	108
Negative	1	891	892
Total	10	990	1000

$$\text{Accuracy for Positive Prediction} = \frac{9}{9 + 99} = .08$$

$$\text{Accuracy for Negative Prediction} = \frac{891}{891 + 1} = .99$$

prediction. Two computational methods are available for calculating the accuracy of test prediction. The first, in which a 2 × 2 contingency table is employed, is illustrated in Table 1-3. To use this contingency table, one first sets an arbitrary total sample size for the tested population. For example, the sample size in Table 1-3 was assumed to be 1,000 patients; however, any arbitrary size could have been used. After arbitrarily setting this sample size, one uses knowledge of disease prevalence to determine the number of diseased [(prevalence) × (total sample size)] and nondiseased [(1 − prevalence) × (total sample size)] individuals. Values for test sensitivity then allow calculation of the number of true-positive [(sensitivity) × (number of diseased)] and false-negative [(1 − sensitivity) × (number of diseased)] test results. Test specificity allows calculation of the number of true-negative [(specificity) × (number of nondiseased)] and false-positive [(1 − specificity) × (number of nondiseased)] results. In this way, one obtains values corresponding to a, b, c, and d in Table 1-2, with a/(a + b) providing the accuracy for positive test prediction, and d/(c + d) giving the accuracy for negative prediction.

If equations are preferred to contingency tables for the calculation of the accuracy of positive and negative prediction, Bayes' formula may be employed. According to Bayes' formula:

Accuracy for positive prediction =
$$\frac{(\text{sensitivity})\,(\text{disease prevalence})}{(\text{sensitivity})\,(\text{disease prevalence}) + (1 - \text{specificity})\,(1 - \text{disease prevalence})}$$

Accuracy for negative prediction =
$$\frac{(\text{specificity})\,(1 - \text{disease prevalence})}{(\text{specificity})\,(1 - \text{disease prevalence}) + (1 - \text{sensitivity})\,(\text{disease prevalence})}.$$

Although knowledge of disease prevalence in the tested population provides the necessary link between test sensitivity and specificity, on the one hand, and the accuracy for positive and negative test prediction, on the other hand, the clinician rarely has information about the actual prevalence of disease in the patient population being tested. In lieu of data about disease prevalence, a surrogate measure, called "pretest disease likelihood" can be employed. Pretest disease likelihood refers to the physician's estimate of the probability of the disease in the patient, after considering all the historical, physical examination, and laboratory data available at the time that the test is obtained. In a 50-year-old male executive who has exertional substernal pressure and has a history of diabetes mellitus and a family history of multiple myocardial infarctions, the pre-exercise tolerance test (ETT) likelihood of coronary disease is quite high. In contrast, the pre-ETT likelihood would be quite low in an anxious 18-year-old woman who presents with recurrent episodes of right-sided anterior chest pain that is nonexertional and stabbing in character and is associated with perioral paresthesias and hyperventilation. To calculate the ETT accuracy for positive and negative prediction of coronary artery disease, the physician's subjective estimates of the pre-ETT likelihood of coronary artery disease are used as substitutes for the prevalence of coronary artery disease in the two patient populations from which the two patients derive. The first patient population would include patients similar in all respects to the first patient and would be expected to have a high prevalence of coronary disease. The second population would include patients similar in all respects to the second patient and would be expected to have a low prevalence of coronary artery disease. Accordingly, subjective pretest estimates of disease are substituted for disease prevalence in estimating the accuracy of test prediction by either the 2×2 contingency table or the Bayes' formula method. Viewed in this perspective, it is evident that values of the accuracy for positive and negative test prediction represent pretest estimates of disease likelihood that have been *revised* by diagnostic test results, interpreted with knowledge of test sensitivity and specificity. Thus, diagnostic tests are performed to revise pretest estimates of disease likelihood, either in an upward or downward direction, depending on the purpose of the diagnostic test. The magnitude of this revision provides a measure of the efficacy of the diagnostic test.

Since revision of pretest disease likelihood comprises the major objective of diagnostic testing, the clinician should be aware of several important generalizations about the way that the level of pretest disease likelihood constrains the ability of test results to raise or lower the probability of disease. Regardless of the pretest disease likelihood, a perfectly sensitive test guarantees that a negative result correctly predicts the absence of disease, and a perfectly specific test guarantees that a positive result correctly predicts the presence of disease. However, most diagnostic tests are neither perfectly sensitive nor perfectly specific, and pretest likelihood becomes extremely important in the interpretation of the results of these imperfect tests. If the pretest likelihood of disease is judged to be very small, as in the above example of the young woman with atypical chest pain, a positive test result has very little effect in revising the likelihood of disease upward and hence has poor ability to confirm the presence of disease. In contrast, a negative test result confirms the suspicion that disease is absent, but only by a small revision of the pretest estimate in a downward direction. If the pretest likelihood is deemed to be quite high, as in the earlier example of the middle-aged man with classical angina pectoris, a negative test result has little effect in revising this estimate downward and hence poor ability to exclude the presence of disease. A positive result, on the other hand, confirms the pretest suspicion that the disease is present, but only by a slight revision of the estimate in an upward direction. Thus, at the extremes of pretest disease likelihood, tests with sensitivity and specificity values much below 1 add little to our a priori clinical suspicions. On the other hand, as pretest estimates of disease likelihood move to values of greater clinical uncertainty (eg, toward .5), test results have a progressively greater effect in revising the likelihood of disease in an upward or downward direction. For any fixed level of test sensitivity and specificity, a positive test result has a greater effect in revising the pretest disease likelihood in an upward direction, and a negative test has greater effect in revising the pretest disease likelihood in a downward direction, as the pretest likelihood approaches the value of .5. It is thus in this range of greatest clinical uncertainty that diagnostic tests convey the most *additional* information about the presence or absence of disease.

Evaluating Test Performance in the Context of Text Indications

There are at least three different clinical circumstances in which clinicians order tests for diagnostic purposes. When a clinician obtains a test to detect disease in asymptomatic patients, the diagnostic test is referred to as a screening test. For example, when a healthy and asymptomatic airline pilot is asked to obtain an exercise tolerance test to detect unsuspected coronary artery disease, the exercise tolerance test is used as a screening test. A second type of diagnostic activity occurs when, on the basis of symptoms, signs, and previous tests, the clinician has a strong suspicion that a disease is present and orders a test to "rule in" the disease. A test ordered in this circumstance is called a confirmation test. An example of this type of testing occurs when an exercise tolerance test is ordered in a patient with classical angina pectoris. The third major diagnostic use of laboratory tests is to rule out the presence of a disease. In this situation, the clinician does not have a strong clinical suspicion that the disease is present, but judges that adequate patient management requires further reassurance that the disease is indeed absent. Tests ordered in this context are termed exclusion tests. For example, an exercise tolerance test may be ordered to exclude the presence of coronary artery disease when it is ordered for a patient who has atypical chest pain and lacks coronary artery disease risk factors. This classification of diagnostic tests according to their uses for screening, confirmation, and exclusion is important, since many diagnostic tests are useful for one or two, but not all three, clinical purposes.

When considering the desirability of a certain diagnostic test for screening, the clinician must bear several factors in mind. First, the goal of screening is to identify as many patients with disease as possible. Thus, high accuracy for negative prediction is important, and the test must have high sensitivity. Second, screening is often undertaken to detect anatomically localized or functionally mild disease. Consequently, a screening test must have high sensitivity not only for extensive disease, but also for limited disease. Third, since screening tests are applied to asymptomatic patient populations, a screening test must function well under circumstances of low disease prevalence. To avoid large numbers of false-positive tests results among the many healthy patients in populations with low disease prevalence, high test specificity is required. On the other hand, since positive screening test results are usually followed by more definitive tests that eliminate false-positive diagnoses, high specificity is less important than high sensitivity for an adequate screening test.

Since a confirmation test must correctly identify disease when it is present, accuracy for positive prediction is of greatest importance. The accuracy of positive prediction, in turn, is augmented by ordering tests in patients with a high pretest likelihood of disease and by employing tests with high specificity. High pretest likelihood of disease reduces the number of nondiseased subjects who are tested, and high test specificity reduces the number of false-positive test results among these nondiseased individuals. As stated above, if the pretest likelihood of disease is low, a positive result has little ability to confirm the presence of disease unless specificity is nearly perfect. Furthermore, if test specificity is low, a positive test result cannot be used to confirm the presence of disease unless the pretest likelihood of disease is quite high—in which case, it may not be justifiable to perform the test in the first place.

An exclusion test must correctly identify the absence of disease. Accordingly, accuracy for negative prediction is paramount. Both low pretest disease likelihood and high test sensitivity increase the accuracy for negative prediction, enhancing the ability of a negative test result to exclude the presence of disease. Low pretest disease likelihood minimizes the number of diseased persons who are tested, and high test sensitivity minimizes the fraction of these diseased persons who give false-negative results. If the pretest disease likelihood is high, a negative test result has little ability to exclude disease unless sensitivity is nearly perfect. Conversely, if sensitivity is low, a negative result cannot exclude a disease unless the pretest likelihood is extremely low—a circumstance in which the test may not be warranted.

In clinical practice, tests rarely have both high sensitivity and high specificity for a disease of interest. As a result, the same test rarely is useful for detecting all cases with the disease and for confirming the diagnosis in these cases. Consequently, tests are frequently used in tandem, with a highly sensitive test used to screen for disease, followed by a highly specific test to confirm the diagnosis in subjects with positive results by the screening test.

Thus, in the diagnosis of tuberculosis, one might choose the convenient and highly sensitive tuberculin skin test to screen for disease and more expensive but more specific microbiologic cultures to confirm tuberculosis in subjects with positive tuberculin reactions.

Even with the availability of tandem tests to perform multiple diagnostic functions, it is still important to have at least one test that is highly sensitive for use in disease screening and exclusion and at least one test that is highly specific for use in disease confirmation. To augment values for test sensitivity and specificity, several strategies are employed. The first strategy exploits the properties of the test receiver-operator characteristic described above. By moving the test cutoff value for "abnormality" to a more stringent level, a test frequently can be made more specific, and by choosing a more lenient cutoff value, a test often can be made more sensitive. For example, in the diagnosis of diabetes mellitus, one might choose a lenient, but sensitive, random blood glucose level for screening purposes and a more stringent, but more specific, criterion for blood glucose using formal glucose tolerance testing to confirm the diagnosis.

An alternative strategy for augmenting test sensitivity and specificity simultaneously considers the results of more than one test for the same disease. The positive results of one test may identify portions of the disease spectrum that are not detected by positive results of another test. Under these circumstances, more diseased subjects are identified by the aggregate of positive results of both tests than by the positive results of each test by itself. Consequently, if a positive result by either test is regarded as "positive," sensitivity will be augmented. Conversely, the negative results of one test may identify portions of the nondiseased spectrum that are not detected by the negative results of a second test. Because more nondiseased patients will be identified by the aggregate of negative results of the two tests than by the negative results for either test taken alone, specificity will be increased by accepting a negative result by either test as "negative." Using this strategy in the diagnosis of coronary artery disease by noninvasive tests, sensitivity would be increased by accepting either a positive exercise tolerance test (ETT) or a positive radionuclide scan. In contrast, specificity would be augmented by accepting either a negative ETT or a negative radionuclide scan (this is equivalent to demanding that both the ETT and the radionuclide scan be positive). It should be recognized that each of these strategies for aggregating test results carries a price. Aggregating positive results to increase test sensitivity will generally diminish test specificity, and aggregating negative results to increase test specificity will often diminish test sensitivity. Nonetheless, when augmentation of either sensitivity or specificity is desired, aggregation of test results may be a useful strategy.

Summary

Clinicians must often use surrogate or imperfect diagnostic tests to distinguish health from disease. The interpretation of quantitative test results thus often relies upon a "range of normal" provided by clinical laboratories. Although useful as a rough guide, the concept of a range of normal suffers because it is based on the range of test values for healthy (not diseased) persons. Deriving a range of normal only from test values in

16

healthy persons may result in excessive false labeling of the healthy as "diseased," particularly when multiple tests are performed. There will also be considerable uncertainty about the likelihood of specific diseases when abnormal results are obtained. Additional problems with the range of normal for many tests include inadequate adjustments of normal limits according to demographic, clinical, and laboratory error factors that affect test variability and improper statistical assumptions about the Gaussian distribution of test values in the healthy population.

When diagnostic tests are evaluated according to their ability to separate patients with a specific disease from patients without that disease, several indexes are available. Test sensitivity denotes the fraction of diseased persons with abnormal test results, and test specificity describes the fraction of nondiseased persons with normal test results. Since the clinician does not know the final disease status of the patient at the time the test is performed, however, the accuracy for positive test prediction—the fraction of positive test results that correctly identify diseased subjects—and the accuracy for negative test prediction—the fraction of negative test results that correctly identify nondiseased subjects—are more useful in a clinical setting. To calculate these latter indexes, disease prevalence, as well as test sensitivity and test specificity, must be taken into account. Each of these indexes of test performance provides a measure of how well a test will function in the three major types of diagnostic activities. In screening for a disease, as well as in excluding a disease, high accuracy for negative test prediction is paramount, and test sensitivity should be high. In contrast, to confirm the presence of a disease, high accuracy for positive test prediction is most important, and hence test specificity should be high.

■ Selected Readings

Bradwell AR, Carmalt MHB, Whitehead TD: Explaining the unexpected abnormal results of biochemical profile investigation. *Lancet* 1974;II:1071–1074.

Feinstein AR: The derangements of the "range of normal." *Clin Pharmacol Ther* 1974;15:523–540.

Galen RS, Gambino SR: *Beyond Normality, the Predictive Value and Efficiency of Medical Diagnosis.* New York, John Wiley & Sons, 1975.

Griner PF, Mayewski RJ, Mushlin AI, et al: Principles of test selection and use. *Ann Intern Med* 1981;94:559–600.

Murphy EA: *The Logic of Medicine.* Baltimore, Johns Hopkins, 1976, pp 117–160.

Ransohoff DF, Feinstein AR: Problems of spectrum and bias in evaluating the efficiency of diagnostic tests. *N Engl J Med* 1978;299:926–930.

All branches of science and technology are interdependent. They rely on each other as sources of basic knowledge to help the development of their own subject, and advances in one subject can be applied practically in another. Modern medicine could not have progressed without taking in knowledge and concepts from the basic sciences as they developed. Each basic science accompanies its expertise with specialist terminology, including symbols and units, and this is accepted by international agreements drawn up by organizations to which all major scientific nations contribute.

■ Development of the Système International d'Unités (SI)

The international organization responsible since 1875 for weights and measures is the Conference generale des Poids et Mesures (CGPM), whose recommendations are now accepted for medicine as a whole by the World Health Organization. The initial metric system, introduced about 1800, was based on the meter as the unit of length and the gram as the unit of quantity of matter, derived then from measuring the circumference of the earth and from weighing a standard volume of water. Many extensions and modifications of this first metric system were introduced over the next 150 years as science and technology progressed. A major revision about 1870 proved unable to encompass many newly developing fields of science.

In 1960 CGPM codified the current revisions and extensions of the metric system as 'Système International d'Unités' (abbreviated as SI in all languages), to include agreed later modifications. This is now the internationally accepted "language" for measurement throughout science and technology.

In the 1970s the relevant international organizations in pathology and laboratory medicine reviewed SI and recommended its adoption. They drew up guidelines for the use of SI in laboratory reporting and made recommendations on the introduction of "amount of substance" (unit: the mole) and the preferred use of molar concentration for measurement of components of known relative molecular mass ("molecular weight") in body fluids.

The Introduction of SI to Medicine In Britain and the USA

In Britain a small working party was set up in 1970, with the author as chairholder and containing representatives of all relevant laboratory organizations. Its recommendations were

D. N. Baron

accepted, with minor modifications, by the parent organizations, by the Department of Health, and by the "consumer" organizations such as the Royal College of Physicians and were finally agreed upon in 1974. They were circulated in 1975 by the Department of Health and by the professional organizations to all hospitals, doctors, and laboratories in the country and included guidelines on recording of patients' temperature, height, etc, in SI units. By 1977 the changeover had been completed peacefully, with no major problems reported, all over the country. Prospective medical students were already being taught their science in High School only in SI units: at that time I noticed J mol^{-1} K^{-1} in one of my daughter's textbooks.

Many factors eased the task of national introduction of SI to laboratory reporting. They include a national steering group accepted for its authority both by laboratory workers and by clinicians; a laboratory system in which almost all analyses (including private work) are done in large laboratories, specialist controlled, either in the National Health Service (NHS) or in medical schools (NHS-linked); an intensive educational campaign by heads of laboratories to clinician and nursing colleagues, including distribution of conversion charts; the refusal by laboratories after the changeover to quote results in both systems; all major journals accepting the need for change.

It is an interesting problem in the sociology of medicine why full change-over to SI, readily accepted in Britain and many other countries, has so far been resisted in the United States. I think that some factors are the isolation-ism of American medicine in that new ideas are not so readily accepted if they originate abroad or from international medical and scientific organiza-tions; the large number of small laboratories in which the different sections (especially clinical chemistry and hematology) are not supervised by single-discipline specialists, medical or nonmedical, who would understand the purpose and value of the new system, but by general pathologists who may be primarily anatomic pathologists, or even by clinicians; and the distribu-tion of authority between the clinical and the laboratory specialist—in the United States clinicians order tests, in Britain they request tests.

■ SI in Relation to Medical and Laboratory Practice

SI, as well as being *decimal* and *metric* (and using approved prefixes for multiples and submultiples), is *coherent*. This means that the unit for any physical quantity can be derived from the units for other physical quantities without the use of numerical factors; a quantity is a physical property that can be measured in terms of a number and a unit. For example, the unit of force (newton) is that which gives to a unit of mass (kilogram) a unit of accel-eration (1 meter per second per second).

The Units and Their Presentation

The current base units are listed in Table 2-1.

Derived units, for more complex quantities, are formed from the base units by simple multiplication and division. Many of these have special names and symbols, an example being the unit of force, the newton (symbol: N), derived as kg•m•s^{-2}. When one unit is divided by another (eg, grams per liter), this may be expressed either by using a solidus (g/1), or by a negative exponent (g•1⁻¹). The use of negative exponents is desirable, to avoid ambiguity, for all complex symbols containing more than two units. To include raised multiplying points within complex symbols is not essential, but makes for clarity. There are many other derived units that do not have special names and symbols, an example being the unit of velocity, derived as m/s.

Decimal multiples and submultiples of the units are formed by prefixes (Table 2-2).

Compound prefixes must never be used as they cause confusion; for example, 10^{-9} g is a nanogram (ng) and not a millimicrogram (mμg).

Length
The SI unit is the meter (m).

The ångstrom (Å) should not be used, and the measurement should be converted to nanometers (1 Å = 10^{-1} nm).

The micron (μ) as a name for a unit of length is obsolete; the correct name for this unit is the micrometer (μm).

Volume
The SI unit is the cubic meter (m³). Because this is inconvenient and unfamiliar the working unit that is accepted for medicine and related sciences

Table 2-1
The Independent Base Units of SI

Physical Quantity	Name of SI Unit	Symbol for SI Unit
Length	Meter	m
Mass	Kilogram	kg
Time	Second	s
Electric current	Ampere	A
Thermodynamic temperature	Kelvin	K
Luminous intensity	Candela	cd
Amount of substance	Mole	mol

There are also the supplementary units of radian (plane angle) and steradian (solid angle).

Table 2-2
Prefixes for Multiples and Submultiples

Multiple	Prefix	Symbol	Sub-multiple	Prefix	Symbol
10^1	deca	da	10^{-1}	deci	d
10^2	ecto	h	10^{-2}	centi	c
10^3	kilo	k	10^{-3}	milli	m
10^6	mega	M	10^{-6}	micro	μ
10^9	giga	G	10^{-9}	nano	n
10^{12}	tera	T	10^{-12}	pico	p
10^{15}	peta	P	10^{-15}	femto	f
10^{18}	exa	E	10^{-18}	atto	a

is the liter (l), which is an alternative special name for the cubic decimeter ($dm^3 = 1,000 \ cm^3$), with its submultiples. The very small difference in the pre-SI metric system between the liter and the cubic decimeter has been abandoned, and the liter has been redefined. The widely used 100 ml is a deciliter (dl).

In American laboratories and clinical journals there is a tendency to use L as the symbol for liter, to avoid possible lack of distinction between l and 1. Perhaps this originated with the popularity of certain typewriters that caused confusion by providing a single key and symbol to serve both for letter "el" and for number "one"; instruments should follow users and not vice versa. The use of L as an alternative to l is now accepted internationally.

The lambda (λ) as a name for a unit of volume (10^{-6} l) is obsolete; the correct name for this unit is the microliter (μL).

Percent (%) means "per hundred parts of the same." Thus "mg%" means "milligrams per hundred milligrams" and must *never* be used to mean "milligrams per hundred milliliters," which differs by a factor of the order of 1,000, depending on the relative density of the solvent. If in doubt, use % only for numbers.

Mass

The SI unit is the kilogram (kg); the working unit is the gram (g). Multiples and submultiples are expressed in terms of the original metric unit, the gram, and not in terms of the SI base unit; otherwise the gram would have to be called the millikilogram.

The gamma (γ) as a name for a unit of mass (10^{-6} g) is obsolete: the correct name for this unit is the microgram (μg).

Amount of Substance

The SI unit is the mole (mol). This is the amount of substance that contains a standard number of specific particles (referred to the mole of ^{12}C atoms, which has a mass of exactly 12 g) whether atoms, ions, radicals, or molecules. This new unit has sometimes been found confusing: 1 mol of H^+ (hydrogen ions) has a mass equal to 1.008 g (usually taken in medicine as 1 g), 1 mol of H_2 (molecular hydrogen) has a mass of about 2 g, 1 mol of H_2O (water) has a mass of about 18 g, and 1 mol of glucose has a mass of about 180 g.

Concentration

SI includes several types of concentration, and particularly relevant to medicine and laboratory analyses are mass concentration (derived unit kg/m^3, working unit g/L) and amount of substance concentration (derived unit mol/m^3, working unit mol/L).

All concentrations of components are to be expressed per liter. Mole (substance) concentrations are to be used to express the results of analyses of all components of known relative molecular/ionic/atomic mass that are measured in blood plasma and other body fluids, and mole quantities will similarly be used for timed excretions and other amounts. Protein measurements continue to be expressed in mass/volume units when they are measured in mixtures (eg, total immunoglobulin G) or when their exact relative molecular mass is unknown. However the quoting of protein analytical results as mole concentrations is beginning as specific protein analyses become more common and is already in use by some laboratories for albumin. Mass concentrations are used for some other mixtures, such as plasma total lipids; for many mixtures, however, results are given as moles of a predominant constituent, such as stearic acid for fecal fat. The traditional way of expressing hemoglobin concentration in blood is as g/dL: there is now an agreed international recommendation to national organizations that the change should be made to g/L.

The change from mass to substance amounts and concentrations requires more than just a change in numerical values (as, for example, from °F to °C) as it involves a conceptual change in dimensions: there is a parallel situation in the change from weight to mass. As the chemical physiological and pharmacological activity of a component is normally proportional to the concentration of molecules or ions present and not to the mass concentration, the use of the mole expresses amounts or concentrations in biologically relevant terms.

To balance a party in biologically relevant terms one might invite 10 mol of men (mass 700 kg) and 10 mol of women (mass 500 kg), not 600 kg of men and 600 kg of women. The mole avoids certain ambiguities in the use of the equivalent and brings in nonionized components whose concentration could not be expressed on the equivalent scale. For monovalent ions—for example, Na^+—1 mol is numerically the same as one equivalent, so for sodium 140 milliequivalents per liter becomes 140 mmol/L: 1 mol of NaCl contains 1 mol of Na^+ and 1 mol of Cl^-. As the molar mass of glucose is 180 g, a plasma glucose concentration of 90 mg/dL becomes 5.0 mmol/L; as the molar mass of thyroxine is 777 g, a plasma thyroxine concentration of 10 μg/dL becomes 130 nmol/L; and as the molar mass of phenobarbitone is 232 g, a plasma phenobarbitone concentration of 4.6 mg/dL becomes 0.2 nmol/L.

Introduction of the molar system for drug concentration in plasma is under discussion. Moles are used for prescription of electrolytes and often for intravenous nutrients, but not for other therapy.

Particle Counts
Particle counts will be expressed per liter. For example, a blood erythrocyte count of $4.5 \times 10^6/mm^3$ becomes $4.5 \times 10^{12}/L$: leucocyte and platelet counts are to be expressed as $\times 10^9/L$.

Time
The SI unit is the second (s).

Working units are minute (min), hour (h), day (d), and year (a; yr is conventional, but it is better not to abbreviate). Note that "24 h" may be necessary when "day" is contrasted with "night," as for urine volumes.

Frequency
The SI unit is the hertz (Hz).

This replaces cycles per second for frequency of periodic phenomena. It should not be used for discontinuous events such as dispensing of doses of medicine or urinating.

Temperature

The SI unit, for thermodynamic temperature and for temperature interval, is the kelvin (K), which is the approved name both for the former degree Kelvin (°K) for scale, and Kelvin degree (degK) for interval. The working unit (for customary temperature) is the degree Celsius (°C).

The kelvin thermodynamic temperature scale starts at absolute zero (− 273.16°C). This is inconvenient, so the familiar Celsius scale, starting at the freezing point of water (0 °C), will be retained in medicine for all clinical purposes. The kelvin temperature *interval* is identical with the degree Celsius temperature *interval.* Note that C here is the symbol for Celsius, not for Centigrade.

Pressure

The SI unit is the pascal (Pa).

In medicine, pressure is most often measured as the height of a liquid column, either as millimeters of mercury (mmHg) or as centimeters or millimeters of water (mmH$_2$O): 1 mmHg = 1 Torr. These measures are not SI and so cannot be used without conversion in calculations involving pressure (such as flow rate), are artificial when applied to instruments such as transducers that do not involve a column, and vary with height above sea level (gravitational acceleration) and with column temperature. However, as there are so many existing clinical sphygmomanometers, column measurements will remain in clinical use for a very considerable time, until new ideas are accepted and new instruments are available. It would be a great convenience if the manufacturers would make stick-on scales graduated in kilopascals for their current instruments.

Although the pascal has been readily accepted, because of its advantages, by laboratory workers and medical research scientists, it has been accepted by few clinicians. In Britain a group of physicians set up a Society for the Preservation of the Millimetre of Mercury!

Energy

The SI unit is the joule (J).

This is to be used for all forms of energy, including heat energy. The traditional unit for heat energy, the calorie (cal: strictly the gram-calorie), was used in nutrition as the kilocalorie (kcal), often called the Medical Calorie (Cal), or, to everyone's confusion, just Calorie: this is to be abandoned. For general use we should refer, for example, to a low-energy instead of a low-calorie diet. However it will be a long time before the food manufacturers agree to change and the public learns to change.

Enzyme Activity

Originally, units for measurement of enzyme activity, particularly in body fluids, were arbitrary. They were usually named after the originators of the analytical method, such as the King-Armstrong unit for alkaline phosphatase and the Somogyi unit for amylase. International agreement led to a unit applicable to any enzyme, which is the amount that will catalyze the transformation of 1 μmol of substrate per minute, under defined conditions. This enzyme unit is used in laboratories now for most enzymes and has the symbol U. Plasma enzyme activities are generally quoted as U/l.

■ Advantages and Disadvantages of SI

SI units have the following specific advantages, especially for results of pathology laboratory investigations. They have general long-term benefits of promoting logical thought about the meaning of measured values.

They are uniform and have been accepted for all branches of science and technology. Medicine thereby becomes more closely linked with its background.

They are international and standard. The units traditionally used for expressing measurements made in medicine have developed empirically and chaotically over many years. Thus results may be misunderstood by those not familiar with any particular scale of units, until a uniform system is used by most laboratories.

They reveal close relationships between components that are present in the body fluids and take part in biochemical and other metabolic processes. The important change has been the adoption of the mole and of the liter; unfortunately enzyme units have not yet been completely standardized.

The disadvantage is the need to remember new reference values and to establish new thought patterns which link certain sets of numbers (for example, plasma urea, calcium, and phosphate concentrations) to a given clinical situation (for example, hyperparathyroidism). In practice, despite their initial worries that this would disrupt patient care, my senior clinical colleagues tell me they soon adapted, although a few admitted to looking occasionally, for two or three years, at conversion charts: the new generation of English doctors have been taught only in SI units as medical students.

Many doctors in clinical practice, and even a few laboratory workers, questioned the value of introducing SI to medicine. They claimed that there was nothing wrong with the old units, that patients would be killed because physicians and nurses would not understand the new laboratory results (which never happened), and that the expense would be immense (which was not so). Many of these doctors were practicing, in respect to quantitative tests, what I call "black-box" medicine—ask for a test and a magic number appears, and if it is higher or lower than another magic number, then take certain actions.

There are some of our number in Britain who still would be using grains per fluid ounce for measurement of urine sugar (*Lancet:* 100 years ago), unless a two-thirds majority of the whole profession had approved the change by a referendum, and even so this would be infringement of their professional freedom! The bacteriologists and the anatomists seem to change their nomenclature every generation, and doctors accept this without much complaint. Conversely, physicians would be appalled if, say, pharmacists used antiquated and misleading medical terminology such as "catarrhal jaundice."

Those who do medical research, or even just think about the scientific basis of disease, all now welcome the added insight given by the universal use of moles per liter for concentrations in body fluids.

■ Selected Readings

Baron DN, Broughton PMG, Cohen M, et al: The use of SI units in reporting results obtained in hospital laboratories. *J Clin Pathol* 1974;27:590–597.

Baron DN (ed): *Units, Symbols, and Abbreviations,* ed 3. London, Royal Society of Medicine, 1977.

Lowe D: *A Guide to International Recommendations on Names and Symbols for Quantities and on Units of Measurement.* Geneva, World Health Organization, 1977.

The SI for the Health Professions. Geneva, World Health Organization, 1977.

Lipper H, Lehmann HP: *SI Units in Medicine: An Introduction to the International System of Units with Conversion Tables and Normal Ranges.* Baltimore and Munich, Urban & Schwarzenberg, 1978.

This chapter presents diagnostic approaches to common hematologic findings. These findings are discussed as laboratory phenomena, but of course most abnormal test results turn up in patients with symptoms. I assume the reader is a clinician who has to deal with unexpected and unexplained abnormalities such as anemia. I also assume that the subject is an adult patient and that the reader is able to go to more detailed accounts than this one as the problem is defined. Some diagnostic approaches are illustrated by decision-tree flow charts.

I intend to focus on presentation and diagnosis of common blood problems and also urgent problems for which timely, expert help may be unavailable. Detailed discussions of specialized topics like red cell enzyme deficiencies and myeloid metaplasia will not be found here.

Diagnostic approaches are affected by technology. The chapter ends with a brief discussion of methods used to perform certain hematology tests: the emphasis is on the most commonly used tests, which have received the most attention from purveyors of new technology.

Normal values for common hematology tests referred to throughout the chapter are presented in Table 3-1.

Anemia

The most common causes of anemia are chronic inflammatory disease and bleeding (Chart 1).

Chronically ill patients become anemic by suppression of normal erythropoiesis and failure to replace senescent red cells. Thus, many sick, hospitalized patients, especially if they have generalized or even localized inflammation, are marginally anemic. The anemia usually progresses as one could calculate from a red cell lifespan, normally 120 days, by the loss of 1% of the red cell mass, represented by the hematocrit, or about 0.4 hematocrit points per day. Thus, in a week the patient who has chronic fever suppressing erythropoiesis loses 7 × 0.4, or about 3 hematocrit points. This decline stops at a hematocrit level of about 25. If the inflammatory state is not obvious, the anemia may be an early and important clue to chronic illness. There are usually few hematologic clues to the nature of this anemia. There is usually no abnormality in red cell size or color, though about one-fourth of anemias of chronic disease are accompanied by mild hypochromia or microcytosis. The reticulocyte count is usually reduced. There usually is not much to pick up on bone marrow evaluation; the erythroid marrow may be hypoplastic, but usually cannot be told from "normal," and red cell precursors just are not increased to compensate for anemia. There *is* an increase in bone marrow iron stores.

25

Table 3-1
Normal Values for Common Hematology Tests*

Test		Range of Normal
Hemoglobin:	Men	14–18 g/dL
	Women	12–16 g/dL
Hematocrit:	Men	40–52%
	Women	37–47%
Red Cell MCV		78–94 fL
Reticulocytes		0.6–2.7%
Platelets × 1000		150–350 Cells/μL
White Cells × 1000		4.0–10.0 Cells/μL
Differential		
Segmented Polymorphonuclear leukocytes		38–70%
Banded Polymorphonuclear leukocytes		0–13%
Lymphocytes		14–46%
Monocytes		2–15%
Eosinophils		0–5%
Basophils		0–2%
Atypical Lymphocytes		0–7%
Metamyelocytes		0–1%
Coagulation		
Partial Thromboplastin Time (APTT)		25–45 Seconds
Prothrombin Time (PT) (Also: less than 1 second over control)		11–13 Seconds
Thrombin Time (Also: less than 5 seconds over 20-second control)		20–25 Seconds
Fibrinogen		
Healthy young adults		150–350 mg/dL
Hospital patients		250–450 mg/dL
Bleeding Time		2–8 Minutes
Ivy, Template		
Antithrombin III		70–130%

*Results obtained in adults in the Clinical Hematology Laboratory, Yale-New Haven Hospital.

This condition, the anemia of chronic disease, is discussed first since in a large proportion of patients with acquired anemia it is easy to diagnose if one remembers that fever or even localized inflammation suppresses erythropoiesis.

The other most common cause of anemia in adults is blood loss: increased vaginal bleeding in menstruating women or gastrointestinal bleeding in either sex. The menstrual history is the first matter to investigate in an anemic woman, whereas questions about melena and hematochezia are important in either sex.

If anemia is not attributable to obvious chronic disease or bleeding, determination of the cause may be approached in several ways. These approaches involve both clinical and laboratory considerations. Certain segments of the population are vulnerable to specific types of anemia: menstruating women and milk-fed infants are candidates for iron deficiency. People in either of these groups, if only mildly anemic, are given iron without further testing. However, treatment without evaluation leaves the doctor with an obligation to check the hematocrit a month or so later. The erythroid response to replacement of needed iron, like the response to needed vitamin B_{12} or folate, may be perceptible at four to five days and leads to marked reticulocytosis at seven to ten days. The hematocrit rises over several weeks. The reponse to the needed iron is blunted or absent if there is a complicating illness, such as an inflammatory state. In addition, there are often problems with compliance in taking prescribed iron. However, if the major cause of

Chart 1

FINDING THE CAUSE OF <u>ANEMIA</u> IN AN ADULT:

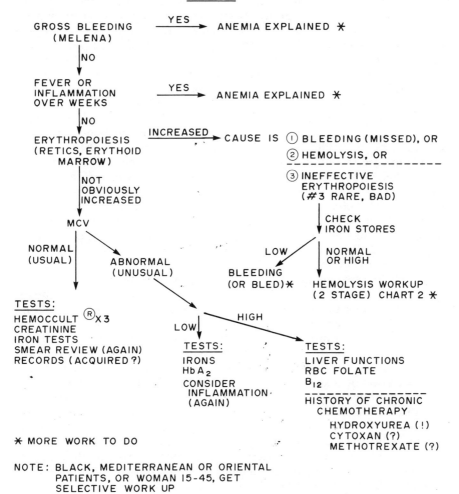

NOTE: BLACK, MEDITERRANEAN OR ORIENTAL
      PATIENTS, OR WOMAN 15-45, GET
      SELECTIVE WORK UP

anemia is iron deficiency, at least partial correction should be clear in three to four weeks.

Another demographic feature that can be helpful in finding the cause of anemia is race. Hemoglobinopathies are likely causes of any anemia found in black or Oriental patients; G6PD deficiency is likely in black and Mediterranean patients.

The laboratory considerations most helpful in the initial analysis of anemia are red cell size and turnover: mean corpuscular volume (MCV) and reticulocyte count. Other initial findings that may indicate the cause, although less commonly, are abnormal red cell shapes such as spherocytes and schistocytes. Workup of anemia from the MCV will be discussed first.

Anemia associated with *large* red cells is most commonly caused by deficiency of folic acid, alcoholic liver disease, or by deficiency of vitamin B_{12}. These three cause 75% of instances of marked macrocytosis (MCV of 115 fL or higher). Other less common causes include the use of oral, chronically ingested anticancer drugs, especially hydroxyurea and cyclophosphamide. Other anticancer drugs may cause megaloblastic change (methotrexate, cytosine arabinoside), but are less likely to cause peripheral macrocytosis.

Marked macrocytosis may precede anemia. The presence of polymorphonuclear leukocytes with six or more lobes suggests folate or B_{12} deficiency. The folate deficiency and liver disease etiologies of macrocytosis commonly occur together. Vitamin B_{12}–deficient patients often are elderly and usually have had a good diet. In patients suspected of folate or B_{12} deficiency it is still valuable to follow up the observation of macrocytosis, the review of the smear for polymorphonuclear leukocytes with six or more lobes, and the vitamin assays with a bone marrow examination; if the bone marrow is megaloblastic, a Schilling test and a gastric aspirate for acid after histamine stimulation are recommended. If a Schilling test is done, care in collecting the ensuing 24-hour urine sample is important. In carrying out this test the patient takes isotopically labeled vitamin B_{12} by mouth. If his or her stomach is normal and secretes intrinsic factor (IF) this labeled vitamin B_{12} binds to his IF, and is absorbed and carried in the blood stream. About an hour after ingestion of the labeled vitamin B_{12}, the patient is given a large amount (1 mg) of *unlabeled* vitamin B_{12} by injection. This "cold" vitamin B_{12} will saturate the serum and tissue binding sites to an extent that most of the previously ingested vitamin B_{12}, if it was picked up by IF and absorbed, will then be excreted in the urine. Laboratories that do this test look for the excretion into the urine of greater than 10% of the ingested "hot" vitamin B_{12} over a 24-hour period in normal persons. Many patients have trouble collecting a 24-hour urine sample, usually because their cooperation has not been enlisted beforehand. The physician trying to interpret an apparent low excretion of B_{12} *must* ask the laboratory to report the urine volume. I have often seen doctors excited about a 3 to 5% B_{12} excretion, ignoring the fact that the "24-hour" urine sample volume was only a few hundred milliliters!

With accurate MCVs and B_{12} and folate measurements available, the bone marrow and Schilling tests are frequently skipped. I believe this to be an error; patients with marked macrocytic anemia deserve at least one complete evaluation. Confirmation of deficiency of folic acid or vitamin B_{12} is important since diagnosis of pernicious anemia commits the patient to monthly injections of B_{12} for the rest of his or her life, and since misdiagnosis of pernicious anemia as folate deficiency leads to progressive nervous system damage.

If the MCV reveals that the red cells are *small,* the possibility that chronic bleeding is causing iron deficiency, or that beta thalassemia minor is present, becomes important. If the microcytosis is marked, but the anemia is slight, thalassemia minor is likely. In the first instance one can confirm iron deficiency by determining the serum iron and iron-binding capacity, looking for percent saturation of the iron-binding protein under 15% (normal is 30%). However, these tests have many problems. Chronic inflammation decreases the iron value, as does drawing the test in the evening (serum iron is subject to marked diurnal variation). An iron pill an hour or two before drawing the sample corrects a low serum iron level. Pregnancy makes the iron-binding capacity high. If locally convenient, it may be better to test for iron deficiency by measuring serum ferritin. This test, when low, is more specific for iron deficiency.

A screening test useful in microcytosis is measurement of free erythrocyte protoporphyrin (FEP). FEP is a heme precursor that builds up if heme cannot be made, as occurs in the presence of lead poisoning or iron deficiency. The FEP test requires extraction of protoporphyrin from red cells before reading in a fluorometer. Recently, rapid whole blood fluorometers have been developed for lead screening. These devices also pick up iron deficiency. Among patients with elevated erythrocyte protoporphyrin, iron-deficient subjects are more likely than lead-poisoned people to have anemia and microcytosis. An important caution is that bilirubin interferes with measurement of erythrocyte protoporphyrin in whole blood fluorometers. The patient with anemia, microcytosis, elevated erythrocyte protoporphyrin, and nonicteric plasma, has iron deficiency diagnosed by two one-minute tests (a serum ferritin would be appropriate for confirmation). If iron deficient, males and nonmenorrhagic females should have barium studies of the gastrointestinal tract.

The person with microcytosis and less severe anemia (hematocrit in the mid-30s), especially if Italian or Greek, deserves tests for hemoglobins A_2 and F (fetal). A_2 is elevated in beta thalassemia minor. The test is not always accurate when done by electrophoresis on cellulose acetate. It can be done accurately by most laboratories with minicolumns or by gel densitometry (if your laboratory is uncertain about an A_2 result, state and federal reference laboratories do this test). Hemoglobin F is elevated in half of patients with beta thalassemia minor. This diagnosis is useful in (1) obviating the two-stage iron deficiency workup and preventing inappropriate iron therapy, (2) explaining mild anemia, and (3) pointing to a need for genetic counseling for young adults.

Most patients with moderate microcytosis who do not have iron deficiency or thalassemia minor have the anemia of chronic disease. These patients usually have only a borderline low MCV (70–80) when microcytosis is present.

When an anemic patient proves to have polychromatophilia or reticulocytosis, he is bleeding, has bled, or has hemolysis. The choice between bleeding and hemolysis, assuming the stool is not black, may be most efficiently made by determining the patient's iron status with serum iron, ferritin, or, if speed is important, with a bone marrow iron evaluation. Like all laboratory tests, evaluation of iron in marrow can be wrong; reported iron stores may be falsely low if not much marrow is put on the slide stained for iron and falsely normal if iron drops on the marrow slide from iron-contaminated glassware. An experienced marrow reader helps here.

If there is reticulocytosis and erythroid hyperplasia and iron is depleted, then the patient has been bleeding and it is important to find the source. Although established iron deficiency due to blood loss is indicated by a low MCV and a hypochromic blood smear, the patient with early blood loss anemia evolving toward iron deficiency may have a normal MCV and smear, or only a few hypochromic red cells. If, on the other hand, iron stores are normal or increased in the patient with increased erythropoiesis, the problem is likely to be hemolysis. One can confirm that suspicion with chemical tests; elevations in indirect bilirubin or lactic dehydrogenase, or absent haptoglobin, would support an impression of hemolysis. If hemolysis is chronic, hemosiderin in renal epithelial cells found in a first morning urine sample may also be present.

The attempt to prove that anemia is hemolytic is followed or sometimes accompanied by identification of the cause of hemolysis. On reevaluation of the blood smear, after learning that the reticulocytes and chemical tests indicate hemolysis, spherocytes or schistocytes may become obvious. Other blood smear findings indicating other causes of hemolysis would include numerous elliptocytes, numerous targets, or any sickle cells. These findings will be discussed further in a later section (Poikilocytosis).

Whatever the morphologic findings, newly suspected hemolysis in an adult is greeted first with a direct Coombs test (the choice of the direct Coombs test for evaluation is reasonable only if numerous spherocytes are present). If the anemia, now known to be hemolytic, is established as long standing or recurrent, evaluation for hemoglobinopathies or red cell enzyme disorders is appropriate. Tests for hemoglobinopathies should include electrophoresis by a sensitive method (unstable hemoglobins may be present in minor percentages) and a stain for Heinz bodies or precipitated hemoglobin. Recent onset of anemia associated with morning dark urine, *or* marrow hypoplasia accompanied by iron deficiency, suggests the rare acquired intrinsic red cell defect, paroxysmal nocturnal hemoglobinuria.

If the anemic patient does not have fever, bleeding, abnormal MCV, or obvious reticulocytosis, a senior technologist, pathologist, or hematologist should take a look at the blood smear. In the patient whose anemia is still obscure we come to difficult problems, and the amount of work required can be greatly shortened by this new evaluation. The person reviewing the smear might, even in the absence of prior evidence of hemolysis, see previously undetected poikilocytes.

The adult with anemia still obscure after the above evaluation should, if it has not already been done, have renal function tested by serum creatinine and creatinine clearance. Tests for occult blood in the stool and a serum ferritin should be done if they have not been done already. The patient's records with previous physicians should be evaluated to see whether the anemia is long standing. Discovery that anemia is unexpectedly long standing channels the workup into arcane studies such as evaluation of red cell enzymes and for hemoglobinopathies.

The evaluation of anemia should be pursued in an orderly fashion. Some of the clues emphasized here, such as fever, abnormal MCV, polychromatophilia, and renal impairment, are often ignored. It is common practice in our hospital to respond to newly discovered anemia by ordering tests for iron, B_{12}, and folate and even a direct Coombs test. This kind of vitaminology (plus) only leads to delays, confusion, and expense, especially if inappropriate tests give borderline results. The MCV, for example, can be a helpful predictor. Patients with high MCVs commonly have folate deficiency, whereas people with normal or low MCVs rarely do. The rare patient with anemia and small red cells who *does* turn out to have folate deficiency has a "dimorphic" anemia, which is obvious on the blood smear. The patient with folate and iron deficiency, for example, has normochromic macrocytes and hypersegmented polymorphonuclear leukocytes (folate lack), accompanied by hypochromic microcytes (iron lack) on the blood smear. However, these dimorphic states are rare. In the literature, and in the very few patients I have seen with dimorphic anemia, the MCVs have turned out to be low. On the other hand, patients can have iron *depletion* without much anemia and with a normal MCV. People with chronic blood loss use up their bone marrow iron stores before serum iron drops and small red cells are made. A sensitive way to identify early iron deficiency is to look at the blood smear for a few hypochromic red cells. If there are a few of these then it may be worth ordering a serum iron or ferritin test even if the MCV is normal.

There are rare people who are iron deficient with a low MCV but a *normal hematocrit*. Such a patient may have polycythemia and have been phlebotomized, or have a duodenal ulcer and have phlebotomized himself. In this situation, an unexpected low MCV with a normal hematocrit, testing for iron deficiency and also for thalassemia is appropriate.

Polycythemia

The patient with a high hematocrit is usually assumed to have a real increase in red cells, but may turn out to have a decrease in plasma (Chart 2). If the red cell mass is increased, the patient may have pure erythrocytosis, which could be due to many things, or may have increased numbers of white cells and platelets as well, which would indicate polycythemia vera. Patients with a true increase in red cell mass are usually referred to as having "polycythemia" whether or not white cells and platelets are also elevated. An upper-normal hematocrit does not require diagnosis and treatment. An elevated hematocrit associated with an increased red cell mass does require treatment, and a reduced plasma volume may also require treatment.

The easiest cases of polycythemics to diagnose are in patients with definite increases in red cell measurements (Hb 20 +, Hct 60 +) *and* any combination of high white cell count, platelet count, and splenomegaly. These patients have polycythemia vera. Further laboratory evaluation shows an elevated red cell mass, elevated leukocyte alkaline phosphatase (LAP), and often basophilia. The initial therapy chosen is often phlebotomy, and it is characteristic of patients with large red cell mass for several phlebotomies to be required before there is any decline in the hematocrit. The patient whose high hematocrit drops markedly after the first phlebotomy or two (one unit off dropping the hematocrit from 55 to 48, for example) does not have

Chart 2

"POLYCYTHEMIA"

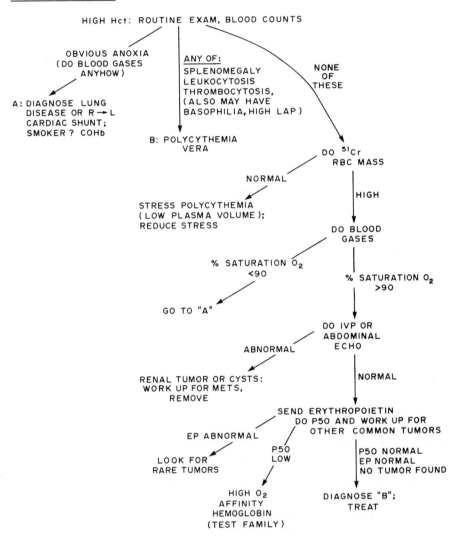

HIGH Hct: ROUTINE EXAM, BLOOD COUNTS

OBVIOUS ANOXIA
(DO BLOOD GASES
ANYHOW)

ANY OF:
SPLENOMEGALY
LEUKOCYTOSIS
THROMBOCYTOSIS,
(ALSO MAY HAVE
BASOPHILIA, HIGH LAP)

NONE
OF
THESE

A: DIAGNOSE LUNG
DISEASE OR R → L
CARDIAC SHUNT;
SMOKER ? COHb

B: POLYCYTHEMIA
VERA

DO ^{51}Cr
RBC MASS

NORMAL

STRESS POLYCYTHEMIA
(LOW PLASMA VOLUME);
REDUCE STRESS

HIGH

DO BLOOD
GASES

% SATURATION O_2
<90

% SATURATION O_2
>90

GO TO "A"

DO IVP OR
ABDOMINAL
ECHO

ABNORMAL

RENAL TUMOR OR CYSTS:
WORK UP FOR METS,
REMOVE

NORMAL

SEND ERYTHROPOIETIN
DO P50 AND WORK UP FOR
OTHER COMMON TUMORS

EP ABNORMAL

P50
LOW

P50 NORMAL
EP NORMAL
NO TUMOR FOUND

LOOK FOR
RARE TUMORS

HIGH O_2
AFFINITY
HEMOGLOBIN
(TEST FAMILY)

DIAGNOSE "B";
TREAT

much increase in red cell mass. Even patients with obvious polycythemia vera deserve further documentation with blood gases (percent O_2 saturation over 90% is expected here) and deserve an IVP or abdominal ultrasound test to exclude renal tumors and cysts.

More difficult to classify are patients with high hemoglobin and hematocrit, but no elevation of white cell count or of platelet count and no splenomegaly. As already indicated, a hemoglobin of 20 or over and a hematocrit of 60 or over always means increased red cell mass; however, values lower than these require *measurement* of red cell mass for confirmation polycythemia. The easiest test of red cell mass for a laboratory to do is plasma volume by radioactive iodine-tagged albumin injection and blood sampling after 10 minutes. Red cell mass is estimated from this plasma volume as follows:

$$\text{Plasma volume in liters} \times \frac{100}{\text{venous plasmacrit (100-Hct)}} = \text{red cell volume in liters}$$

Next, the red cell volume is converted to milliliters, divided by body weight in kilograms, and compared with normal values (34 ml/kg of body weight would be upper normal). This test is commonly offered by nuclear medicine laboratories. However, this test ignores the variable discrepancies between venous hematocrit and body hematocrit (the body hematocrit is lower than the venous hematocrit, but persons with large muscles or spleens will have more red cells than will asthenic or hyposplenic patients). Direct measurement of red cell mass by withdrawing blood, labeling the *red cells,* reinjecting, and sampling gives a more reliable red cell mass. This is usually done with ^{51}Cr isotope, which attaches to β globin chains. If the red cell mass turns out to be normal, the high hematocrit indicated a low plasma volume. This is usually labeled "stress polycythemia." If the cause of the low plasma volume is not due to something obvious like a diuretic (which should have been withdrawn before deciding to do a red cell mass test, but might not have been), the situation may warrant psychological consideration. If the ^{51}Cr red cell mass is high, a search is made for the cause.

Red cell production is normally amplified by renal erythropoietin, which is in turn controlled by oxygenation of unidentified cells in the kidneys, which secrete erythropoietin. If these cells do not get enough oxygen because of anemia, red cell oxygen desaturation, or interference with their blood supply (by vascular abnormality or tumor or renal cyst), they increase erythropoietin production. Erythrocytosis, if due to increased erythropoietin production, is termed "secondary"; if it is due to bone marrow misbehavior (polycythemia vera), it is termed "primary." If there is an increase in erythropoietin and this increase is due to renal anoxia, the resultant erythrocytosis is termed "appropriate"; if increased erythropoietin is coming from a tumor, it is termed "inappropriate."

The patient with proven erythrocytosis, but no increase in white cells or platelets and no splenomegaly, should be checked for unsuspected anoxemia by testing blood gases; if these are normal, he should have his kidneys evaluated. Possible renal causes for polycythemia include tumors and cysts and are readily detectable by IVP or echo studies. There is a long list of tumors that *can* cause erythrocytosis, but only four appear to be common among patients with erythrocytosis: hypernephroma, hepatoma, cerebellar hemangioblastoma and uterine fibroids. These associations have been documented as causes by detection of increased erythropoietin in the blood, urine, or tumor of affected patients or by remission of erythrocytosis after tumor removal. Erythrocytosis in hepatoma may not be at all obvious, because such patients are likely to have cirrhosis, ascites and increased plasma volume, and sequestration of part of the "erythron" in the spleen.

The great majority of cases of erythrocytosis will have been documented and explained by the tests already mentioned, namely, (1) careful examination and reexamination for splenomegaly, (2) routine blood counts (WBC, platelets), (3) red cell mass ^{51}Cr, (4) LAP, (5) blood gases, and (6) IVP or abdominal ultrasound.

Patients with definite erythrocytosis still resisting classification should have their plasma or urine erythropoietin measured done. Reliable radioimmunoassay is not yet available, and the test must be done by bioassay, available only at a few centers.

A low erythropoietin with a high hematocrit supports the diagnosis of polycythemia vera; increased erythropoietin would indicate the presence of an erythropoietin-secreting tumor still to be found.

One category of polycythemia of special interest to hematologists is erythrocytosis due to high-oxygen-affinity hemoglobin. The renal oxygen sensor presumably detects reduced availability of oxygen from the patient's hemoglobin and causes increased erythropoietin secretion. This increases marrow red cell output and adjusts the hematocrit upward to a level where the oxygen supply is adequate. Abnormal hemoglobins associated with high oxygen affinity and high hematocrit are detected by hemoglobin electrophoresis or by direct study of hemoglobin oxygen affinity. The result of the latter evaluation is reported as the "P50": the PO_2 at which the patient's red cell oxygen capacity is 50% saturated with oxygen (normal being 26 mm Hg [ca. 3.47 kPa], and lower values indicating increased affinity). Such erythrocytosis is lifelong and is present in half of the first-degree relatives.

Leukopenia

"Leukopenia," "neutropenia," and "granulocytopenia" are terms commonly used interchangeably. "Leukopenia" refers to a reduced total white cell count. "Neutropenia" refers to a reduction in leukocytes containing small, lilac-colored neutrophilic granules, the segmented and band polymorphonuclear leukocytes. These are usually decreased in leukopenia and increased in leukocytosis. Most discussions of leukopenia are about neutropenia. The term "granulocytes" adds eosinophils, basophils, and monocytes. Neutropenia is sometimes referred to as granulocytopenia, and these two terms *are* interchangeable, since eosinopenia (with the exception of the "Thorn test"), basopenia, and monocytopenia are not clinical entities. On the other hand, the patient with drug-induced leukopenia who develops monocytosis has a hopeful sign for control of infection and recovery from his leukopenia.

A normal, healthy person's white cell count varies during the day and from day to day, so it is wise to repeat a mildly reduced white cell count before getting too concerned about it. However if a person has a white cell count repeatedly below 3500, it is appropriate to give some attention to the leukopenia. If this is accompanied by a neutrophil (seg plus band) percentage that gives an absolute neutrophil count below 1800/μL, the leukopenia is caused by an absolute neutropenia.

The neutrophil lower limit of 1800 is derived from surveys of white male medical students. Other segments of the population have different normal ranges; 25% of black subjects have absolute neutrophil counts below the 1800 count limit. This finding is not associated with increased numbers of infections in blacks. A neutrophil count unexpectedly below 1800 has therapeutic and diagnostic implications which should be considered in that order. Marked neutropenia can make the subject vulnerable to bacterial infection; the potential seriousness of the situation is qualified by the absolute level. Generally, we are concerned about and would consider hospitalizing an individual with a newly identified absolute neutrophil count under 500, and we are particularly concerned about someone with a neutrophil count under 100. In one special category of neutropenic patients, patients with acute leukemia who are also immunosuppressed, neutrophil counts at this level are associated with a *high* rate of serious infection. Patients with less than 100 neutrophils require hospital surveillance for serious infection and, if signs such as chills and fever occur, immediate culturing and broad-spectrum antibiotic coverage until the cause of the fever as well as the neutropenia is uncovered.

Beyond these considerations of protecting the patient, the diagnostic problem of neutropenia may be best addressed by dividing the patients between those with neutropenia of less than one month's duration ("acute") and those with neutropenia of more than one month's duration ("chronic"). Some patients with acute neutropenia are at the onset of either viral or bacterial infections and respond with leukocytosis in a few hours. In some individuals neutropenia of this type implies a compromised marrow neutrophil reserve. People with compromised neutrophil reserve, such as alcoholics, may not rebound with leukocytosis in a few hours as normal persons do, but may remain neutropenic or with "normal" absolute granulocyte count even during severe pneumonia when granulocytosis would be expected. In the infected patient who fails to develop leukocytosis, but develops an infiltrate on chest x-ray, for example, it is often speculated that the compromised marrow is making enough white cells to mobilize to the site of the infection, but that there are not enough left to be measured as an increment in the blood.

Infections causing neutropenia are always obvious. *Drugs* which cause neutropenia can be overlooked. If a patient is receiving a drug for cancer chemotherapy which always causes reduction in normal cell counts the situation is easy to understand, and usually the cell count recovers during observation. Patients who are receiving drugs which only occasionally cause neutropenia may fail to report them to their physician initially. Drugs commonly causing such unexpected or idiosyncratic reactions are phenothiazines and propylthiouracil. However, if the patient has become leukopenic after starting to use *any* new drugs and while still taking the drug, and it is the only drug being taken, that medicine should be assumed to be the cause of the neutropenia and discontinued.

Chronic neutropenia, that is, neutropenia persisting for more than a month, is usually just a low normal value. Ninety-five percent of healthy white adults have absolute granulocyte counts between 7000 and 1800, but 2.5% have values below 1800. Such constitutional or "chronic idiopathic" neutropenia is, however, a diagnosis of exclusion. It is supported by tracking down any earlier low neutrophil counts that had no other explanation and by ruling out the common causes of neutropenia. In our experience these are (1) splenomegaly, or, surprisingly, liver disease without proven splenomegaly; (2) systemic lupus or rheumatoid arthritis; and (3) hematologic neoplasm.

Patients with chronic neutropenia who do not have any of these conditions may rarely have preleukemia, but this should not be assumed. In local experience, most patients have constitutional ("chronic idiopathic") neutropenia and do not go on to leukemia.

Chronic neutropenia does require a workup. Likely mechanisms are splenic sequestration, autoimmunity, and marrow failure. Careful palpation for splenic enlargement is particularly important. A liver-spleen scan may be necessary. Because of our own experience with liver disease we also do liver function tests. Antinuclear antibody and rheumatoid factor address the collagen-vascular diseases likely to be important here. A bone marrow aspirate would detect the presence of any hematologic neoplasm and the rare possibility of preleukemia, the latter suggested by megaloblastoid change or ringed sideroblasts. The possibility of preleukemia can be further investigated by doing chromosomal analysis looking for the abnormal chromosome marker of an abnormal clone.

A review of earlier white cell counts, if such are available, is desirable. Earlier neutropenia would give positive support to a diagnosis of chronic idiopathic neutropenia or to splenomegaly as the cause.

Finally, the person who has very marked neutropenia, generating concern about risk of infection, may benefit from the performance of a leukocyte mobilization study. The best of these tests is done by injecting 100 mg of intravenous Solu-Cortef and comparing preinjection absolute neutrophil counts with those obtained at 2, 3, 4, and 5 hours after the injection. A normal neutrophil reserve allows mobilization of 2000 neutrophils (a 2000-fold increase in absolute neutrophils above the baseline) at one of these times. This normal response is reassuring if the person happens, for example, to be a kidney dialysis patient with a scheduled date for transplantation. This event is necessarily followed by the use of immunosuppressive drugs, which are also marrow suppressive. If the marrow reserve is poor to begin with, or the spleen is detaining too many neutrophils, severe neutropenia will recur after transplantation, requiring discontinuation of the immunosuppressive drug and resulting in loss of the transplanted organ.

When a patient has chronic, marked leukopenia it is important to monitor him or her especially in the early months after discovery of the cytopenia. The monitoring may show worsening of the neutropenia or emergence of the cause or, more likely and important, the occurrence of serious bacterial infection. Any suspected bacterial infections (chills, or fever over 38.5 °C) should be reported and should lead, within an hour or two, to hospitalization, culturing, and treatment with parenteral antibiotics. Although periodic cycling of the neutrophil count ("cyclic neutropenia") was an early described type of neutropenia, cyclic neutropenia appears less common than stable neutropenia.

Lymphopenia is usually found in patients treated with steroids, and these individuals usually also have leukocytosis, so would not be found within the low white count category. Another group of lymphopenic patients are patients with aplastic anemia and marrow panhypoplasia. Adult patients with a selective, true lymphopenia (ie, total lymphocyte counts less than 1000) should probably be investigated further, particularly if they are having trouble with recurring infections. In such patients it might well be worth studying antibody globulins for hypogammaglobulinemia, and perhaps in a research context, looking at lymphocyte subpopulations (T and B cells, and T cell subpopulations).

Leukocytosis

Leukocytosis is commonly found in various acute illnesses and other stresses. If it is accompanied by neutrophilia, and especially by increased band neutrophils, leukocytosis is taken to imply an infectious and bacterial etiology for an illness. With increases in neutrophils and band neutrophils, the other major component of the normal differential, the lymphocyte family, makes a relative decline. Thus, the lymphocyte percentage offered on the new Coulter counters is a useful, if inverse, sign of neutrophilia.

Several changes in cytoplasmic contents often accompany leukocytosis in infection. Unusually dark and coarse cytoplasmic granules ("toxic granulation") and indistinct, light blue Döhle bodies may be seen. If special cytochemical stains are done, leukocyte alkaline phosphatase is consistently increased. If Wright-stained neutrophils should contain cytoplasmic vacuoles, bacteremia is suggested. (Note that cytoplasmic vacuoles are normally found in monocytes in ethylenediaminetetraacetic acid (EDTA)-anticoagulated blood.) A search for bacteria in the smear, usually seen as 1-μm, encapsulated blue dot inclusions in neutrophil cytoplasm, is worthwhile. These may be more readily found in buffy coat smears.

Bacteria are only rarely found in Wright-stained blood smears, but are important when present, as they indicate a septic emergency. If they are found, it is important not to fall into the trap of identifying such inclusions, blue on Wright stain, as "gram positive." Also beware of precipitated stain, which can resemble bacteria but is easily distinguished, since the stain is extracellular and scattered all over the smear, whereas bacteria are intracellular and rare.

Aside from its occurrence in acute bacterial infection, leukocytosis develops in various kinds of physical stress including major abdominal and thoracic surgery. Leukocytosis, neutrophilia, and increased bands are noted within 30 minutes of induction of general anesthesia and persist for two to three days after an operation without indicating any infection. This point is frequently forgotten, as early postoperative fever is often evaluated for infection with white cell count and differential. Examples of other noninfectious stresses that cause neutrophilia include athletic exertion and labor and delivery. Similar degrees of leukocytosis can be induced experimentally by injection of bacterial pyrogen or corticosteriods or epinephrine. Pyrogen and corticosteriods mobilize bone marrow neutrophils, and steroids also prevent egress of neutrophils from the blood. Epinephrine acts by recruiting the "marginal" granulocyte pool from blood vessel walls. Corticosteroids administered chronically produce a neutrophilia with very few bands. Most cases of leukocytosis are not obscure, nor do they require specialized hematology laboratory workup.

Another, less commonly important point in trying to explain leukocytosis, is that increases in cell count can be observed after splenectomy (after splenectomy, leukocytosis, thrombocytosis, lymphocytosis, and eosinophilia are all possible). These increases may persist for only weeks to months after the surgery or for much longer. A patient with unexplained leukocytosis with an upper abdominal scar may have had a splenectomy incidental to other surgery.

In the absence of any of these causes, unexplained leukocytosis calls for a sophisticated blood smear review. The purpose of this review is to look for cells not noted in the routine differential. If blasts are present among the leukocytes, a bone marrow aspiration may be desirable. However, a blast or two accompanying leukocytosis at the onset of an acute infection may indicate an activated lymphocyte, rather than evidence of leukemia, and require no special attention. If leukocytosis includes myelocytes and metamyelocytes, the patient should be evaluated for chronic myelocytic leukemia. The appropriate evaluation includes reexamination for splenic enlargement and leukocyte alkaline phosphatase and, if the blood picture is impressive, bone marrow aspiration with chromosome studies. If the smear review does not reveal any immature forms, it may be useful to repeat the blood cell count in a week to two. If neutrophilia is persistent, especially if the patient is apparently healthy, certain other unusual conditions should be considered. One of these is congenital asplenia. This is indicated by the presence of solitary inclusions in red cells (Howell-Jolly bodies) in the absence of any past splenectomy. A liver-spleen scan shows the lack of reticuloendothelial function in the left upper quandrant. Another reported cause of chronic neutrophilia is "neutrophilic leukemia." This condition was associated with a persistent high white cell count with increased segmented and banded polymorphonuclear leukocytes, tissue infiltration with segmented and banded polymorphonuclear leukocytes, and hyperuricemia. There really is no specific way to diagnose this entity, but it would be appropriate to do a bone marrow analysis and look for chromosome abnormalities here as well. Of course, one should review the history carefully for chronic illness or an inflammatory state being ignored by the patient. Looking at any prior records at this junction might be reassuring. If the leukocytosis is only mild and has persisted for a long time it could be the normal value for the individual.

Lymphocytosis

Children between the ages of approximately one week and four years normally have more lymphocytes than neutrophils. Lymphocytosis over $4000/\mu L$ in an adult is usually transient and disappears unexplained. Patients recovering from the stresses of infection or surgery may have mild transient lymphocytosis instead of the more common neutrophilia. One unusual cause for a mild increase in normal-appearing lymphocytes that does not always go away is splenectomy. Lymphocytosis may persist for years in such patients, although it usually subsides after weeks to months.

When mild lymphocytosis develops in an adult, and the lymphocytosis is accompanied by an acute or subacute illness with or without fever and lymphadenopathy, a spectrum of infections should be considered. These include toxoplasmosis, cytomegalovirus infection, infectious hepatitis, and infectious mononucleosis. All of these are likely to be accompanied by increase in normal lymphocytes and "atypical" lymphocytes. An atypical lymphocyte resembles a normal lymphocyte, with several important modifications. The cell is large and has abundant, often "foamy" cytoplasm which is indented by surrounding red cells. The nucleus, compared to normal mature lymphocytes, appears young, with unclumped chromatin. If a large fraction of the lymphocyte increment is composed of atypical lymphocytes, workup for these conditions is appropriate. Such workup can be focused toward toxoplasmosis in the presence of fever and lymphadenopathy, toward cytomegalovirus infection in patients who are immunosuppressed or have received fresh blood transfusions, toward hepatitis in transfused or jaundiced patients, and toward infectious mononucleosis in previously healthy young adults.

Lymphocytosis not accompanied by any acute illness may represent chronic lymphocytic leukemia. This condition is not considered strongly unless there is a rather marked lymphocytosis, over an absolute 10,000 (more convincing if over 15,000), and unless the lymphocytosis is persistent. In the past, lymphocytosis of marked degree was observed in certain "leukemoid" reactions, especially in advanced tuberculosis.

A reported marked increase in small lymphocytes needs morphologic review. Sometimes the small lymphocytes are accompanied by large ones and clefted ones, suggesting an aggressive variant of chronic lymphocytic leukemia called lymphosarcoma cell leukemia. Rarely, cells of myeloblastic leukemia may resemble small lymphocytes, the so-called "micromyeloblasts." These cells contain nucleoli and will usually stain with cytochemical stains such as Sudan B and peroxidase. Finally, the blood smear review may show that the lymphocytes really are all small ones, and that they are accompanied by numerous spherocytes, indicating that the patient has chronic lymphocytic leukemia (CLL) that is complicated by hemolytic anemia (which happens at some point in the course in 25% of CLL cases). A positive direct Coombs test would confirm the presence and pertinence of the spherocytes.

If, on review, the reported lymphocytosis consists of small, normal-looking lymphs, the patient is over 40, and lymphocytosis persists, it is appropriate to consider the patient as having chronic lymphocytic leukemia. Physical examination may deserve repetition for lymphadenopathy and splenomegaly. Also to be noted are the person's hematocrit and platelet count, as anemia or thrombocytopenia have an unfavorable impact on stage and prognosis (CLL with anemia: Rai stage III; CLL with thrombocytopenia: Rai stage IV). It is appropriate, if sometimes difficult, to wait a week to a month to assure oneself that the lymphocytosis is really persistent. If the lymphocytosis disappears, especially if there was a suspicion of fever, stress, or sweats at the onset, it is reasonable to accept lymphocytosis as the product of an unidentified infection.

If the lymphocytosis is marked and persistent, and the patient shows no sign of infection, the diagnosis is chronic lymphocytic leukemia. At this point to check quantitative immunoglobulins to predict and prepare for complications in the event of hypogammaglobulinemia. An occasional patient, 1 in 20 with CLL, will have a monoclonal gammopathy. Bone marrow aspiration and biopsy is not essential for diagnosis, but correlates with the Rai staging system. A marrow with diffusely increased cellularity consisting of small lymphocytes is typical of stage III and stage IV of CLL. If available, T- and B-cell quantitation of circulating lymphocytes will be helpful. In the usual case of chronic lymphocytic leukemia, 80 or 90% of circulating lymphocytes are B cells, faintly staining with fluorescein-tagged anti-immunoglobulin M (IgM). In chronic lymphosarcoma cell leukemia, exposure to fluorescein-labeled anti-IgG will show brightly staining surface immunoglobulin. T- and B-cell typing in normal patients shows 60 to 70% T cells and about 20% B cells, with the rest being null cells.

Eosinophilia

Eosinophilia is more likely to be explained by findings of history and physical examination than by laboratory investigation. The differential diagnosis stated here is based on local clinical experience and on a survey carried out on patients with subacute and chronic eosinophilia sufficiently persistent to have bone marrow aspiration carried out.

When eosinophilia appears in a patient who is taking medicine, days to weeks after the start of the exposure, it is reasonable to presume that eosinophilia has been caused by the drug; discontinue the drug and observe. Although antibiotics and psychotropic medications are likely culprits, any medicine that has been taken for a period of days to weeks before the eosinophilia is noted should be considered a possible cause. If the medicine is deemed essential, the eosinophilia is usually ignored and the patient is observed. However, there is probably some risk of other kinds of allergic reactions, and it is preferable to discontinue any possibly offending drug.

In addition to drugs, allergy, pulmonary disorders, and skin disorders in various overlapping arrays are sometimes associated with eosinophilia. The eosinophilia in these situations is usually more chronic. Pulmonary symptoms such as wheezing, cough, and dyspnea point to asthma, Löffler's pneumonia, or the pulmonary infiltration with eosinophilia (PIE) syndrome as causes of eosinophilia. Asthma is usually obvious from history and examination. The others are accompanied by lung infiltrates on x-ray. Löffler's pneumonia is usually transient and steroid responsive, whereas PIE is chronic and only partially steroid responsive. The presence of rash in a person with eosinophilia suggests that both the eosinophils and the rash are due to allergy, but some dermatoses associated with eosinophilia are not necessarily allergic. Skin disorders associated with eosinophilia in the past have included pemphigus, urticaria, and dermatitis herpetiformis.

If the patient with eosinophilia has obvious cancer or lymphoma, it is reasonable to presume that the condition is the cause of the blood change. Effective treatment of the neoplasm causes the disappearance of the eosinophilia. An individual with eosinophilia sufficient to cause leukocytosis and associated splenomegaly may have eosinophilic leukemia. This is probably the same condition as the "hypereosinophilic syndrome." The eosinophils in these patients are sometimes abnormal or immature; characteristically, the eosinophils are not as packed with granules like normal eosinophils. Associated clinical findings of fever, pulmonary infiltration, cardiac murmurs, and wasting all contribute to the diagnosis of this syndrome.

A history of residence in the tropics or recent consumption of raw pork suggests parasitism as the cause of eosinophilia. Parasites invading tissues, rather than merely resident in the gastrointestinal tract, are considered likely causes of eosinophilia.

There are numerous other conditions occasionally associated with eosinophilia. As reported by others, we have seen eosinophilia associated with peritoneal dialysis; the mechanism is not clear.

There are also many patients who have eosinophilia of totally unknown cause, which may or may not be persistent. Consideration of allergy, cancer, lymphoma, hypereosinophilic syndrome, pulmonary infiltration, and skin disorders may be desirable. However, it is not clear whether investigation of patients with eosinophilia will turn up occult cases of any of these entities at the time, or whether any are likely to emerge in patients under surveillance for eosinophilia.

Patients with peripheral eosinophilia also have eosinophilia in their marrow, and doing a marrow analysis does not advance the workup. Other special hematology studies such as leukocyte alkaline phosphatase and chromosome analysis also do not add anything. Careful examination of the blood smear for hypogranular eosinophils and echo and scan studies for splenomegaly may be useful in patients with possible eosinophilic leukemia.

Monocytosis

Monocytosis is often an enigmatic finding. Mild monocytosis, ie, 15 to 20% monocytes associated with a normal white cell count or mild leukocytosis, seems to be about as specific as an elevated erythrocyte sedimentation rate. This degree of monocytosis has been reported to occur in cancer patients more often than in healthy persons, but has not been shown to be useful in prospective studies.

The 15 to 20% monocytosis is commonly noted in our hospital in persons recovering from drug-induced neutropenia. It is seen after cancer chemotherapy and can also be seen with recovery from idiosyncratic neutropenias. In the latter setting it is taken as a favorable prognostic sign.

Most commonly, mild monocytosis is unexplained and transient. Long-term follow-up data on patients with this abnormality are not available. Presumably it is a variant of a neutrophil response to noxious stimuli. Like neutrophilia, monocytosis seems to be a nonspecific clue to diagnosis. The two cells may respond to the same spectrum of stimuli because of a close family relationship. The presence of monocytes in neutrophilic granulocyte colonies grown from single cells in agar suggests that monocytes arise from myeloblasts, as does the evolution of myelomonocytic acute leukemia from a single cell.

In the rare instances of high-level (50%) monocytes associated with leukocytosis, the diagnosis is often acute monocytic or myelomonocytic leukemia. Occasionally, reports of monocytosis will be made in error, and the reported monocytes are blasts. In the past, high-level monocytosis was described in leukemoid reactions to tuberculosis.

Red Cell Morphology

Many interesting things have been found in blood smears, and Wright-stained blood smears may afford diagnostic clues to a wide range of diseases (Figure 3-1). However most blood smears are either normal or abnormal in limited, stereotyped ways.

In trying to organize the range of possible red cell morphologic abnormalities it is convenient to classify red cell abnormalities as changes in red cell (1) size, (2) color, (3) shape, (4) inclusions, and (5) rouleaux. The size changes of interest include macrocytosis, microcytosis, and anisocytosis (variation in red cell size). Most of these abnormalities are identified by abnormal MCVs, discussed in a previous section, which are more reliable although not more sensitive than microscopic evaluation of cell size. One additional comment about the relationship between high MCVs and the smear: macrocytosis which is consistent and involves all red cells is likely to be due to liver disease or antimetabolites. Macrocytosis associated with anisocytosis may indicate folate or vitamin B_{12} deficiency.

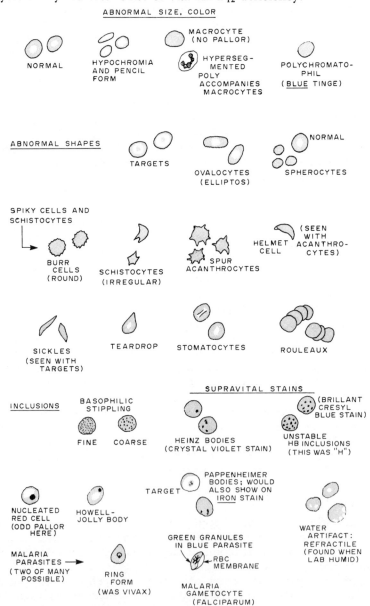

Figure 3-1 Schematic drawings of some red cell morphologic variants.

In our laboratory we try to minimize use of the general terms "anisocytosis" and "poikilocytosis," as they convey very little to the clinician except the technician's inability to identify a specific abnormality. However, a reading of "marked anisocytosis" merits careful consideration and review.

Color abnormalities recognized as useful are hypochromia, meaning more than one-third of the red cell diameter is pale, and polychromatophilia. Hypochromia usually correlates with microcytic anemia, although target cells may also appear hypochromic. Polychromatophilia reflects, but underestimates, reticulocytosis.

Abnormal red cell shapes will be discussed in the next section.

Red cell inclusions frequently seen on Wright-stained smears include nucleated red cells, basophilic stippling, Howell-Jolly bodies, and Pappenheimer bodies. Nucleated red cells are seen in the blood in severe hemolytic states, in severe acute illnesses such as life-threatening infections, and in leukemias. Rare nucleated red cells in otherwise normal smears suggest a myelophthisic state (marrow invasion by tumor, fibrosis, or tuberculosis). Basophilic stippling, a more common and often trivial observation, is usually fine and is usually found in polychromatophilic red cells. It has no meaning beyond polychromatophilia. *Coarse* basophilic stippling in erythrocytes is more suspicious and suggests lead poisoning or hemoglobinopathy. However, coarse basophilic stippling, like fine stippling, can also be found in high-grade reticulocytosis. Howell-Jolly bodies, seen as 1-μm solitary blue dots, are morphologic hallmarks of splenic absence or dysfunction. Pappenheimer bodies, which are smaller, clustered, multiple blue dots, represent iron combined with precipitated ribonucleic acid in the red cell. Like Howell-Jolly bodies, these are found in splenic hypofunction, but the carriers of Pappenheimer bodies are usually also iron loaded. Conditions associated with Pappenheimer bodies include hemoglobinopathies and sideroblastic anemias. The unexplained presence of Pappenheimer bodies might lead to some combination of hemoglobin electrophoresis, bone marrow aspiration, serum ferritin, and liver-spleen scan (if the status of the spleen is not known).

Note that reports of these two red cell inclusions, Howell-Jolly bodies and Pappenheimer bodies, are often in error due to the artifact of refractile intraerythrocytic bodies caused by water in the stain. We commonly see this in humid seasons in our laboratory. Water artifacts are identified with the microscope as being refractile as one focuses up and down, rather than flat and only in focus with the rest of the red cell, as authentic red cell inclusions are.

There are of course other red cell inclusions which could be mentioned, but they do not turn up on routine Wright-stained peripheral blood smears. These include Heinz bodies, which are precipitated hemoglobin attached to the red cell membrane. These are found in unstable hemoglobin hemolytic anemias and reportedly in hemolytic anemia in G6PD deficiency. Despite a long-standing interest in G6PD deficiency, I have not seen Heinz bodies in that condition.

Rouleaux are red cells stacked like coins. When a smear is made with too much blood, rouleaux are not meaningful, but if they are found in thin areas of the smear they are important. If one suspects the presence of rouleaux one usually reviews the whole blood smear to look for relatively thin areas. When red cells persistently cluster in groups of two, three or more in these areas, rouleaux are present. This implies that the patient has a high level of serum proteins (globulins or fribrinogen), which in turn indicates a febrile or inflammatory illness lasting days to weeks, or longer. Recall that the increase in proteins causing rouleaux is the same phenomenon that causes an increase in the erythrocyte sedimentation rate.

Marked rouleaux are also found in people with marked hyperglobulinemia due to chronic liver disease or multiple myeloma. Hemolytic anemias associated with a positive direct Coombs test may also be associated with marked rouleaux formation. Clumps of red cells that one can see before putting the slide under the microscope are sometimes noted in conditions associated with cold agglutinins, such as mycoplasma pneumonia, infectious mononucleosis, and idiopathic cold agglutinin disease.

Microorganisms in the peripheral smear are uncommon, but are extremely important when present. Malaria parasites of any species are usually found as ring forms within red cells. These ring forms are usually 3 to 4 μm in diameter with a bright red jewel of perhaps 1 μm in diameter somewhere on the ring. In the commonest malaria that is caused by *Plasmodium vivax*, red cells containing the parasites are commonly spiky and may have little red inclusions (Schüffner's dots). Vivax gametocytes, granule-containing nuclear bodies the size of a red cell, are often present along with the ring forms. They are sometimes confused with giant platelets, but the malaria gametocyte has greenish granules, whereas giant platelets have purple and red-purple granules. The presence of another important malaria species, falciparum, is indicated by large, banana-shaped gametocytes. Malaria parasites usually are brought to our laboratory in a Vacutainer tube carried by a suspicious clinician, often an infectious disease expert.

Poikilocytosis

Common abnormal red cell shapes can be grouped, in approximate order of frequency in our laboratory, as follows: target cells; a group consisting of ovalocytes, elliptocytes, and pencil forms; spherocytes; spiky red cells including acanthrocytes and burr cells; sickle cells; teardrops; and stomatocytes.

The presence of target cells suggests a limited set of possible interpretations which are listed here in order of frequency (Chart 3). Nearly all patients with target cells have liver disease, have hemoglobinopathy, have had a splenectomy, or have iron deficiency. Liver disease is known from the history or can be identified by liver function tests. If liver disease is not present and if the patient is black or of Mediterranean or Asian ancestry, hemoglobin electrophoresis may identify sickle thalassemia, SC, CC, or EE (Asian) hemoglobinopathies, or C trait. Any of these conditions can be unsuspected in adult life. Other hemoglobinopathies causing target cells, thalassemia major, and sickle cell disease, are usually known to the patient. Splenectomy, if the cause of the targets, is usually known from history and physical examination and is confirmed on the smear by the observation of Howell-Jolly bodies. Patients who have target cells due to iron deficiency usually have microcytosis and prominent hypochromia, and the true diagnosis can be confirmed by iron or ferritin studies.

Chart 3

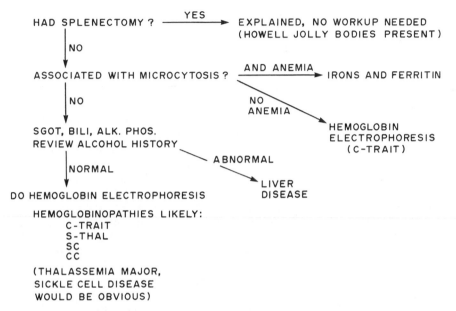

TARGETS (HYPOCHROMIA OFTEN REPORTED, TOO):

HAD SPLENECTOMY? ──YES──► EXPLAINED, NO WORKUP NEEDED
(HOWELL JOLLY BODIES PRESENT)

│ NO

ASSOCIATED WITH MICROCYTOSIS? ──AND ANEMIA──► IRONS AND FERRITIN

│ NO   NO
              ANEMIA

SGOT, BILI, ALK. PHOS.   HEMOGLOBIN
REVIEW ALCOHOL HISTORY   ELECTROPHORESIS
                                          (C-TRAIT)

│ NORMAL   ABNORMAL

DO HEMOGLOBIN ELECTROPHORESIS   LIVER
                                 DISEASE
HEMOGLOBINOPATHIES LIKELY:
    C-TRAIT
    S-THAL
    SC
    CC
(THALASSEMIA MAJOR,
SICKLE CELL DISEASE
WOULD BE OBVIOUS)

Ovalocytes, elliptocytes, and pencil forms are progressive elongations of the round to slightly oval red cells seen on normal blood smears. Although the presence of a few ovalocytes is normal, the presence of numerous ovalocytes, approaching 50% of separately spread red cells, usually indicates hereditary ovalocytosis (elliptocytosis). These ovalocytes are normal in size. This condition, inherited as an autosomal dominant, is usually just a blood smear finding with no clinical implications. However, about 10% of patients with ovalocytosis have a hemolytic anemia resembling that seen in spherocytosis and confirmed by the same test, the osmotic fragility test. If the blood smear shows marked anisocytosis including a few ovalocytes which are very large, the picture suggests megaloblastic anemia. This situation will be accompanied by high MCV in the Coulter counter. Very long, thin ovalocytes, also referred to as pencil forms, are commonly associated with microcytosis and hypochromia in iron deficiency.

Spherocytes, if few, can be present due to artifact. We see this frequently in anemic smears in our laboratory; it is associated with a local habit of making "pulled" rather than the usual "pushed" blood smears. Small numbers of nonartifactual spherocytes, which would be seen on a pushed smear or a saline-diluted "wet preparation," can be found in various hemolytic states. When spherocytes are numerous, approaching 50% of red cells, there are only three likely diagnoses: hereditary spherocytosis (HS), Coombs positive hemolytic anemia as a separate entity, and Coombs positive hemolysis occurring in a patient with chronic lymphocytic leukemia. HS is usually found in children and young adults, whereas either of the Coombs positive hemolytic anemias is seen in older adults. Some patients with hereditary spherocytosis have only minimal anemia because of the ability of their bone marrows to compensate for the increased cell turnover, and they unexpectedly decompensate in the presence of a febrile illness that would cause little anemia in another person not dependent on a constant high level of red cell output. Other patients with spherocytosis have been incorrectly classified as iron deficient and treated with iron supplements. *Acquired* spherocytosis, which is accompanied by a positive direct Coombs test, is seen on the blood smear as marked polychromatophilia. The diagnostic test that confirms either form of spherocytosis is the red cell osmotic fragility test (fragility is increased). This test is most sensitive when carried out after the blood has been incubated for 24 hours at 37 °C ("incubated osmotic fragility").

The presence of many spiky red cells is an important finding usually reflecting hemolysis, but here we encounter problems in both recognition and nomenclature (Chart 4). Most of us are confused about how to name and classify these cells, unless the patient's diagnosis is already known. The terms frequently used for these poikilocytes are "acanthrocyte," "burr cell," "crenated cell," "echinocyte," "schistocyte," and "spur cell." One patient's spiky cells are rarely labeled with the same term by any two observers. However, the problem can be simplified by noting that, for a given patient, these cells are either basically round with numerous evenly spaced small protrusions, resembling a sea urchin (echinocytes) or basically irregular in shape with irregularly placed, often large protrusions (acanthrocytes). Irregular spiky cells are smaller-than-normal fragments in some conditions (schistocytes).

Round spiky cells can be artifacts and can be reproduced by exposing normal red cells to unphysiologic conditions of pH or osmolality in vitro. Irregular spiky cells, if numerous, always represent in vivo abnormalities. If the report or your blood smear review indicates that there are many *round*

Chart 4

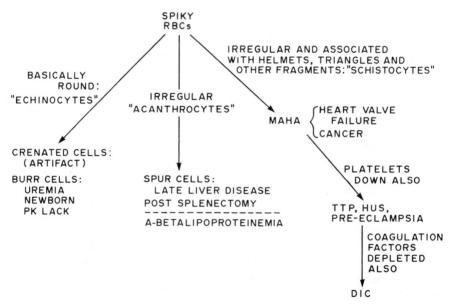

spiky red cells (proper terms are burr cells, crenated cells, and echinocytes) the next step is to obtain a fresh blood sample and repeat the blood smear. If the observation is not repeated on the fresh blood smear, the spiky red cells were probably artifacts. The original crenated cells may have suffered from delay between blood drawing and making the smear. Overnight-stored red cells in EDTA anticoagulant are all crenated. If, on the other hand, the basically round, spiky cells are also seen in a fresh sample it is reasonable to assume that the abnormality is pathological (burr cells). Tests of renal function should be reviewed, as renal failure is a prominent cause of burr cells. Pyruvate kinase deficiency is reported to cause burr cells, so it may be worth testing for this if the patient has anemia and reticulocytosis. Round spiky cells are a normal finding in newborn infants.

Conditions commonly causing *irregular* spiky cells include microangiopathic hemolytic anemia and disseminated intravascular coagulation (DIC). In both of these disorders the irregular spiky cells are referred to as schistocytes, implying mechanical damage within the blood stream as the cause of shape change (and hemolysis). The irregular spiky cells are likely to be associated with helmet-shaped cells, triangles, and other little fragments. The concept and the term "microangiopathic" for this kind of red cell fragmentation were first applied to patients with malignant hypertension, renal failure, and hemolysis. Other causes of microangiopathic change include disseminated cancer, failing prosthetic heart valve ("Waring blender"), thrombotic thrombocytopenic purpura (TTP), and preeclampsia. TTP and preeclampsia are accompanied by thrombocytopenia, whereas the others usually are not. These four entities usually do not cause accompanying coagulation abnormalities.

Irregular spiky red cells are, however, also found in disseminated intravascular coagulation, in which case the schistocytes (spiky forms and helmet cells) are accompanied by thrombocytopenia and changes in clotting tests. The easiest tests to check for support for this diagnosis include the prothrombin time, fibrinogen, tests for fibrin split products, and the platelet count. DIC can occur in sepsis, complications of pregnancy, and cancer, and in any terminally ill patient.

Other conditions in which irregular spiky cells are found are liver disease and abetalipoproteinemia. The liver disease that is associated with irregular spiky cells (here called spur cells) is usually late and ominous. The patient is likely to be deeply jaundiced, ascitic, and comatose. Irregular spiky cells termed acanthrocytes were early found in neurologically impaired children with abetalipoproteinemia.

Splenectomy leaves behind a few irregular spiky red cells as well as red cell inclusions. Many patients will have a few spiky erythrocytes in their blood smear, and no specific cause will be found.

When sickle cells are found in stained blood smears, one of three symptomatic sickling disorders is likely: sickle cell anemia, sickle-thalassemia, or sickle-hemoglobin C hemoglobinopathy. The sickle cells are banana shaped and do not show the sharp protrusions seen in sickle preparations made with sodium metabisulfite. Also present in the smear in any of these conditions are numerous target cells. In sickle cell anemia, one also sees polychromatophilia and nucleated red cells, and, in autosplenectomized (spleen-infarcted) adults, Howell-Jolly and Pappenheimer bodies. Sickle thalassemia is associated with microcytosis (low MCV); sickle-C hemoglobinopathy is associated with especially prominent targeting, but no signs of spleen dysfunction (no Howell-Jolly or Pappenheimer bodies). Note that sickle cells are *not* found in the smear in sickle trait, although they can be produced in sickle cell preparations done with sickle trait blood.

Teardrop-shaped red cells are found in large numbers in myeloproliferative disorders associated with myelofibrosis, including myeloid metaplasia. In myeloid metaplasia, the teardrop-shaped red cells are accompanied by various combinations of nucleated red cells, immature granulocyte precursors, and giant platelets. A few teardrops without these other monsters may be found in iron-deficient blood.

Finally stomatocytes, which are red cells showing a slot-shaped instead of round central pallor, have gained interest and credibility from a few case reports and from electron microscopic studies. These cells have been observed and reported in drinking alcoholics with hemolytic anemia. In this situation they persisted for only a few days. Stomatocytes have also been reported in a few subjects with high-sodium red cells, and a few others with abnormal red cell antigens, specifically the absence of Rh antigens (Rh null). We pursue observed stomatocytes by making repeat smears from the blood sample, obtaining repeat blood samples, and looking at "wet preparation" morphology as well as more stained smears. In our laboratory, stomatocytes have consistently been due to artifact. They have generally been regional on the slide, or, if all over the slide, have not been found on repeat blood sampling. If the stomatocytes persisted, we would review the history for alcoholism, look for hemolysis, check the patient's Rh antigens, and test the electrolyte content of the red cells.

Thrombocytopenia

Newly found, isolated thrombocytopenia in an ambulatory adult suggests a limited array of possible causes. If viral infection is present, and if the thrombocytopenia is mild, it is reasonable simply to observe the patient for early recovery. The marrow is usually looked at if the thrombocytopenia is marked or does not recover in days to weeks. Alternatively, there may be a history of taking medicines that can cause thrombocytopenia. Drugs in current use which are particularly likely to do this include thiazides (usually mild thrombocytopenia) and quinidine (sometimes marked thrombocytopenia). Again, if the thrombocytopenia is mild one can simply discontinue the drug and observe the patient. Another possible cause is hypersplenism. If splenomegaly is present and the thrombocytopenia is mild, the latter is considered explained. However, one should check the marrow aspirate to look for the cause for both the splenomegaly and thrombocytopenia, to rule out hematologic neoplasm and direct attention to the liver, and also to ensure that platelet production is normal (the presence of normal numbers of megakaryocytes assures this).

If the thrombocytopenic patient has no history of viral infection, no recent drug ingestion, and no splenomegaly, the likely diagnosis is idiopathic thrombocytopenic purpura (ITP). Bone marrow aspiration should be done. It will show megakaryocytes in normal or increased numbers, indicating that the cause is ITP. Normal maturation in erythroid and granulocyte series indicates that the cause of the thrombocytopenia is not hematologic neoplasm.

One can further support the diagnosis of ITP by testing or having tests done for platelet-associated IgG (antibody) and perhaps by looking at platelet size. It is not really established that platelet sizing is a sensitive test for immune thrombocytopenia, but ITP is associated with high output and turnover of platelets, and young platelets are known to be larger than other platelets. Demonstration of platelet antibody and increased numbers of large platelets confirms the diagnosis of ITP. *Large* amounts of platelet-associated IgG predict splenectomy failure. If these tests are unavailable, simply finding normal or increased numbers of megakaryocytes in the presence of marked thrombocytopenia is sufficient to make a diagnosis of ITP.

Occasionally, the patient with idiopathic thrombocytopenia will be found to have megakaryocytopenia. This ominous finding can occur on a congenital basis, after some drugs, or as a precursor to bone marrow neoplasm.

High Platelet Count

Elevation of the platelet count is commonly observed with inflammatory states and malignancies associated with tissue destruction and fever, and with gastrointestinal bleeding, when these disorders occur over a period of weeks. In these situations the high platelet count is called "thrombocytosis" and is considered to be secondary to the inflammation or bleeding. The platelet count is usually less than 1 million. In the patient with thrombocytosis but no inflammation or gastrointestinal bleeding, it is worth looking at the MCV. If the MCV is low in a patient with marked thrombocytosis and normal hematocrit, it is quite possible that one is dealing with polycythemia vera with an associated duodenal ulcer. Polycythemia can be confirmed by administering iron and observing the hematocrit to climb to polycythemic levels, or, more efficiently, by checking the ferritin level and showing iron depletion at a normal hematocrit level.

In the absence of these causes for the elevated platelet count one is justified in suspecting the myeloproliferative disorder called primary "thrombocythemia." The findings usually consist of a platelet count over 1,000,000 with normal hematocrit and white cell count. Splenomegaly, basophilia, and an elevated leukocyte alkaline phosphatase may be found. Platelet dysfunction (abnormal aggregation to epinephrine or adenosine diphosphate [ADP]) is sometimes demonstrated. Episodes of hemorrhage or thrombosis are characteristic. The key test for diagnosis is a persistently markedly elevated platelet count with no obvious cause. One patient with G6PD heterozygosity was shown to have only one of the two possible G6PD enzyme types in her platelets, confirming that the entity is clonal. However this is not a practical test for diagnosis unless your patient with possible thrombocythemia happens to be a black woman heterozygous for G6PD enzyme type. Tests for in vivo platelet clumping, said to be characteristic of thrombocythemia, have not been helpful in our hands.

Pancytopenia

The first questions are, "How bad is it?" and, if the counts are not very low, "Is there a spleen?" In the presence of mild pancytopenia and splenomegaly it is reasonable to assume that the cytopenias are caused by hypersplenism. It is usual to document normal bone marrow cellular components by doing a bone marrow aspiration and biopsy. If there is hypersplenism, meaning pancytopenia, splenomegaly, and a normal or hyperplastic bone marrow, one should still question the etiology of the splenomegaly and consider liver disease.

The person with mild, unexplained pancytopenia but *no* splenomegaly, and no history of exposure to marrow suppressive drugs, may have a myelophthisic picture, that is, a marrow space packed with cancer, granulomas, or fibrosis. Such patients are always sick with fever and wasting and often have an identified focus of their disease elsewhere. Circulating nucleated red cells may be a clue to myelophthisis. These entities require marrow *biopsy* for diagnosis.

In the patient with marked pancytopenia and no splenomegaly, bone marrow aspiration and biopsy are the keys to the evaluation. A bone marrow that is hypoplastic or aplastic is the likely finding. The usual mechanism is probably toxic or immune destruction of marrow stem cells, but aplasia can also be produced by damage to marrow vasculature. Drugs are apparent causes in more than half of the patients with aplastic anemia. A role for cellular immunity in marrow aplasia is suggested by the occasional presence of clumps of lymphocytes in an otherwise hypoplastic marrow. It is also suggested by the apparent effectiveness of cyclophosphamide and antithymocyte globulin in promoting recovery from aplasia in some patients.

Occasional patients with pancytopenia will have normal or only mildly reduced marrow cellularity. This has been referred to as "pancytopenia with a cellular marrow." This may be observed as a transition to aplasia or to leukemia. When seen in a single bone marrow aspirate it may rarely represent an island of persistent marrow function in a generally aplastic organ. The reasonable workup in this kind of situation is a repeat marrow aspiration. Because pancytopenia with a cellular marrow can be a preleukemic state, the repeat marrow should be accompanied by chromosome studies. A preleukemic state may also be indicated by the presence of megaloblastoid precursors and ringed sideroblasts in the marrow.

Neutropenia and thrombocytopenia, if marked, require immediate attention in pancytopenic patients. Neutrophil counts below 500, and especially below 100, require hospitalization and aggressive investigation with appropriate cultures and, if there are chills or fever, immediate treatment. Waiting for a positive culture result can be fatal. A platelet count below 10,000 in the presence of gross gastrointestinal bleeding, headache, or extensive skin hemorrhage is an indication for platelet transfusion. Unless there is bleeding, thrombocytopenia is not an indication for replacement of platelets, especially before the hypoproliferative etiology of the thrombocytopenia is documented. However, when platelets *are* first used in such patients, counts should be checked at one hour, three hours, and the next morning to assess the yield of the transfusion and the possible presence of antibody. When there is no platelet increment at one hour the infused platelets were nonviable. When the one-hour increment approached $7000/\mu L$ per unit infused, but the three-hour increment is down, there is probably recipient platelet antibody present.

Abnormal Screening Clotting Tests: Prothrombin Time (PT) and Partial Thromboplastin Time (PTT)

Although blood cell counts and differentials are done on most new patients, coagulation screening is not for everyone. The availability of citrate-containing blood drawing tubes and semiautomated machines giving reproducible results have made it customary for some house officers to do these tests on *all* admissions, although the yield here will be low. If one tests patients with significant history and patients about to be challenged, coagulation screening pays off. Worthy of hemostasis testing are patients who are actively and abnormally bleeding, especially from minimal lesions or bleeding from more than one location, patients with a history of abnormal bleeding, and patients about to undergo surgery that is an exceptional threat to hemostasis. Pathological bleeding suggesting "hemostatic" disorder would include extensive bruising after minor trauma or no trauma and prolonged hemorrhage after tooth extraction. Operations in the "exceptional threat" category include minor procedures such as percutaneous liver biopsy and tonsillectomy, because the operative sites cannot be compressed, and major surgery such as open heart operations and prostatectomy. The latter is particularly challenging because the raw prostate bed will be bathed with a natural fibrinolytic activator, urokinase, postoperatively.

Patients in all of these categories can be screened for hemostatic disorders by carrying out a battery of four tests (Chart 5). These tests are the PT, PTT, platelet count, and bleeding time. Special care needs to be taken in obtaining blood samples for clotting tests, especially the PTT. The sample will be satisfactory if drawn into the *second* syringe or *second* Vacutainer tube filled after the venipuncture, as the first draw is contaminated with thromboplastic tissue juices. If the sample must be obtained from an indwelling intravenous line, the line must be carefully cleared of intravenous fluid and heparin, and this material must be discarded before using anything for clotting studies. If a good sample is obtained, the PTT is the best coagulation screening test. It is generally sensitive to clotting factor deficiencies in the range of 30% or less. Clotting factor levels less than 50% are generally considered abnormal, but results in the 50 to 30% range are not clinically important.

If the patient has a long PTT with a normal PT, the disorder is likely to be due to congenital deficiency of a single clotting factor. Identification of which clotting factor is aided by knowledge of the clotting "cascade" (Figure 3-2) and relative frequencies of the congenital disorders. Before making any such analysis, one should recheck the PT on a fresh blood sample of good quality. If the PTT is still prolonged we commonly double check for the presence of heparin by checking the thrombin time, which is even more sensitive to heparin than the PTT. This precaution is not necessary for outpatients or patients whose blood you drew from a vein yourself, but hospitalized patients with intravenous lines in or a need for blood gas monitoring commonly have confusing traces of heparin in their coagulation samples.

With the PTT prolonged and the PT and thrombin time normal, a presumptive diagnosis of congenital clotting disorder can be made. A good

HEMOSTATIC DISORDER OR HEMOSTATIC THREAT

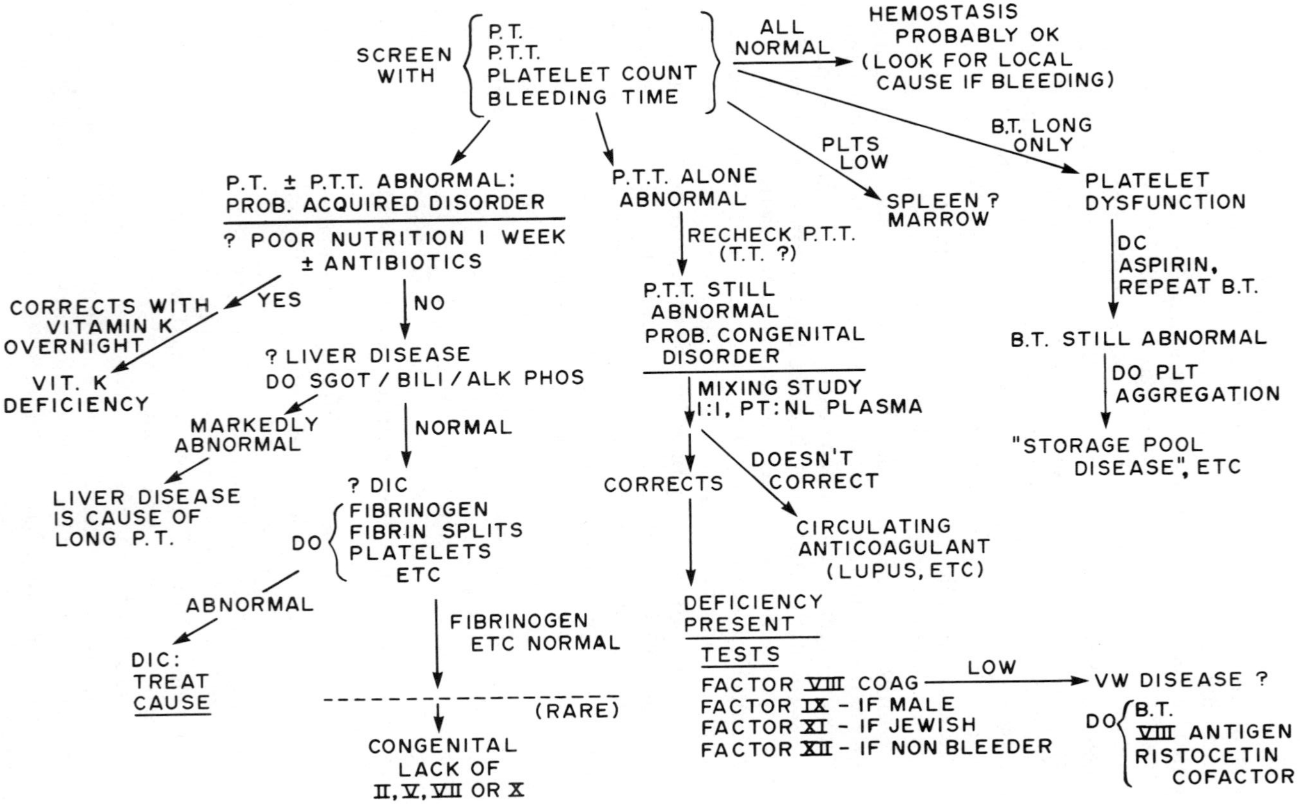

Chart 5

SCREEN WITH { P.T., P.T.T., PLATELET COUNT, BLEEDING TIME }

ALL NORMAL → HEMOSTASIS PROBABLY OK (LOOK FOR LOCAL CAUSE IF BLEEDING)

B.T. LONG ONLY → PLATELET DYSFUNCTION → DC ASPIRIN, REPEAT B.T. → B.T. STILL ABNORMAL → DO PLT AGGREGATION → "STORAGE POOL DISEASE", ETC

PLTS LOW → SPLEEN? MARROW?

P.T.T. ALONE ABNORMAL → RECHECK P.T.T. (T.T. ?) → P.T.T. STILL ABNORMAL PROB. CONGENITAL DISORDER → MIXING STUDY 1:1, PT:NL PLASMA
- DOESN'T CORRECT → CIRCULATING ANTICOAGULANT (LUPUS, ETC)
- CORRECTS → DEFICIENCY PRESENT

TESTS:
FACTOR VIII COAG LOW – IF MALE
FACTOR IX – IF MALE
FACTOR XI – IF JEWISH
FACTOR XII – IF NON BLEEDER

VW DISEASE ? DO { B.T., VIII ANTIGEN, RISTOCETIN COFACTOR }

P.T. ± P.T.T. ABNORMAL: PROB. ACQUIRED DISORDER → ? POOR NUTRITION I WEEK ± ANTIBIOTICS
- YES → CORRECTS WITH VITAMIN K OVERNIGHT → VIT. K DEFICIENCY
- NO → ? LIVER DISEASE DO SGOT / BILI / ALK PHOS
  - MARKEDLY ABNORMAL → LIVER DISEASE IS CAUSE OF LONG P.T.
  - NORMAL → ? DIC DO { FIBRINOGEN, FIBRIN SPLITS, PLATELETS, ETC }
    - ABNORMAL → DIC: TREAT CAUSE
    - FIBRINOGEN ETC NORMAL → (RARE) → CONGENITAL LACK OF II, V, VII OR X

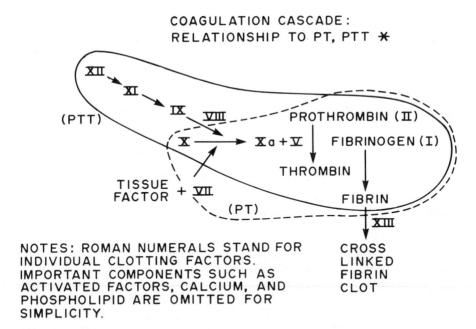

COAGULATION CASCADE:
RELATIONSHIP TO PT, PTT *

NOTES: ROMAN NUMERALS STAND FOR INDIVIDUAL CLOTTING FACTORS. IMPORTANT COMPONENTS SUCH AS ACTIVATED FACTORS, CALCIUM, AND PHOSPHOLIPID ARE OMITTED FOR SIMPLICITY.

Figure 3-2

next step is to mix some of the patient's plasma with an equal volume of normal plasma. If the patient has a *deficiency* of a clotting factor, the normal plasma mixed with the patient's will supply enough of that factor to correct the PTT. (The "normal plasma" is made by pooling five or more fresh plasma samples giving normal PT and PTT results and will usually have assay values near 100% for all clotting factors; a 1:1 mixture of this pool with any deficient plasma will thus have a 50% level of the clotting factor deficient in the patient. The mixture will therefore give a normal PTT.) If, however, the patient has a *circulating anticoagulant,* the PTT will not be corrected. This simple mixing study becomes more sensitive if the mixture is incubated for an hour at 37°C before repeating the PTT on it. Significant anticoagulants will lengthen the screening test done on this mixture by 10 seconds longer than at zero time (Table 3-2) and also much longer than a control mixture not containing the patient's plasma. If, in addition, an abnormal PTT can be corrected by increasing lipid in the clotting activator system, a diagnosis of "lupus anticoagulant" is suspected.

Inspection of the clotting cascade (Figure 3-2) shows that the clotting factors involved in the PTT that are not involved in the prothrombin time are factors VIII, IX, XI, and XII. Deficiencies of clotting factors VIII and IX are most common in males, since hemophilia A and B are sex-linked disorders. If a patient with a long PTT has a low factor VIII the workup is pursued for the important differential diagnosis between classical hemophilia and von Willebrand's disease by checking bleeding time, factor VIII antigen, and ristocetin cofactor (von Willebrand's factor). If any of these follow-up tests is markedly abnormal, accompanying a low coagulant factor VIII, von Willebrand's disease is diagnosed. Factor XI deficiency is most common in

Table 3-2
Typical Mixing Study for Long PTT*

	PTT of Mixture (Seconds)	
Plasmas	At Zero Time	After 60 min at 37°C
Patient and control (1 + 1)	38	52†
Control and VIII deficient (1 + 1)	35	37

*In the example, the patient's initial PTT was 60 seconds, the normal range being 25–45 seconds.
†This lengthening would be suggestive of an anticoagulant in the patient. Specific clotting factor assays could also be done on the zero time and 60-minute patient and control mixtures.

Jewish subjects. Patients who are found to have an isolated long PTT but are *not* bleeders may be factor XII (Hageman factor) deficient.

The patient with a long prothrombin time, usually accompanied by a long PTT, usually has an *acquired* coagulation disorder. The most common of these are vitamin K deficiency, liver disease, and DIC. A patient dependent on intravenous intake for a week or more, especially if previously malnourished and especially if receiving broad spectrum antibiotic coverage while on intravenous is a candidate for vitamin K deficiency. If the diagnosis is correct, the administration of parenteral vitamin K corrects the prolonged PT overnight. If there is no correction, or if liver function tests are abnormal, the next consideration is the presence of hepatocellular disease. In the absence of hepatocellular disease, or sometimes even in its presence, a long PT may be due to DIC. The presence of DIC is supported if the fibrinogen is under 100 mg/dL, fibrin split products are over 40 μg/mL, and the platelet count is below 100,000/μL. If several of these tests are abnormal, especially in the setting of sepsis or a complication of pregnancy, DIC is very likely.

Less common is the patient with a long PT or PTT, or both, who has a positive "mixing study," meaning persistent prolongation of the affected test after mixing patient plasma with normal plasma, indicating the presence of an anticoagulant. The anticoagulant is most sensitively detected if the mixture of plasma is incubated for an hour and *then* tested with a PT or PTT, whichever was longer.

Long PT and PTT tests can sometimes be found in surgical patients who have been vigorously transfused. During storage of bank blood, clotting factors V and VIII decline. Deficiency of these factors in stored blood may contribute to pathological oozing during surgery in heavily transfused patients. However, the volume of distribution of many coagulation factors is large, and the patient's liver replaces coagulation factors fast. We have not seen this kind of hemostatic failure due to transfusion of less than 30 units of blood. The decline of platelets and of platelet function is of much greater concern in patients given massive transfusions of stored blood (figure the preoperative platelet count to halve after each eight units).

If the patient with a present or past hemostatic disorder or impending surgery is merely thrombocytopenic, then the same considerations apply as were discussed in the section on thrombocytopenia. The evaluation should proceed through reviewing the examination for splenomegaly, rechecking histories of recent infection or drug exposure, checking the bone marrow for megakaryocytes, and possibly testing for antibody on the patient's platelets and for abnormal-sized platelets. This collection of tests will usually direct one to the cause of the thrombocytopenia.

If the patient has normal screening clotting tests and a normal platelet count, the bleeding time may still be abnormal. When the bleeding time is the only abnormality, one's attention should turn to the possibility of platelet dysfunction. The first question is whether platelet-inhibiting drugs are involved. If so, and if the patient is bleeding, platelet transfusions will correct the defect. If the patient is not bleeding, the pertinent drug is discontinued, and the bleeding time is tested again after a lapse of time. The adverse affect of aspirin on thromboxane A_2 synthesis persists for a week. If the bleeding time is still prolonged, the next step in the workup is platelet aggregation with platelet activators such as ADP, epinephrine, and perhaps arachidonic acid. Frequently, the platelets will exhibit a poor release reaction to ADP and epinephrine, leaving unreported aspirin ingestion or storage pool disease (SPD) as possible causes. Arachidonic acid aggregates, platelets of patients with SPD, but not aspirinated platelets. Another way of confirming the diagnosis of SPD is to demonstrate an abnormal ADP/adenosine triphosphate (ATP) ratio (reduced ADP), or reduced platelet serotonin. Other patients with prolonged bleeding time have normal aggregation to ADP and the others. Despite a normal PTT, such a patient, if a bleeder, deserves testing for factor VIII coagulant and perhaps ristocetin cofactor levels for the possible presence of mild von Willebrand's disease.

If all four of the screening tests are completely normal in a bleeder, the bleeding is attributed to local causes such as trauma, an ulcer, etc, depending on the bleeding site, rather than abnormal hemostasis. If the patient is a candidate for surgery one can conclude that he is as safe as can be determined by laboratory screening.

In an alert, intelligent patient, *questions* about past experiences with dental extractions and minor injuries are better than laboratory tests for hemostatic screening. Reviewing the patient's experience with dental extraction is most useful, because the patient is usually able to tell whether there was excessive bleeding. The family history may also be quite helpful in this kind of workup.

Hypercoagulable States

This aspect of hematology must be approached clinically since there are no screening laboratory tests.

Most clinically important thrombotic episodes are believed to be caused by local pathology in the endothelium of an artery or vein. However, occasional patients have recurring episodes of venous or arterial thrombosis based on abnormalities in the blood itself. A variety of abnormalities have been reported to cause hypercoagulable states, but the only one that is generally accepted as prognostically meaningful is deficiency of antithrombin III (AT III). This physiologic clotting inhibitor has been shown to take up activated clotting factors including thrombin and, much more sensitively, clotting factor Xa. The binding of AT III to these clotting intermediates is greatly accelerated by the presence of heparin. A deficiency state for AT III has been described in certain families. Patients who have 30% to 40% AT III (70% to 130% being normal) have an increased frequency of thrombophlebitis and thromboembolic phenomena (pulmonary emboli). The pattern of inheritance of the deficiency is autosomal dominant, and the clinical manifestations begin in young adults.

Although the significance of congenital AT III deficiency is well documented by the impressive histories of some of the patients, the inheritance pattern, and the test, it is puzzling to physicians interested in coagulation that deficiency of this factor allows thromboses when there is residual 30% of normal activity present. In contrast, most coagulation factor deficiencies do not cause spontaneous bleeding unless the factor missing is less than 10%.

A practical problem in diagnosis is that AT III deficiency is often thought of in somebody with thrombophlebitis or pulmonary emboli after anticoagulant therapy has begun. The problem is that heparin infusion causes a marked decrease of AT III activity in normal persons, a decrease seen within 24 hours of starting heparin treatment.

Other abnormalities in clotting factors have been described in patients with recurring thromboembolic (TE) phenomena. Most familiar is the postoperative situation in which patients are likely to have episodes of venous thromboembolism after a surgical procedure, coinciding, perhaps by chance, with a time when fibrinogen and platelets are often elevated. It is impossible to be sure at present whether the TE phenomena and the increase in fibrinogen and platelets are all results of a single cause, or whether the increase in fibrinogen and platelets causes the occasional TE episodes. An increase in blood viscosity due to high hematocrit, especially if associated with a high platelet count, also appears to cause increased TE phenomena.

Recent Important Changes in Hematology Methods

During the 1970s, advances in technology made a set of red and white blood cell counts and other measurements rapidly available as a battery. This came about as machines capable of automatic sample dilution, rapid cell counting, and red cell sizing were built and sold. The more prevalent Coulter counters do cell counts and cell sizing by detecting the impedance of cells sucked through a small aperture; the less prevalent Ortho cell counters do the same tests by measuring light scattering by cells flowing through a laser beam. The early models of these machines offered seven parameters. These were hemoglobin, hematocrit, red cell count, white cell count, and red blood cell indices (mean corpuscular volume [MCV], mean corpuscular hemoglobin [MCH], mean corpuscular hemoglobin concentration [MCHC]). White cell count, red cell count, hemoglobin, and MCV are measured, and the others are calculated, but all are reproducible with a coefficient of variation of less than 1% of the values reported. The seven parameters are now standard reporting for blood cell counts. Thus one is confronted with the list of these seven numbers plus a test number and a date, and it takes time to find the single test, the hematocrit or white cell count, that was really desired.

The major contribution of this technology is the speed and reproducibility of the results and the availability of an accurate MCV, so useful in some anemic persons. While the red blood cell count, the MCH, and the MCHC have some utility inside the hematology laboratory, they are really not useful to clinicians and probably should not be reported outside the laboratory. Physicians should not be put in the position of religiously pondering the MCH when it really follows MCV.

More recently these cell counters, and some competitors, have added a platelet count to the automatic battery. This addition had been slow in coming because electronic noise made the counting of these smallest formed elements difficult, and because the diluent used in the cell counter had to be free of small particles. Platelet counts from automatic cell counters should still be treated with skepticism (*not* ignored, just checked by other methods) when (1) the reported platelet count is low or (2) there is any tendency to red cell fragmentation. Red cell fragments can make a low platelet count appear normal.

In addition to cell counts, these automatic machines are now offering red cell, white cell, and platelet histograms, a separate curve for each cell type showing the number of cells in the vertical axis and the size of the cells on the horizontal axis. For red cells in healthy persons this is a Gaussian "normal" curve with the peak at the MCV of 90; for white cells the curve should be double humped with lymphocytes on the low side and granulocytes on the high side; for platelets the curve is at the low end of the scale and skewed toward the right. The Coulter machines also present statistics related to these curves on the report: the red cell distribution width (RDW) and the mean platelet volume (MPV). Histograms may become useful in differential diagnosis of the causes of cytopenias, since the MCV is useful in anemia diagnosis, and since increased numbers of large platelets are known to indicate increased bone marrow platelet output. One might suppose that a patient evolving from a normal red cell size distribution with a peak at 90 fL into iron deficiency might develop a minor peak on the left-hand side of the red cell curve showing the change in red cell population even before the MCV changes. Abnormal red cell histograms *have* been recorded and published in a few remarkable cases. However, it appears that mere widening of the red cell curve is more common in microcytic anemias. The RDW statistic offered by Coulter reflects this observation. However, neither histograms nor RDWs have been shown to be of value in the differential diagnosis of anemia. As for the platelet histograms, the market leader presents these only for platelets below 20 fL and corrects the observed distribution to a log-normal curve. Neither the platelet size curve nor the derived MPV has been shown to be of value in the differential diagnosis of thrombocytopenias or other abnormal platelet states.

The contribution of electronic and laser beam cell counters lies primarily in the accuracy, speed, and reproducibility of the cell counts and in the availability of an accurate MCV. The other measurements are not yet proven to be of value in clinical medicine and should not be considered in choosing a laboratory or a machine to do blood counts. Physicians should not waste their attention on measurements, such as the MCH, that have no independent diagnostic value.

Also during the 1970s several manufacturers developed new technology for doing the white blood cell differential, a widely used test which is indispensable for certain diagnoses. It has of course been done by the technologist tallying cells on a microscopic slide. The results are not very reproducible from technologist to technologist. Because the test is so time consuming and subjective, it was a natural target for attempts at newer methods. Since the early 1970s, one manufacturer (Technicon) has built and sold a multichannel machine able to do crude white blood cell differentials by discriminating white blood cells according to size and stainability with peroxidase and other cytochemical stains. Thus the Technicon Hemalog offered a blood cell differential consisting of granulocytes (segs plus bands, bands not discriminated), monocytes, lymphocytes, and eosinophils. If other kinds of white cells are present they are reported as "other." This evaluation does not answer questions about abnormal red cell morphology raised by hematocrit or MCV; it does not provide an independent smear type evaluation of the platelet count, as a routine differential would. This multichannel size and cytochemical differential is primarily of value in a population where nearly all of the test results are expected to be normal.

Several other methods for determining differentials became available during the late 1970s. These were based on pattern recognition techniques; blood smears are evaluated by machines able to recognize nuclear shapes and cytoplasmic density of various normal and abnormal white cells. The pattern recognition machines built by three different manufacturers were able to give more detailed white cell differentials than was the multichannel machine, including such things as bands and atypical lymphocytes, platelet estimates, and red cell morphology, although readings differed from technologists' evaluations of blood smears.

The automatic differential techniques are generally more reproducible than routine evaluation of routine smears, but cannot make as wide a range of observations as an experienced technologist with a microscope. Machine reports of red cell morphology are less specific about abnormal shapes than those of technologists; the machines cannot identify red cell inclusions (Howell-Jolly bodies, malaria parasites), and they cannot use (cannot see) white cell granules or nucleoli. For these reasons, and because of the large initial investment required, these techniques of doing white cell differentials have not been widely adopted by hospital laboratories. They seem to have been more successful in commercial laboratories geared to the outpatient measurement of normal differentials.

Routine clotting tests and clotting factor assays were helped during the 1970s by the introduction of at least three different versions of semi-automatic clot timers. These machines allow the technologist to set up a series of plasmas for testing and walk away. The machine adds thromboplastin, partial thromboplastin, or calcium and observes the mixture for changes in turbidity indicating clotting. The technologist returns to be presented with a list of accurate and reproducible PTs and PTTs. This of course is done without the necessity of tilting the tube and watching for a gel to form.

Some problems have been encountered with clotting activators for PTTs in automated machines. These activators have not consistently been sensitive to the wide variety of possible clotting factor deficiencies or to heparin. More recently we have found commercial activators able to detect levels of 20% or less of most clotting factors. Current commercial PTT activators are also sensitive to heparin. However, it is important for the physician who is depending on a clotting laboratory to screen patients who are reportedly bleeders, especially if they are to undergo surgery, to have a good knowledge of the sensitivity of the semiautomatic screening tests done by this laboratory. This kind of information should be generated by the laboratory by making artificial dilutions of normal plasma in factor VIII deficient plasma and other deficient plasmas. The laboratory offering such tests should be able to tell clinicians what clotting factor levels the tests are sensitive to, and what array of clotting factor deficiencies their PTT will pick up.

■ Selected Readings

Specific Subjects

Barrett O Jr: Monocytosis in malignant disease. *Ann Intern Med* 1970;73:991.

Beck EA (ed): Mild bleeding disorders II. *Semin Hematol* 1980;17:215–305.

Beeson PB: The clinical significance of eosinophilia, in Mahmoud AAF, Austen KF (eds): *The Eosinophil in Health and Disease.* New York, Grune and Stratton, 1980, pp 313–321.

Garrey WE, Bryan WR: Variations in white blood cell counts. *Physiol Rev* 1935;15:597.

Kyle RA: Natural history of chronic idiopathic neutropenia. *N Engl J Med* 1980;302:908–909.

Lipson RL, Bayrd ED, Watkins CH: The post splenectomy blood picture. *Am J Clin Pathol* 1959;32:526.

Maldonado JE, Hanlon DG: Monocytosis: A current appraisal. *Mayo Clin Proc* 1965;40:248.

Ottesen EA, Cohen SG: The eosinophil, eosinophilia and eosinophil related disorders, in Middleton JRE, Reed CE, Ellis EF (eds): *Allergy, Principles and Practice.* St. Louis, CV Mosby Co, 1978, pp 584–632.

Todd D: Diagnosis of hemolytic states. *Clin Haematol* 1975;4:63–82.

General Sources

Henry JB (ed): *Todd-Sanford-Davidsohn. Clinical Diagnosis and Management by Laboratory Methods.* ed 16. Philadelphia, WB Saunders Co, 1979.

Miale JB: *Laboratory Medicine: Hematology.* ed 6. St. Louis, CV Mosby Co, 1982.

Williams WJ, Beutler E, Erslev AJ, et al (eds): *Hematology.* ed 2. New York, McGraw-Hill Book Co, 1977.

Over the last 10 to 15 years, analytical techniques for measurement of drug concentrations in biologic specimens have become increasingly available to practicing physicians. Concurrently, the relationships between drug concentrations and pharmacological effects and adverse effects for many drugs have been documented. These developments have led to the wide use of drug concentration measurement to aid the therapeutic monitoring of patients. This chapter offers a rationale and plan for obtaining drug levels, points out some common errors in their use, and offers specific recommendations for monitoring the use of a number of drugs for which levels are particularly useful and widely available.

Rationale for Drug Level Measurement

Drug levels have several important clinical uses. The most common application is to confirm clinical impressions of therapeutic or adverse effects. It is also appropriate to use drug levels to (1) establish a baseline for future decisions and to guide dosage adjustments, (2) determine compliance with prescribed regimens, (3) assess the effects of disease states on drug effect or drug elimination, (4) document efficacy or lack of efficacy at commonly accepted therapeutic ranges, and (5) assess whether antibiotic doses are producing plasma or serum concentrations in excess of the minimal inhibitory concentration (MIC) of a given organism. Drug levels may also aid the management of patients with drug overdoses.

To utilize drug levels in any of these ways, the relationship between concentration and pharmacologic effect or adverse effect must be known. For most drugs there is a range of serum concentrations in which therapeutic but not toxic effects occur—the therapeutic range of the drug. Some drugs, such as digoxin and the aminoglycoside antibiotics, have narrow therapeutic ranges, whereas others, such as the penicillins, have wide therapeutic ranges. The former groups exhibit little difference in concentrations that cause therapeutic and toxic effects, and it is in monitoring this type of drug that drug levels are particularly helpful.

The relationship between levels and effect has been elucidated for many commonly used drugs. Note that most assays are for drug levels in plasma or serum, whereas the site of action for most drugs is in a particular tissue. Although tissue level measurements are feasible, they are not widely available. Fortunately, the plasma levels of many drugs correlate well with pharmacologic action and side effects.

Drug levels should not be thought of as substitutes for the clinical evaluation of drug action. As with other laboratory tests, drug levels are costly and should be used when they are warranted and justifiable.

4

Utilization of Drug Levels

Jean M. Nappi
John A. Bosso

The pharmacokinetics of numerous commonly used drugs have been elucidated, and the relationships between dose, time course in the body, and effect are known. At the same time, it should be remembered that the pharmacokinetics of many drugs may be altered by disease, age, or the concurrent use of other medications. The bioavailability (amount of a given dose reaching the site of action) of drugs may vary from one manufacturer's product to another, and problems have been encountered when switching brands. Additionally, variations exist in the rate of drug detoxification and/or elimination throughout the population. An example is the presence of fast and slow acetylators of procainamide, a characteristic which is genetically determined.

Thus, drug level monitoring, when performed appropriately, is a useful tool to confirm clinical impressions relating to drug action or side effects and to aid in dosage adjustment. Further, monitoring may be used in efforts to prevent toxicity by ensuring that levels are below those associated with adverse effects. Drug levels are particularly helpful in evaluating the adequacy of a given dosage when the disease state or the concurrent use of other medications is known to alter the normal disposition of a drug in the body.

As with any laboratory test, there are always exceptions to the rules. These are often the result of interpatient variations in drug disposition or response. For example, the accepted therapeutic range for digoxin is 0.7 to 2 ng/mL, yet patients are encountered in whom the drug is toxic within that range or in whom there is no response when levels exceed 2 ng/mL.

These generalizations should be kept in mind when ordering and utilizing drug levels.

Pharmacokinetics

Some knowledge of the discipline of pharmacokinetics is exceedingly helpful in the utilization of drug levels. Pharmacokinetics is the science of using mathematical models to describe the processes of drug absorption, distribution, metabolism, and elimination, thus allowing predictions about drug levels at various sites in the body as a function of dose or dosing regimen. Although a thorough explanation of pharmacokinetics is beyond the scope of this chapter, some general concepts should be useful.

Rate of Elimination

Perhaps the most commonly used pharmacokinetic parameter is a drug's elimination rate. This is usually expressed as an elimination rate constant or as half-life. A drug's half-life is that time for a given concentration to be reduced by one half. Therefore, it follows that if 50% of a drug is eliminated in one half-life, 75% is eliminated in two half-lives, and 97% is eliminated in five half-lives. Knowledge of a drug's elimination rate or half-life is helpful in planning a therapeutic regimen and in timing the measurement of drug concentrations. Although the concept of drug clearance is becoming increasingly popular in describing a drug's elimination from the body, we will discuss only half-life because this parameter is more readily available for most drugs and perhaps easier to utilize clinically.

A drug's elimination may be mathematically described as first order, zero order, or a combination of the two. The clinical relevance of these different rate processes can be stated simply. A drug with first-order elimination has a half-life that is constant and is not affected by the size of the dose. Most drugs fit into this category. The half-life of a drug eliminated in zero-order fashion varies with the size of the dose. For example, the half-life of phenytoin increases with increasing doses. In some cases in which a drug is eliminated by multiple pathways (eg, salicylic acid), first-order or zero-order elimination kinetics may be manifested, depending on the size of the dose.

Compartments

It is common to describe the pharmacokinetic characteristics of drugs by representing the body as a system of compartments with the simplest form being a one-compartment model which depicts the body as a single homogenous unit. The pharmacokinetics of most drugs can be described by a one- or two-compartment model. It should be realized that compartments have no direct anatomic or physiologic correlation and can be thought of as mathematical conveniences. One-compartment models are only valid for drugs that are eliminated from the body in a linear fashion. Multicompartment models are used to describe the pharmacokinetics of drugs that are distributed to a number of tissues in addition to the blood and other rapidly equilibrating fluids and/or tissues. The time course of a single intravenous dose of a drug with two-compartment characteristics in the body is graphically depicted in Figure 4-1. As can be observed, this line has two distinct segments with different slopes. The first segment, termed the "α phase," predominantly reflects drug distribution between the two compartments, whereas the second segment, termed the "β phase," predominantly reflects elimination. Although there are some exceptions to this basic rule, it holds for most cases. The important fact to keep in mind when dealing with drugs whose elimination is best characterized by a two-compartment model is that drug levels obtained during the distribution phase usually correlate poorly with effect and elimination. It is therefore generally recommended that drug levels be drawn after the distribution or α phase is completed.

Steady State

Most drugs are used therapeutically in multiple-dose regimens. Under these circumstances, the drug will accumulate in the body, reflected as increasing levels, until that time when the amount entering the body in a given time equals the amount removed from the body in that same time. This situation is known as steady state. Once steady state has been achieved, the maximum, minimum, and mean concentrations of a drug during any given dosing interval are theoretically always the same. Ideally, drug concentrations are determined at steady state. Steady state is achieved after a period of time equal to approximately five half-lives of a given drug. Therefore, for a drug with a half-life of four hours, steady state would be reached in 20 hours after starting therapy. If you want to confirm toxicity of a drug, it would be unnecessary and unwise to wait until steady state is achieved.

Plasma Protein Binding

Most drugs are partly bound in the blood to proteins (chiefly albumin) to some extent. It is the unbound or free fraction of the drug that is active, however. The degree of binding is critical for drugs that are highly (greater

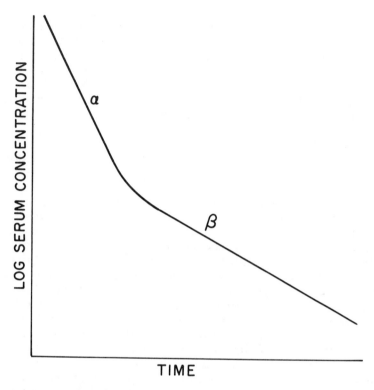

Figure 4-1 Log serum concentration versus time curve for drug elimination characterized by a two-compartment model.

than 90%) plasma protein bound. One can see that a change in binding from 99% to 98% essentially doubles the concentration of free or active drug and may result in an increased effect or toxicity. The degree of plasma protein binding may be affected by various diseases or the concomitant use of two or more highly bound drugs.

General Recommendations for Obtaining Drug Levels

Drug concentration data are used to monitor therapy, confirm clinical impressions, avoid toxicity, and to guide dose adjustments. Assuming that a valid reason exists for obtaining drug levels, some prior planning and knowledge is required to optimize their use. General knowledge of a drug's pharmacokinetic properties is necessary for the proper timing of samples and the subsequent alteration of dosage. Knowledge of the relationship between level and effect/side effect is necessary to evaluate the appropriateness of a given dose.

The most common times for sampling drug levels during a dosing interval are those associated with the maximum (peak), minimum (trough), and mean concentrations. However, when assessing drug toxicity, levels should be obtained at the time the patient is exhibiting side effects. Although the time for the peak concentration varies from one drug to another, the trough level occurs immediately before the next dose. It is best to determine drug concentrations during steady-state conditions as this situation best describes drug behavior over extended use.

The half-life of a drug may be approximated by using peak and trough levels. For example, if a drug has a peak level of 8 μg/mL and a trough level of 4 μg/mL at one and six hours, respectively, after a dose, one-half of the drug has been eliminated in that time and the half-life must be five hours. A more general rule to use to determine half-life is:

$$t_{1/2} = \frac{\ln C_1 - \ln C_2}{t_2 - t_1}$$

where $t_{1/2}$ is the half-life and $\ln C_1$ and $\ln C_2$ are the natural logarithms of the concentrations at the sampling times t_1 and t_2, respectively.

It must be pointed out that since it takes five half-lives to approximately achieve steady state, once a change in the dose is made, it takes an additional five half-lives to achieve the new steady-state situation. A common error in using drug concentration data is to overlook this requirement. A drug with a long half-live, such as digoxin (1.6 days), takes eight days to achieve steady state after a dose adjustment.

Common Errors in the Use of Drug Concentration Data

There are two broad classes of errors in the use of drug levels. These are in obtaining the levels and in interpreting them.

Orders for drug levels must be precise. The exact time of the last dose and the sample(s) must be known for proper interpretation. This must be emphasized to the personnel administering the drug and obtaining the samples. Errors resulting in toxicity or subtherapeutic response easily result from reactions to imprecise values. Samples should be obtained from a different vein from that used to administer the drug to avoid misleading results. The proper handling of biologic specimens is also vital. Many drugs or their metabolites are unstable at physiologic pH and/or at room temperature. Prior knowledge of proper handling should minimize this source of error. The laboratory should be able to provide this information as well as that relating to the sensitivity of the assay. Additionally, laboratory personnel should be informed of concomitant medications being administered to avoid this potential source of error in the assay. This is especially important when bioassays are used to measure antibiotic concentrations.

Drug levels must be cautiously interpreted and acted upon. The clinician should avoid the pitfall of treating laboratory values rather than the patient. Drug levels are not a substitute for clinical evaluation and judgment. When levels do not correlate well with dosage or clinical response, a number of things should be considered. One should expect to encounter variations from normal or average pharmacokinetic parameters and sensitivity to drugs. The fact that other medications or disease states can alter drug response or pharmacokinetics should be kept in mind. Patient non-compliance with physician's instructions for drug therapy is a very common reason for the lack of correlation between dosage and drug level or response. It should always be suspected in the outpatient setting. The possibility of interference with drug assays by other drugs should also be kept in mind.

Once the above sources for error have been ruled out, it is reasonable to adjust dosage, if necessary. Adjustments should be made cautiously for drugs with a narrow therapeutic range and, at times, should be followed with subsequent drug level determinations.

Pharmacokinetics of Commonly Used Drugs

The remainder of this chapter is dedicated to commonly used drugs for which the relationship between serum concentration and pharmacologic effect has been established. The generic names are followed by American trade names in parentheses and British trade names in brackets. All brands are not listed. Listed in Table 4-1 is some information that is useful in drug monitoring.

Kanamycin/Amikacin (Kantrex/Amikin) [Kannasyn]
Kanamycin and amikacin are similar pharmacokinetically and will be discussed together.

Peak concentrations are reached at one hour after an intramuscular dose. Although the highest plasma levels occur at the end of an intravenous infusion, the therapeutic peak levels should be obtained at the end of the distribution phase, which lasts 30 to 60 minutes after the end of infusion.

The half-life of kanamycin averages four hours, whereas that of amikacin ranges from 1.4 to 2.3 hours. Half-lives in newborn infants are significantly longer. These drugs are almost exclusively eliminated by the kidneys, and dosages must be adjusted in the presence of renal impairment. In patients with severe renal failure, the half-life of kanamycin becomes 70 to 80 hours, and that of amikacin is 86 hours. Additionally, half-lives may increase in the presence of gram-negative sepsis. Both drugs exhibit low plasma protein binding.

The therapeutic range for these agents is from 1 to 25 μg/mL but will vary depending on the MIC of the organism being treated. Peak concentrations above 20 μg/mL are generally preferred, whereas toxic effects are likely with peak levels greater than 30 μg/mL or trough concentrations greater than 10 μg/mL. Peak and trough levels should be obtained 30 to 60 minutes after the intravenous infusion and immediately before the next dose, respectively, at steady state.

Gentamicin/Tobramycin (Garamycin/Nebcin) [Cidomycin, Genticin/Nebcin]
Peak concentrations of gentamicin and tobramycin given intramuscularly occur 30 to 60 minutes after the dose. Similarly to kanamycin and amikacin, therapeutic peak levels occur after the distribution phase, which is 30 to 60 minutes after the end of the intravenous dosage infusion.

The normal half-lives of gentamicin and tobramycin range from 2.5 to 4 hours and 1.9 to 2.2 hours, respectively. Both drugs are excreted unchanged by glomerular filtration. As with the other aminoglycoside antibiotics, half-lives are longer in newborn infants and in patients with renal impairment. Half-lives in patients with severe renal failure are 40 to 50 hours for gentamicin and 54 hours for tobramycin. Gram-negative sepsis may also increase the half-lives of these agents. Plasma protein binding is negligible.

The therapeutic range for these drugs depends on MICs of the organisms being treated, but is generally between 0.5 and 10 μg/mL. Peak concentrations of 6 μg/mL or greater are generally preferred. Toxic side effects are associated with peak levels of 12 μg/mL and greater and with trough levels of 2 μg/mL or greater. Peak levels should be obtained 30 to 60 minutes after the drug infusion, whereas trough levels occur immediately before the next dose. Ordinarily, levels should be obtained during steady-state conditions.

Chloramphenicol (Chloromycetin) [Animycetin, Ertilen, Intramycetin, Leukamycin, Kemicetine, Salophen]

Chloramphenicol is well absorbed from the gastrointestinal tract with peak levels occurring two hours after the dose. Intramuscular doses are associated with peak levels at two hours, whereas intravenous peak levels occur immediately after the dose. Chloramphenicol is chiefly eliminated by hepatic metabolism and is about 50% plasma protein bound.

The half-life of this drug ranges from 1.6 to 3.3 hours, but is longer in neonates and in patients with hepatic cirrhosis.

The MICs of the organisms commonly treated with chloramphenicol are generally less than 8 μg/mL, and serious toxic effects are uncommon with levels below 25 μg/mL. Peak and trough levels should be obtained during steady state immediately after an intravenous dose or two hours after an oral or intramuscular dose and immediately before the next dose, respectively.

Primidone (Mysoline)

Primidone is well absorbed from the gastrointestinal tract. Peak levels occur at one to three hours after oral administration. The drug is metabolized to phenobarbital and phenylethylmalonamide, both of which possess anticonvulsant properties. These metabolites are subsequently eliminated from the body through metabolism and renal excretion.

The half-life of primidone varies between five and 11 hours and is probably prolonged further in patients with hepatic disease. The therapeutic range for primidone is 5 to 12 μg/mL, and toxic effects are associated with levels in excess of 15 μg/mL. Primidone levels may be altered by the concurrent use of other drugs, including other anticonvulsants. Plasma protein binding is not significant (less than 20%).

Primidone levels should be obtained at steady state, immediately before a dose. Phenobarbital levels are usually monitored concurrently with primidone therapy.

Phenobarbital (Luminal) [Phenobarbitone]

Phenobarbital, one of the most commonly used anticonvulsants, is well absorbed after oral or intramuscular administration. It is eliminated from the body by metabolism (65%) and renal excretion. Peak levels are achieved at two to 18 hours after oral or intramuscular administration.

The half-life of phenobarbital ranges between 40 and 120 hours, but tends to be in the lower end of this range in children. The half-life may be prolonged in patients with hepatic and/or renal disease. Phenobarbital levels may be

Table 4-1
Guide to Drug Monitoring

Drug	Half-Life (h)	Elimination	Therapeutic Range (µg/mL)	Recommended Sampling Times	Additional Comments
Amikacin	1.4–2.3	Renal	Peak 20–30, Trough 10	Peak and trough	30- to 60-min distribution phase
Carbamazepine	10–30	Metabolism	3–12	Trough	
Chloramphenicol	1.6–3.3	Metabolism	Peak ≤ 25 Trough ≤ 1	Peak and trough	
Digoxin	38	Renal (85%), metabolism	0.7–2†	Trough	6-h distribution phase
Disopyramide	4–10	Metabolism, renal	3–5	Trough	Active metabolite, variable binding
Ethosuximide	30–60	Metabolism	40–80	Trough	
Gentamicin	2.5–4	Renal	Peak 6–10, Trough 0.5–2	Peak and trough	
Kanamycin	4	Renal	Peak 20–30, Trough < 10	Peak and trough	

Lidocaine	1.2–2.3	Metabolism	1.5–5	12 h after infusion	Active metabolites
Phenobarbital	40–120	Metabolism (65%), renal	15–40	Trough	
Phenytoin	20–40	Metabolism	10–20	Trough	High plasma protein binding
Primidone	5–11	Metabolism	5–12	Trough	Active metabolites
Procainamide	2.7–5.2	Metabolism	4–10	Trough	Active metabolites
Quinidine	6–7	Metabolism (60–80%), renal	2.5–5	Trough	
Salicylate	2.4–19*	Metabolism	100–300	Trough	High plasma protein binding
Theophylline	4–16	Metabolism	10–20	Peak and trough	
Tobramycin	1.9–2.2	Renal	Peak 6–10 Trough 0.5–2	Peak and trough	
Valproate	6–15	Metabolism	50–100	Trough	High plasma protein binding

*See text.
†Digoxin concentrations are reported in nanograms per milliliter.

altered by the concomitant use of other drugs, including other anticonvulsants. Phenobarbital is about 50% plasma protein bound.

The therapeutic range of phenobarbital is 15 to 40 μg/mL, but significant interpatient variations occur. Side effects commonly occur at levels above 60 μg/mL. Phenobarbital levels should be drawn sometime between four hours after a dose and the next scheduled dose.

Ethosuximide (Zarontin) [Emeside]
Ethosuximide is well absorbed after oral administration with peak levels at two to four hours post dose. It is eliminated by metabolism.

The half-life of ethosuximide is between 30 and 60 hours, but is often less in children. Plasma protein binding is insignificant.

Therapeutic levels range from 40 to 80 μg/mL, and side effects occur at levels over 100 μg/mL. Levels should be obtained just before a scheduled dose at steady state.

Carbamazepine (Tegretol)
Carbamazepine absorption from the gastrointestinal tract after oral dosing is slow and variable. Peak concentrations occur at six hours after an oral dose. It is eliminated by metabolism.

The half-life of carbamazepine varies between 10 and 30 hours, but may decrease with chronic use due to stimulation of its own metabolism. The half-life may also decrease with concurrent use of phenytoin or phenobarbital. Concurrent use of propoxyphene may increase carbamazepine's half-life. Carbamazepine is 75% plasma protein bound.

The therapeutic range of carbamazepine is 3 to 12 μg/mL, and side effects are associated with levels above 9 to 12 μg/mL. Levels should be obtained immediately before a scheduled dose at steady state.

Valproic Acid (Depakene)
Valproic acid is well absorbed from the gastrointestinal tract. Peak levels occur at 30 minutes with the syrup formulation and at two hours with the capsule. As with other anticonvulsants, valproic acid is extensively metabolized. It is about 90% plasma protein bound.

The half-life of valproic acid ranges from six to 15 hours, but may be less in children. Additionally, the half-life may be decreased by the concurrent use of other anticonvulsants that induce hepatic enzymes.

The therapeutic range for valproic acid is poorly defined, but generally believed to be between 50 and 100 μg/mL, with side effects occurring with levels above 100 μg/mL. Levels should be obtained at steady state just before a scheduled dose.

Phenytoin (Dilantin) [Epanutin]
Phenytoin (formerly diphenylhydantoin) exhibits slow but relatively complete absorption from the gastrointestinal tract. Peak concentrations are reached three to 12 hours after oral administration depending on the product used. Parke-Davis kapseals are more slowly absorbed than those of other manufacturers. Intramuscular administration is not recommended due to poor solubility. Phenytoin exhibits a 30- to 60-minute distribution phase after intravenous administration.

Phenytoin is eliminated by capacity-limited metabolism and thus exhibits nonlinear or zero-order elimination kinetics. Thus, there is a lack of predictability between the dose and the concentration versus the time profile of the drug. The half-life of phenytoin varies between 20 and 40 hours at therapeutic concentrations, with children metabolizing the drug more rapidly. The drug is highly plasma protein bound (90%), but binding is decreased two- to threefold in renal failure and also diminished with hyperbilirubinemia and in neonates. Phenytoin levels may be altered by the concurrent administration of a number of other drugs, including other anticonvulsants.

The therapeutic range for phenytoin (anticonvulsant or antiarrhythmic) is 10 to 20 μg/mL, and side effects occur with levels over 20 μg/mL. Peak levels of phenytoin should be obtained 30 to 60 minutes after an intravenous dose, but it is difficult to recommend a time after oral dosing because of the wide variability of time to reach peak concentrations with this route of absorption. Trough levels should be obtained immediately before a scheduled dose. As with the other drugs discussed, levels should be obtained during steady-state conditions.

Quinidine Sulfate (Cin-Quin, Quinora, Quinidex Extentabs) [Quinicardine, Kiditard, Kinidin], Quinidine Gluconate (Duraquin, Quinaglute Dura-Tabs), and Quinidine Polyglacturonate (Cardioquin)
Quinidine absorption is rapid, but highly variable (40% to 80%). Between 80% and 90% is bound to plasma proteins. Quinidine is metabolized in the liver to a significant extent (60% to 80%). At least two of the metabolites appear to have some antiarrhythmic activity. The metabolites of quinidine are excreted by the kidneys along with up to 25% of the parent drug. Renal excretion of quinidine is increased by acidification and decreased by alkalinization of the urine. Dosage adjustments may be necessary in patients with reduced renal function. In most patients, the elimination half-life is between six and seven hours.

Some assays of quinidine measure its metabolites as well. Therefore, it is possible that therapeutic serum levels will vary between laboratories. Generally, levels between 2.5 and 5 μg/mL are considered to be in the therapeutic range. A slightly lower range may be observed when a more specific assay method that measures only quinidine is used.

Peak levels of quinidine sulfate occur one hour after an oral dose, whereas peak levels of quinidine gluconate occur five hours after an oral dose. The rate of oral absorption is decreased in patients with congestive heart failure; however, the extent of absorption is usually not affected. Unless one suspects toxicity, a trough level is most useful. This level should be drawn immediately before the next oral dose. Levels should be obtained when the drug has reached steady state. For most adults this will be between 30 and 35 hours after initiating therapy, or just before the sixth dose.

Different quinidine salts contain different amounts of quinidine. Quinidine sulfate contains 82% quinidine, whereas quinidine gluconate contains 62% quinidine. Since quinidine gluconate is absorbed more slowly, there will be less variation between peak and trough levels.

Procainamide (Pronestyl, Procan, Procan SR)
Under usual circumstances, procainamide is absorbed rapidly and completely from the gastrointestinal tract. About 15% of an oral dose is extracted

during its first pass through the liver, resulting in a bioavailability of 85%. With plasma levels encountered clinically, only 15% of the drug is bound to plasma proteins. Normally, between 40% and 60% of the systemically available dose of procainamide is excreted unchanged by the kidneys. The major metabolite of procainamide is the N-acetylation product commonly referred to as N-acetylprocainamide (NAPA). NAPA appears to be pharmacologically active although its electrophysiologic properties may differ from that of the parent compound. The half-life of procainamide averages 2.7 and 5.2 hours, respectively, in fast and slow acetylators. The half-life of NAPA is two to four times longer than the parent compound, usually six to 10 hours.

The most reliable method for evaluating the plasma levels of procainamide are the assays that measure the parent drug as well as the active metabolite, NAPA. The therapeutic range for procainamide is generally considered to be between 4 and 10 μg/mL, with the sum of procainamide and NAPA being between 10 and 30 μg/mL.

With an oral dose of procainamide, the peak plasma level occurs between one and 1.5 hours after administration. However, there are some individuals who have a delayed absorption with peak concentrations occurring two to four hours after an oral dose. A sustained release preparation of procainamide is also available. There should be less fluctuation between peak and trough levels with this dosage form.

Although steady-state concentrations are usually obtained within 24 hours after initiating procainamide, steady-state concentrations of NAPA take longer to achieve. In a patient with normal renal function, NAPA levels should reach steady state within 48 hours. Patients with renal dysfunction need more time.

Disopyramide (Norpace)
Disopyramide absorption is rapid and complete. The drug undergoes apparent first-pass metabolism by the liver, resulting in a bioavailability between 78% and 91%. Disopyramide is eliminated by both renal and hepatic mechanisms. The N-monodealkylated metabolite exhibits approximately 25% of the antiarrhythmic activity of the parent compound. The elimination half-life of disopyramide in healthy adults ranges from four to 10 hours. The half-life increases significantly in patients with severe renal dysfunction (eight to 43 hours) and acute myocardial infarction (20 to 40 hours).

The protein binding of disopyramide varies and is concentration dependent, with lower binding at higher plasma concentrations. At levels associated with normal doses, 55% to 80% of the drug is protein bound. The pharmacokinetics of disopyramide are complex. The currently available assay methods measure total (free and bound) disopyramide levels. However, only the free or unbound portion of disopyramide follows first-order kinetics. Therefore, it is possible that a doubling in the total plasma concentration could represent a fourfold increase in the free disopyramide.

Patients with altered protein binding states, such as hypoalbuminemia or uremia, may exhibit toxicity at normal therapeutic plasma concentrations secondary to increased amounts of free drug.

Peak plasma levels are reached between two and three hours after an oral dose. Trough levels should be obtained immediately before the next oral dose. Without a loading dose, steady-state levels will be reached within 48 hours in persons in whom the drug has a normal half-life. In those persons with renal dysfunction or an acute myocardial infarction, steady-state levels may not be reached until one week after the initiation of disopyramide treatment. The usual effective plasma concentration is between 3 and 5 μg/mL.

Lidocaine (Xylocaine) [Xylocard, Lidocaton, Lignol, Xylotox, Lignostab, Lidothesin, Versicaine]

Lidocaine is usually given intravenously, although it can also be given by intramuscular injection. Peak levels from the deltoid muscle occur 10 to 20 minutes after injection. With other injection sites, peak levels are obtained within 30 to 45 minutes.

Lidocaine is predominantly metabolized by the liver to monoethylglycinexylidide and glycinexylidide. Monoethylglycinexylidide has approximately the same antiarrhythmic potency as lidocaine, whereas glycinexylidide seems to have 25% of the potency of the parent compound. Some laboratories routinely report lidocaine and metabolite levels, which is valuable in patients who may accumulate these metabolites.

At the usual therapeutic plasma concentrations, approximately 70% is bound to plasma proteins. Binding occurs to alpha-1-acid glycoprotein (approximately 70% of the total binding) and albumin (30% of the total binding). The amount of alpha-1-acid glycoprotein varies considerably between individuals, so that the amount of free or unbound lidocaine can vary from 20% to 40%. Plasma alpha-1-acid glycoprotein levels rise in patients with acute myocardial infarctions. The percentage of free lidocaine is increased by 17% in females who take oral contraceptives. The elimination half-life of lidocaine is between 70 and 140 minutes. Without a loading dose, it would take 6 to 12 hours to reach a steady-state level. Plasma lidocaine concentrations between 1.5 and 5 μg/mL are considered to be therapeutic.

Since lidocaine is usually given as a loading dose followed by a constant infusion, the following guidelines can be used in monitoring plasma concentrations. Monitoring drug levels is useful (1) when toxicity is suspected, (2) when ventricular arrhythmias occur despite lidocaine administration, (3) 12 hours after starting therapy when a myocardial infarction is suspected and daily as long as the drug is administered, and (4) every 12 hours in patients who have cardiac or hepatic insufficiency.

Since current laboratory assays measure total drug and not free drug concentrations, it is possible that some patients with increased plasma binding of lidocaine will not show signs of toxicity in the face of high plasma concentrations.

Digoxin (Lanoxin) [Diganox]

Digoxin absorption from tablets varies between 60% to 80%, with peak serum concentrations occurring 60 to 90 minutes after administration. Some differences may exist between different manufacturers, and for this reason, patients should be maintained on the same brand. Absorption from the oral elixir is about 10% greater than that from the tablet, whereas absorption from intramuscular injections is often erratic, incomplete, and painful.

Digoxin is eliminated from the body by the kidneys as unchanged glycoside and metabolites. Patients with normal renal function eliminate 60% to 80% of digoxin via the kidneys. For some patients, especially those with severe renal dysfunction, metabolism plays a significant role in the overall elimination of the drug.

Only 25% of serum digoxin is bound to albumin, but digoxin is extensively bound to tissue. The distribution of digoxin to the various body tissues where it is bound takes several hours to complete. When plasma concentrations are determined for the purpose of evaluating therapeutic response, the blood samples must be drawn at least six hours after drug administration. Samples drawn before this time may be misleading if the drug has not finished its distribution phase.

The therapeutic range for digoxin is 0.7 to 2 ng/mL. There are several factors that appear to predispose patients to toxicity even though their plasma concentrations are in the therapeutic range. Hypokalemia, hypomagnesemia, hypothyroidism, and hypoxemia are examples of conditions that may increase a patient's sensitivity to the drug. The plasma concentrations required to slow conduction across the atrioventricular (AV) junction are higher than those required for digoxin's inotropic effect. It is common to require plasma concentrations of 1.5 ng/mL or more to control adequately a rapid ventricular response in patients with atrial fibrillation or flutter. The half-life of digoxin is approximately 1.6 days in patients with normal renal function.

When therapy is started with a maintenance dose, the time to reach 97% steady state will be five half-lives (about one week) in an adult with normal renal function. In patients with renal dysfunction, the half-life can be as long as five days, in which case the time to reach steady state could be as long as three weeks.

When therapeutic doses of quinidine are added to an existing digoxin regimen, plasma concentrations of digoxin may double within five to seven days. Patients should be monitored very closely for toxicity.

Salicylic Acid

The most common drug given for salicylate therapy is aspirin, which is rapidly converted to salicylate in the body. Salicylic acid is rapidly absorbed from the gastrointestinal tract when administered orally, but slowly and erratically when administered per rectum.

Salicylic acid is eliminated from the body by a number of routes. At least four metabolites are formed via hepatic biotransformation, and a portion is eliminated unchanged by the kidneys. Two of the metabolic pathways are saturation limited, accounting for the somewhat complex pharmacokinetic profile of this drug. At low and high doses of aspirin or salicylate, the drug is eliminated in an "apparent" first-order or linear fashion, although the half-life is quite different. At low doses the half-life averages 2.4 hours, but at high doses (4 g or more daily) the half-life averages 19 hours. The reason for this difference can be explained by the saturation of two of the metabolic pathways. In the intermediate dosage range, as saturation occurs, small dosage changes result in alterations in half-life and perhaps large fluctuations in drug levels. It is therefore prudent to make dosage changes cautiously and to monitor levels frequently. It should be noted that concurrent antacid therapy may increase salicylate elimination. Salicylate is 90% protein bound at concentrations of 100 μg/mL, but this binding decreases at higher levels. Binding is also decreased by conditions associated with low albumin levels.

The therapeutic range for salicylate varies with the condition to be treated. The generally accepted level for analgesia is 100 μg/mL, whereas that for antiinflammatory effects is 150 to 300 μg/mL. Toxicity is associated with levels in excess of 300 μg/mL.

Salicylate levels should be obtained during steady-state conditions (five days after starting therapy or a change in dosage). In an overdose situation, however, levels should be obtained as soon as possible. Levels may be obtained at any time during a dosing interval.

Theophylline (Slo-Phyllin, Theophyl, Elixicon, Theolair, Somophyllin, Theo-Dur, Sustaire, Constant T) [Neulin, Rona-Phyllin, Theograd]

Theophylline, when given as an oral solution or plain uncoated tablet, is rapidly and completely absorbed. There are several products available that decrease the rate of absorption, and some of these have less than complete absorption. Rectal solutions are well absorbed, but absorption from suppositories is erratic. Theophylline can be given intravenously as aminophylline. A few so called "salts" of theophylline, eg, aminophylline and oxtriphylline, are metabolized in the body to theophylline. When making dosage adjustments, consider only the amount of theophylline in each product and not the total of theophylline and its salt; 100 mg of aminophylline is equivalent to 85 mg of theophylline. Dyphylline is a derivative of theophylline that is not metabolized to theophylline. Optimal plasma levels for dyphylline have not been defined.

Theophylline has a rapid distribution phase, with approximately 60% becoming reversibly bound to protein. Binding is reduced in neonates and in the presence of acidemia. Theophylline is metabolized in the liver to relatively inactive metabolites. Some of these pathways appear to be saturable, so that it is possible that small changes in dosage could result in disproportionately large changes in plasma concentrations.

The half-life of theophylline is extremely variable, from four to 16 hours in nonsmoking adults (mean nine hours). The average half-life of the drug is four hours in adult smokers and children, who have an increased metabolism of theophylline. In neonates, the half-life of theophylline is between 24 and 30 hours. The clearance of the drug is decreased by cardiac failure, hepatic dysfunction, sustained fever, macrolide antibiotics, and cimetidine. Cessation of smoking is associated with a gradual increase in half-life of theophylline.

The therapeutic range for plasma theophylline levels is 10 to 20 μg/mL. Seizures and cardiac arrhythmias have occurred at levels greater than 35 μg/mL. These life-threatening side effects may not be preceded by the more common adverse effects of nausea, vomiting, and nervousness.

The peak plasma concentration occurs approximately two hours after oral solutions and solid dosage forms with rapid dissolution characteristics. With slow-release preparations, the peak concentration occurs between three and seven hours after a dose. Peak levels are generally most useful. If a patient experiences a lack of therapeutic effect toward the end of a dosing interval, the same daily dose should be given, but the intervals should be shorter, or the product can be changed to a more slowly absorbed preparation that

76

provides less fluctuation in plasma concentrations. Ideally, all levels should be taken at steady state. With intravenous therapy, a blood sample should be taken 30 minutes after the completion of a loading dose and four to eight hours later to determine whether the maintenance infusion is appropriate. With repeated oral dosing, patients in whom theophylline has a normal half-life should have a stable dosage regimen for 48 hours to ensure that plasma concentrations will represent steady-state levels.

■ Selected Readings

Greenblatt DJ, Koch-Weser J: Clinical pharmacokinetics. *New Engl J Med* 1975; 293:702–705 and 964–970.

Kaufman RE: The clinical interpretation and application of drug concentration data. *Pediatr Clin North Am* 1981;28: 35–45.

Pippenger CE: Rationale and clinical application of therapeutic drug monitoring. *Pediatr Clin North Am* 1980;27: 891–925.

Rowland M, Tozer TN: *Clinical Pharmacokinetics. Concepts and Applications.* Philadelphia, Lea and Febiger, 1980.

■ Blood Gases and Acid-Base Disturbances

The first section of this chapter is for practicing physicians who may want a firmer grasp of the fundamentals of acid-base problem solving. It demonstrates an approach to the laboratory results, but does not require the ability to derive the Henderson-Hasselbalch equation.

Definitions

The terms *acidosis* or *alkalosis* refer to processes that tend to move the pH in one direction or the other. If acidosis is unopposed by another disturbance, *acidemia* (an increase in blood hydrogen ion concentration) will result, and vice versa for alkalosis resulting in *alkalemia*. However, one can have an acidosis (eg, uremic acidosis) and not have acidemia if a second disturbance (eg, metabolic alkalosis from vomiting) opposes the pH change of the first. Respiratory disturbances elicit renal compensation, and metabolic disorders have respiratory compensation. A *simple acid-base disturbance* is the initial process producing the primary change in HCO_3 or PCO_2 and all of the compensatory changes as well. There are six simple disturbances (Table 5-1). A *mixed acid-base disturbance* is present when two or more primary disturbances exist simultaneously in the same patient. Common clinical settings associated with mixed acid-base disorders are listed in Table 5-1.

Analysis of the Blood Gas Values

If your laboratory reports hydrogen (H^+) ion concentration indirectly as pH, an increase in blood concentration of H^+ (acidemia) will be reflected in a lower pH, and a decrease in the blood concentration of H^+ ions (alkalemia) will be reflected in a higher pH. This is because pH is the reciprocal of the common logarithm of the H^+ ion concentration. Some laboratories now report H^+ ion concentration directly as such; if so, you should know this. The body is said to be "neutral" when the blood pH is between 7.35 and 7.45 (H^+ concentration approximately 40 mEq/L). At a glance, if the blood pH is all the information you have, you know whether the patient is alkalemic, acidemic, or "neutral." Arterial blood is usually used for blood gas studies. With minor adjustments of the figures, venous blood can be used if free-flowing venous blood is obtained.

Once you know the patient is alkalemic or acidemic, you need to know whether it is due to metabolic or respiratory causes or to both. To determine the source of the abnormality, it is helpful to look at the simultaneous blood PCO_2 value. If the PCO_2 is below normal and acidemia is present, you know that the patient has a metabolic acidosis. If the PCO_2 is elevated

Interpretation of Blood Gas and Electrolyte Values

Harvey N. Mandell
Margaret Johnson Bia

77

Table 5-1
Types of Acid-Base Disturbances

Simple Acid-Base Disturbances
1. Metabolic acidosis (either hyperchloremic or "anion gap" acidosis)
2. Metabolic alkalosis
3. Acute respiratory acidosis
4. Chronic respiratory acidosis
5. Acute respiratory alkalosis
6. Chronic respiratory alkalosis

Common Mixed Acid-Base Disorders
1. Respiratory alkalosis and metabolic acidosis (eg, septic shock, salicylate, overdose)
2. Metabolic alkalosis and respiratory acidosis (eg, diuretic use in a patient with chronic lung disease)
3. Metabolic alkalosis and metabolic acidosis (eg, vomiting in a uremic patient)
4. Respiratory acidosis and metabolic acidosis (eg, cardiopulmonary arrest)
5. Metabolic alkalosis and respiratory alkalosis (eg, nasogastric suction in a patient on a ventilator)
6. Acute and chronic respiratory acidosis (eg, superimposed infection in a patient with chronic lung disease)

and the pH is decreased, you know the patient has a respiratory acidosis—that for some reason this person is not adequately ventilating his or her alveoli. Alternatively, if the pH is elevated a low PCO_2 suggests respiratory alkalosis, whereas a normal or slightly elevated PCO_2 is found in metabolic causes for alkalemia.

$$\downarrow pH + \downarrow PCO_2 = \text{metabolic acidemia}$$
$$\downarrow pH + \uparrow PCO_2 = \text{respiratory acidemia}$$
$$\uparrow pH + \downarrow PCO_2 = \text{respiratory alkalemia}$$
$$\uparrow pH + \text{normal or } \uparrow PCO_2 = \text{metabolic alkalemia}$$

Analysis of Electrolytes and Anion Gap

Move on to the electrolyte values. Arrange them in a cross, as shown in Figure 5-1A, with the positive-charged ions (cations) on your left and the negative-charged ions (anions) on your right. There are other anions and cations, but they are usually present in very small amounts and are not reported routinely (Figure 5-1B). The serum bicarbonate concentration may be reported as "total CO_2." The total CO_2 includes bicarbonate ions, carbonic acid, and dissolved carbon dioxide. Since the latter two are present in minute amounts, the total CO_2 is a good reflection of bicarbonate level. Add up the cation and anion concentrations. In a normal person, the measured cations outnumber the measured anions because of the negative charge in albumin and other unmeasured anions such as sulfates and phosphates. The difference between the measured cation and anion concentrations is known as the anion gap and should equal 8 to 16 mEq/L. In most instances when calculating the anion gap, physicians ignore the potassium because its presence in extracellular fluid is so limited and changeable as compared with

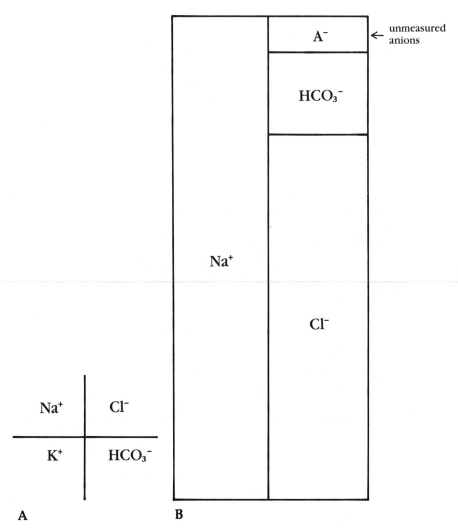

Figure 5-1 **A** Framework for evaluating electrolytes. **B** Approximate proportion of cations and anions in "neutral" body fluid.

sodium that it usually is not vital in anion gap measurements. An elevated anion gap is most commonly found in certain kinds of metabolic acidosis where the H^+ concentration is increased in association with an increase in anonchloride anion (for example, lactate). Therefore, if the anion gap is elevated, a metabolic acidosis should be suspected.

Metabolic Acidosis

If a patient has a metabolic acidosis and acidemia ($\downarrow$pH and $\downarrow$PCO$_2$), the electrolytes will usually fall into one of two patterns. In one pattern, the serum chloride is elevated when the serum bicarbonate is low. This is called hyperchloremic acidosis or "normal anion gap" acidosis and is caused by diarrhea;

interstitial renal diseases (eg, renal tubular acidosis); or drugs (eg, acetazolamide) and urinary diversion procedures such as ureterosigmoidostomy, which leads to bicarbonate losses in the stool.

Another form which the electrolyte pattern may take is "elevated anion gap acidosis" or, in today's jargon, "anion gap" acidosis. Here the difference between the measured serum anion and cation concentrations exceeds 16 mEq/L. In these cases, anions not routinely measured are present in abnormally high quantities. For example, in uremia, accumulation of unmeasured sulfates, phosphates, and other anions will occur in association with uremic acidosis. Diabetic ketoacidosis also raises the anion gap because of the presence of serum ketone bodies. Lactic acidosis, an important and often fatal disorder, is another important cause for anion gap acidosis. With removal of phenformin from the American market, the incidence of lactic acidosis may decrease. Finally, ingestion of toxins such as methanol, salicylates in toxic quantities, ethylene glycol, and paraldehyde can result in an anion gap acidosis because of the generation of organic acids when these drugs are metabolized. When you encounter metabolic acidosis associated with an elevated anion gap, these four major causes (uremia, ketoacidosis, lactic acidosis, and toxin ingestion) should be considered and eliminated one by one with appropriate ancillary data.

Before completing the laboratory evaluation of a patient with metabolic acidosis, you should decide whether respiratory compensation for the metabolic acidosis is appropriate. If you know the blood PCO_2 and the bicarbonate level, a simple formula will tell you whether the degree of hyperventilation (the decrease in PCO_2) is adequate for the degree of metabolic acidosis (the decrease in bicarbonate). If the patient cannot increase ventilation in response to a metabolic acidosis, then you know there is added trouble and you may have to look toward mechanical ventilation. The formula is simple and applies to all cases of metabolic acidosis: $PCO_2 = [1.5 \times (HCO_3^-)] + 8$. Multiply the bicarbonate concentration by 1.5 and add 8. If the measured PCO_2 has not fallen to this calculated level, you may assume that the patient is unable to ventilate the alveoli sufficiently to compensate for the degree of acidemia. Alternatively, if the measured PCO_2 is lower than that predicted from the formula, you can be sure that another stimulus, in addition to metabolic acidosis, is driving respiration.

Respiratory Acidosis

If the problem is respiratory acidosis ($\downarrow$pH and $\uparrow PCO_2$), you need to decide whether it is chronic or acute. Remember that when an acid-base abnormality is due to metabolic causes, the lungs work very fast to compensate. The kidneys, on the other hand, work more slowly in correcting a respiratory problem. Therefore, respiratory acidosis may be "acute" (before renal compensation) or "chronic" (after renal compensation).

When the alveolar and blood PCO_2 rises because of impaired ventilation, the blood H^+ concentration also rises. Serum bicarbonate levels will eventually rise, but at a much slower rate in an attempt by the kidneys to keep the pH normal. When acute respiratory acidosis is present, the pH is depressed and the PCO_2 is elevated. Bicarbonate levels are only slightly elevated during this acute phase. As time goes on and the disturbance becomes chronic, the PCO_2 remains elevated, but renal mechanisms operate to raise the bicarbonate level which returns blood pH toward normal. This process takes time. A patient does not jump immediately from an acute to a chronic respiratory disturbance. In the literature, you may find the term "ventilatory failure" used interchangeably with "respiratory acidosis," since significant elevations in blood PCO_2 produce an acidosis for which compensation is never complete.

Respiratory Alkalosis

If the blood pH is elevated (alkalemia), look again at the PCO_2 value. If this is low, you know that the alveoli are being hyperventilated. This can be due to anxiety or to a normal respiratory response to various insults such as fever, sepsis, and liver failure. It is seen frequently in intensive care units due to "overventilation" by a ventilator. Once again, respiratory alkalosis can be divided into an acute and chronic process. If compensation has taken place, the pH will be near normal while the PCO_2 is still very low because the bicarbonate will also have fallen, producing a chronic respiratory alkalosis. If the PCO_2 is depressed but the bicarbonate level has not yet fallen significantly, the disturbance is still acute.

Metabolic Alkalosis

If alkalemia is present but not due to a respiratory alkalosis, then a metabolic alkalosis must be present. In this case, the serum bicarbonate level is significantly elevated, causing the increase in blood pH. PCO_2 can be either normal or increased due to pulmonary compensatory mechanisms. Major causes for a metabolic alkalosis include vomiting, nasogastric intubation, administration of diuretics, and diseases associated with hypercorticoidism such as hyperaldosteronism. Hypokalemia is frequently present in patients with metabolic alkalosis; in patients who are vomiting or receiving diuretics, the associated chloride losses lead to a decrease in serum chloride concentration as well. The lungs compensate much more poorly for a metabolic alkalosis, by underventilating and retaining CO_2, than they do for a metabolic acidosis, by hyperventilating. As a result, the PCO_2 is elevated in a metabolic alkalosis, but only minimally (frequently < 50 mm Hg).

Mixed Acid-Base Disturbances

So far, we have discussed only the "simple" acid-base problems. Unfortunately, neither life about us nor life in our extracellular fluid or alveoli is usually so pure. Because patients frequently have more than one acid-base disturbance at the same time, it is useful to have an organized approach to acid-base problems so that mixed disturbances can be identified. Appreciating the clinical possibility for a mixed disturbance is important, since correcting only one part of the problem may make the other part worse and well-intended therapy may cause mischief. Clinical settings in which mixed acid base disturbances occur are listed in Table 5-1.

Approach

The best way to identify an acid-base disturbance is to take the clinical approach as outlined in Table 5-2. Begin the analysis by suspecting a disturbance based on the history and physical examination. For example, suspect a

Table 5-2
Clinical Approach to Mixed Acid-Base Disturbances

1. Suspect disturbances based on historical information
2. Suspect disturbances based on signs from the physical exam
3. Evaluate the electrolytes
    ↑HCO₃—Think of metabolic alkalosis or compensated respiratory acidosis
    ↓HCO₃—Think of metabolic acidosis or compensated respiratory alkalosis
    ↑K—Suspect acidemia
    ↓K—Suspect alkalemia
    ↑Cl—Think of hyperchloremic metabolic acidosis
    ↓Cl—Think of metabolic alkalosis
    Calculate the anion gap—if elevated, consider causes for "anion gap" acidosis
4. Evaluate blood gas values—see if compensation is appropriate

metabolic alkalosis in a patient who is vomiting or a lactic acidosis in a patient in shock. Next, proceed to step 3 and analyze the electrolyte values. Remember that there are always two explanations for an increase in serum bicarbonate concentration (metabolic alkalosis and compensated respiratory acidosis) and two explanations for a decrease (metabolic acidosis or compensated respiratory alkalosis). The serum potassium concentration can be used as a clue since potassium can shift in or out of cells with changes in the blood pH. Acidosis is frequently associated with hyperkalemia, and alkalosis frequently occurs with hypokalemia. The electrolyte evaluation is not complete without calculating the anion gap. If it is elevated, the four causes of anion gap acidosis should be considered, and appropriate tests to prove these possibilities should be obtained.

The blood gas values are then evaluated as described in the preceding section. If compensation for a given disturbance is not appropriate (too much or too little), then a mixed disturbance is present. For instance, in a patient with a metabolic acidosis (↓pH and ↓HCO₃), PCO_2 should be decreased as part of the normal respiratory compensation according to the equation $PCO_2 = [1.5 \times (HCO_3^-)] + 8$ as described above. The patient with a metabolic acidosis who has a normal or elevated PCO_2, perhaps due to lung disease, is underventilating. This results in a mixed acid-base disturbance (a metabolic acidosis and a respiratory acidosis). In this example, the respiratory disturbance is adversely affecting the respiratory compensation for the metabolic disturbance and vice versa. Blood pH is lower than would occur with either disturbance alone.

The effects of mixed disorders on blood pH are not always additive but may, in fact, cancel one another, making any acid-base disturbance very difficult to diagnose. For example, blood pH could be normal in the uremic patient who is vomiting because the decrease in blood pH (from the metabolic acidosis of uremia) is opposed by an increase in blood pH (from the metabolic alkalosis due to vomiting). Proper interpretation of the blood pH value will depend on knowing a great deal about the patient's clinical state so that these various possibilities can be considered. Some familiarity with the guidelines for appropriate compensation is necessary for mixed disturbances to be readily appreciated. For instance, in an acute respiratory acidosis ($\uparrow$PCO$_2$, $\downarrow$pH), the bicarbonate should rise very slightly (< 30 mEq/L). If, in this setting, a marked elevation in serum bicarbonate concentration is found, a concomitant metabolic alkalosis should be suspected. Similarly, a bicarbonate level lower than expected is equally inappropriate and indicates a concomitant metabolic acidosis.

A few final points are useful to remember. In the setting of a known primary disorder, the finding of a normal pH usually implies a mixed disorder since *compensation rarely corrects the pH back to normal.* Obviously, the finding of a pH change in a direction opposite to that predicted for a known primary disorder demands the diagnosis of a mixed disturbance. Lastly, in a simple disturbance, the HCO$_3$ and PCO$_2$ move in the same direction as one compensates for the other. Therefore, if the PCO$_2$ and HCO$_3$ move in opposite directions, a mixed disturbance must be present.

In summary, the presence of acid-base disorders is first suspected on the basis of the history and physical examination. The electrolytes are then examined for clues and a calculation of the anion gap. Lastly, the blood gas values are analyzed, remembering the expected degree of compensation for each disturbance. As usual, the more you know about the patient the better.

■ Interpretation of the Serum Sodium Concentration

In analyzing a patient's serum sodium concentration, one must realize that the serum sodium concentration does not reflect the body's total sodium content. The serum levels of most other physiologic ions can be markers for either excesses or deficits of those ions in the body (eg, an excess of total body potassium will generally result in hyperkalemia). In contrast, the serum sodium concentration is regulated, not by the body's sodium content, but by forces, such as thirst, vasopressin levels, and renal water excretion, which control water metabolism and consequently serum osmolality. Because sodium is the main osmotically active solute in the extracellular fluid, it is important to keep its concentration, and therefore serum osmolality, constant to maintain normal physiologic functions. Hyponatremia does not necessarily mean too little sodium in the body, but rather too little sodium *in relation to water.* This results from a defect in water metabolism leading to water retention and a decrease in serum osmolality. Similarly, an increase in serum sodium reflects an excess of sodium in relation to water or a defect in water metabolism leading to an increase in serum osmolality. Both hyponatremia and hypernatremia can occur in disorders associated with either increases or decreases in total body sodium that are not reflected in the serum sodium concentration.

Hyponatremia

Definitions
Hyponatremia is frequently used synonymously with the term hypoosmolality where *osmolality* is defined as the number of milliosmoles per liter in the extracellular fluid. Some molecules which contribute to osmolality, such as urea, will freely cross cell membranes. Changes in the concentration of these

molecules can change serum osmolality without changing *tonicity,* where tonicity reflects the concentration of osmotically active particles which are confined to the extracellular fluid. Thus, an increase in blood urea nitrogen (BUN) produces hyperosmolality without hypertonicity, whereas an increase in sodium, a particle which is confined to the extracellular fluid, changes both osmolality and tonicity. Therefore, hyponatremia is also frequently used synonymously with the term hypotonicity. When evaluating a hyponatremic patient it is useful to remember the two clinical situations in which hyponatremia does not mean hypoosmolality or hypotonicity. Depression in serum sodium in association with hyperglycemia is one clinical setting in which hyponatremia exists but plasma osmolality is actually elevated. In hyperglycemic states, the elevated glucose level raises plasma osmolality but, in doing so, pulls water out of cells to maintain osmotic equilibrium. The movement of water out of cells results in a lowering of the serum sodium concentration at a time when extracellular fluid hyperosmolality is being maintained by a high glucose concentration. It is useful to remember that serum sodium decreases by about 1.6 mEq/L for every rise of 100 mg/dL in plasma glucose concentration. A much rarer cause for hyponatremia without hypoosmolality occurs in clinical disorders associated with severe hyperlipidemia or hyperproteinemia. Sodium is present in the water, not the lipid or protein fraction of plasma. The serum concentration per volume of serum will be depressed if the lipid or protein fractions of serum are markedly elevated. This phenomenon is sometimes referred to as *factitious hyponatremia* or *pseudohyponatremia* since the sodium concentration per amount of serum water, which determines serum osmolality, is normal. When in doubt as to whether the hyponatremia is real, a simple measurement of serum osmolality, which will be elevated with hyperglycemia and normal with hyperlipidemia or hyperproteinemia, will clarify this point. Hyponatremia is harmful only when associated with hypoosmolality.

Measurements

Serum sodium is measured in the chemistry laboratory with a flame photometer and the value is reported in units of milliequivalents per liter. You can calculate plasma osmolality (P_{osm}) from the serum sodium concentration with use of the formula: $P_{osm} = 2 \times [Na] + [glucose]/18 + [BUN]/2.8$, where, [Na] is the measured serum sodium concentration. It is multiplied by two since the anions accompanying sodium (chloride and bicarbonate) also contribute osmotic particles to the plasma osmolality. [Glucose] and [BUN] are the measured values for glucose and blood urea nitrogen, respectively, in milligrams per deciliter. They are divided by 1/10 of their molecular weight to convert milligrams per deciliter to milliosmoles per liter. This calculation should agree, within 10–15 mOsm/L, with the plasma osmolality measured directly with an osmometer. If the measured osmolality is significantly higher than the calculated value, an *osmotic gap* exists. This means that osmotic particles, other than sodium, glucose or urea, are raising plasma osmolality. If you detect an osmotic gap, you should suspect alcohol ingestion since ethanol, methanol, and ethylene glycol can all raise plasma osmolality when ingested.

Under normal conditions, the serum sodium is maintained between 134 and 144 mEq/L, corresponding to a plasma osmolality of 285–295 mOsm/L.

Mild to moderate hyponatremia is present at values between 125 and 135 mEq/L. Hyponatremia is considered severe at values below 120–125 mEq/L. A serum sodium concentration below 115 mEq/L indicates a medical emergency requiring immediate treatment, especially if lethargy, disorientation, seizures, or coma is present.

Causes and Treatment

The causes of hyponatremia are categorized into disorders associated with normal, increased, or decreased extracellular fluid volume (Table 5-3). Since extracellular fluid volume is determined by sodium content, hyponatremia can occur with normal, increased, or decreased total body sodium. Although an impairment in water excretion is present in each case, the etiology of the defect and the preferred treatment of hypoosmolality differ depending on the status of the extracellular volume. Thus, it is helpful to utilize these categories when approaching a patient with hyponatremia. Unless congestive heart failure is present, treatment with hypertonic saline is recommended in all patients with symptomatic hyponatremia, especially if the serum sodium concentration is below 115–120 mEq/L since mortality can be as high as 50% in patients with acute hyponatremia. As a general rule, chronic hyponatremia is associated with fewer symptoms and is better tolerated than acute hyponatremia. However, since the first symptom to appear may be a grand mal seizure, dangerously low levels of hyponatremia must be treated aggressively regardless of symptoms. Although cell swelling due to hypoosmolality from hyponatremia occurs in all cells of the body, the resultant water intoxication in brain cells is particularly devastating and produces the most severe clinical manifestations.

Hypernatremia

Definitions

Clinically significant hypernatremia is always associated with hyperosmolality and hypertonicity. However, not all hyperosmolar conditions are due to elevations in serum sodium concentration. Hyperglycemia is a frequent cause of hyperosmolality and hypertonicity in which the serum sodium concentration can be normal or depressed. *True osmolality* refers to the total

Table 5-3
Major Causes of True Hyponatremia and Hypoosmolality

Normal ECF* Volume	Increased ECF Volume	Decreased ECF Volume
SIADH†	Cirrhosis	Gastrointestinal losses‡
Reset osmostat	Nephrosis	(vomiting, diarrhea)
Renal failure	Congestive heart failure	Skin losses (burns)
Hypothyroidism		Renal losses (diuretics,
		Addison's disease, renal
		salt wasting)
		Losses from fistula

*ECF, Extracellular fluid.
†SIADH, Syndrome of inappropriate antidiuretic hormone secretion.
‡Losses refer to losses of salt and water producing decreases in ECF volume.

measured osmolality. *Effective osmolality*, like tonicity, refers to the concentration (in milliosmoles per liter) of osmotically active particles confined
to the extracellular fluid such as glucose and sodium, but not urea. An increase in these osmotically active particles exerts a pressure on cell membranes to pull water out of cells. Thus, the increase in effective osmolality or
hypertonicity associated with hypernatremia will result in cellular dehydration from which the morbidity of the electrolyte disturbance arises.

Causes and Treatment

Clinically, hypernatremia occurs much less frequently than hyponatremia.
The reason for this difference is that the thirst mechanism becomes activated
by small increases in serum sodium concentration and drives normal subjects to drink and thus correct the hypernatremia by water ingestion. Just as
patients with sustained hyponatremia all have a defect in water excretion,
patients with sustained hypernatremia must have a problem either with
thirst or with the ability to relieve thirst. As a general rule hypernatremia is
seen mainly in subjects who are too young, too old, or too sick to respond to
the normal thirst stimulus. As can be seen in Table 5-4, the causes of hypernatremia are categorized according to how they affect the status of the extracellular fluid volume, which is determined by the body's sodium content.
Hypernatremia can occur after pure water loss or loss of water in excess of
salt loss or salt gain. Again, it should be obvious that hypernatremia can
occur with normal, increased, or decreased total body sodium.

Specific therapy will depend on the underlying cause, but all patients with
severe hypernatremia (serum sodium concentration greater than 160–165
mEq/L) should be treated immediately with fluids which are hypotonic
relative to their plasma. Central nervous system abnormalities due to brain
cell dehydration produce most of the symptomatology. Irritability, disorientation, lethargy, seizures, and coma can all occur and correlate with both the
degree and the rapidity of the rise in serum sodium concentration. It is important to remember that patients with hypernatremia due to pure water
losses (as in diabetes insipidus) usually do not have signs of extracellular
fluid volume concentration or hypotension since only 1/12 of the water lost
comes from the intravascular compartment. In these patients, severe central
nervous system derangements appear before shock from fluid depletion
occurs. Permanent brain damage or death from cerebral edema can also
occur when hypernatremia is corrected too rapidly. To prevent this
phenomenon, a slow restoration toward a normal serum sodium concentration over a 48-hour period is recommended.

■ Interpretation of the Serum Potassium Concentration

Potassium is an extremely important ion since the ratio of intracellular to extracellular potassium concentration determines neuromuscular activity. Extracellular fluid potassium is measured as serum potassium since the serum
compartment is in constant equilibrium with all other extracellular fluid
compartments. Ninety-eight percent of total body potassium remains within
cells and serves as the main intracellular cation. Only 2% of the body's

Table 5-4
Causes of Hypernatremia

Normal ECF* Volume (hypernatremia due to pure water loss)	Increased ECF Volume (hypernatremia due to sodium gain)	Decreased ECF Volume (hypernatremia due to water loss in excess of sodium loss)
Renal water losses (central or nephrogenic DI†)	Hypertonic Na HCO₃ Administration (during cardiac resuscitation)	Renal losses (osmotic diuresis, diuretics)
Skin water loss (burns)	Accidental—hypertonic saline abortion	Gastrointestinal losses, (vomiting, diarrhea, fistulas)
Respiratory water losses (fever, hyperventilation)	Accidental—hypertonic dialysis	Skin losses (excessive perspiration)

*ECF, Extracellular fluid.
†DI, Diabetes insipidus.

potassium stores is found in the extracellular fluid, where its level is finely regulated to maintain a concentration between 3.5 and 5.0 mEq/L. An excess or deficit in total body potassium is reflected in the serum potassium concentration such that total body changes of 100–200 mEq of potassium will generally alter serum potassium concentration by 0.5–1.0 mEq/L. Changes in serum potassium concentration can also occur with cellular shifts of potassium. Factors such as acid-base changes, hypertonicity, cell damage, and alterations in the hormones which regulate potassium can all affect the intracellular/extracellular potassium ratio and thus affect serum potassium concentration. Hyperkalemia can therefore be caused by an excess in total body potassium or by a shift of potassium out of cells. Similarly, hypokalemia can result from a deficit in total body potassium or by a shift of potassium into cells. Moderate increases or decreases in serum potassium levels will significantly affect the cardiac muscle depolarization process producing changes in the electrocardiogram (EKG). These effects on the EKG can be very useful especially in emergencies in which hyperkalemia is suspected, but the value has not yet been reported from the chemistry laboratory.

Hyperkalemia

Definitions
When serum potassium exceeds 5 mEq/L, hyperkalemia is present. Before considering the possible etiologies, *pseudohyperkalemia* should be excluded. Pseudohyperkalemia refers to hyperkalemia occurring not in the patient, but in the test tube. When a blood sample is drawn with difficulty, the resultant hemolysis can release potassium into the serum. Similarly, test tube hyperkalemia can occur when potassium is released from white blood cells and platelets during the process of blood clotting, a significant phenomenon only if the cell count is greater than 600,000–1,000,000. In cases of pseudohyperkalemia from high cell counts, serum potassium is elevated while plasma potassium, measured in plasma from an unclotted blood sample, is normal. You should exclude pseudohyperkalemia as the first step in

evaluating a patient with hyperkalemia. This can be done by avoiding hemolysis and by measuring potassium from a plasma (ie, unclotted) sample, such as one collected in a heparinized tube.

Causes and Treatment

As can be seen in Table 5-5, the causes of hyperkalemia are basically divided into those associated with increased input, decreased output, or changes in the cellular distribution of potassium. Examination of other laboratory results such as BUN, creatinine, serum bicarbonate level, and anion gap can provide useful clues concerning the etiology of the hyperkalemia such as renal failure or acidosis. One test which is not very helpful in evaluating hyperkalemia is a random or "spot" measurement of urinary potassium concentration. This value, measured at one given time, provides no information about the total amount of potassium excreted daily, which is what determines, at least in part, the serum potassium level. A 24-hour measurement of total potassium excreted per day is of somewhat greater value, but only if the intake is known so that intake and renal output of potassium can be compared. Morbidity and mortality from hyperkalemia occur mainly because of associated cardiac toxicity. The earliest EKG signs of hyperkalemia are peaked T waves which are usually seen at a serum potassium of 5.5–6.0 mEq/L. Flattening of the P wave is evident with potassium levels of 7–7.5 mEq/L, and prolongation of the QRS interval usually occurs with levels above 8 mEq/L. While the EKG does not indicate the exact serum potassium level, it does provide an indication of the degree of electrical instability of the heart and danger to the patient. It is generally agreed that hyperkalemia requires immediate medical therapy if EKG changes are present or if the serum level exceeds 6.5–7.0 mEq/L.

Hypokalemia

Causes and Treatment

Hypokalemia can be caused by a total body loss of potassium or by a shift of potassium into cells (Table 5-6). Although a potassium deficit of 100–200 mEq will lower serum potassium by 0.5–1.0 mEq/L, this relationship becomes much less predictable with greater total body potassium deficits. Thus, a serum potassium below 2.0 mEq/L could represent a deficit of as little as 300 mEq or as large as 800 mEq, a factor which must be kept in mind in prescribing replacement therapy in a patient with severe hypokalemia. As with hyperkalemia, careful inspection of other laboratory data will frequently provide clues as to the cause of the hypokalemia. For example, a high serum bicarbonate and low chloride level could represent a metabolic alkalosis. A high blood glucose value could imply that an osmotic diuresis caused by glycosuria resulted in potassium losses. A "spot" urine value for potassium concentration may be helpful here in that high values (> 40 mEq/L) in the setting of hypokalemia (< 3 mEq/L) indicate inappropriate urinary potassium losses. Another useful test to consider while evaluating a patient for hypokalemia is a urine screening test for the presence of diuretics. A patient with occult diuretic abuse can have unexplained hypokalemia. Although hypokalemia adversely affects cardiac muscle, severe cardiac toxicity is not observed as frequently as with hyperkalemia. The correlation between EKG change and serum potassium concentration is not as good as in hyperkalemia. However most patients with a serum potassium below 2.5 mEq/L will have U waves and prolongation of the P-R interval on EKG. Hypokalemia predisposes to arrhythmias, especially in patients on digitalis. Skeletal muscle weakness and paralysis can also occur with severe hypokalemia (< 2.5 mEq/L). In treating the patient with hypokalemia, you should use oral potassium repletion when possible. However, in both severe cases (< 2.0 mEq/L) and in cases associated with muscle paralysis or arrhythmias, intravenous KCl can be administered at a rate not exceeding 40 mEq per hour.

Table 5-5
Causes of Hyperkalemia

1. Factitious
   A. Laboratory error
   B. "Pseudohyperkalemia"—in vitro hemolysis or release of K from white
      blood cells or platelets during the clotting process
2. Increased Input
   A. Exogenous—diet, salt substitutes, low Na^+ diet, K^+-penicillin
   B. Endogenous—hemolysis, GI bleed, catabolic states, burns, rhabdomyolysis,
      cancer cell lysis, exercise
3. Decreased Output—decreased renal excretion
4. Drugs—eg, K^+ sparing diuretics
5. Changes in Cellular Distribution Caused By:
   a. Hypertonicity
   b. pH or HCO_3 changes
   c. Drugs (digitalis, succinylcholine)
   d. Changes in amount or action of hormones known to be important in
      maintaining normal cellular distribution of potassium (insulin,
      ? aldosterone, ? epinephrine)

Table 5-6
Causes of Hypokalemia

1. Decreased Intake—Starvation, alcoholism
2. Increased Output—Renal: Diuretics
                            Osmotic diuresis
                            Vomiting and 2° hyperaldosteronism
                            1° hypermineralocorticoidism
                            Bartter's syndrome
                            Renal tubular acidosis
                     Gastrointestinal: Diarrhea, vomiting
3. Change in Cellular Distribution of Potassium Caused by—
   Alkalemia
   Hypokalemic periodic paralysis
4. Drugs—Alkali treatment
          Corticosteroids
          Diuretics
          Insulin
          Mannitol
          Antibiotics (carbenicillin, Amphotericin B)

■ Selected Readings

Acid-Base Disorders

Andreoli TE: Disturbances in acid-base balance, in Wyngaarden JB and Smith LH (eds): *Cecil Textbook of Medicine.* ed 16. Philadelphia, The W. B. Saunders Co, 1982, pp 486–494.

Bia M, Thier SO: Mixed acid base disturbances: a clinical approach. *Med Clin N Am* 1981;65:347–361.

Cohen JJ, Kassirer JP: *Acid/Base.* Boston, Little, Brown and Co, 1982.

Emmett M, Narins RG: Clinical use of the anion gap. *Medicine* 1977;56:38–54.

Narins RG, Gardner LB: Simple acid base disturbances. *Med Clin N Am* 1981; 65:321–346.

Rose BD: *Clinical Physiology of Acid-Base and Electrolyte Disorders.* New York, McGraw-Hill Book Co, 1977.

Disorders of the Serum Sodium Concentration

DeFronzo RA, Thier SO: Pathophysiologic approach to hyponatremia. *Arch Int Med* 1980;140:897–902.

Feig PU: Hypernatremia and hypertonic states. *Med Clin N Am* 1981; 65:271–290.

Friedler RM, Koffler A, Kurokawa K: Hyponatremia and hypernatremia. *Clin Nephrol* 1977;7:163–172.

Disorders of Serum Potassium Concentration

Cox M: Potassium homeostasis. *Med Clin N Am* 1981;65:363–384.

Nardone DA, McDonald WJ, Girard DE: Mechanism of hypokalemia: Clinical correlation. *Medicine* 1978;57: 435–446.

■ Assessment of Renal Integrity

Urinary Sediment

Examination of the urine is an important part of the evaluation of patients with renal diseases. When performed carefully, this examination frequently provides diagnostic information not available through many more invasive and expensive tests.

Technique of Examination

A fresh, concentrated urine sample with a low pH provides the most information. Patients are instructed to void in the morning after their overnight fast and then come to the office and void again. This second void is collected for examination. Women are instructed to collect a midstream specimen with the labia spread to avoid vaginal contamination. If urinary tract infection is suspected, a small volume of this fresh urine is placed on a slide, stained with Gram stain, and covered with a glass cover slip. The presence or absence of bacteria is then evaluated under the microscope. To perform the remainder of the urinalysis, 15 mL of urine is centrifuged for three to five minutes. The supernatant is tested with a dip stick for protein, pigment (hemoglobin or myoglobin), urinary pH, glucose, and acetone. The supernatant can likewise be tested for bilirubin pigment. The supernatant is then decanted, and the sediment at the bottom of the test tube is resuspended in the small volume of remaining urine. Sediment is then placed onto a glass slide, covered with a cover slip, and examined under the microscope. With the low-power objective, the field is scanned and the edges of the cover slip are completely examined searching for casts. When a cast is found, it is characterized by examination with the high-power objective. After such thorough scanning, several fields are examined with the high-power objective to count the number of formed elements.

Normal Urine Sediments

Several formed elements can be found in normal urine sediment. Erythrocytes may be seen, but are usually low in number in normal urine. Ninety percent of normal urine samples have less than one red blood cell per high-power field. However, up to ten red blood cells per high-power field occasionally can be found in normal urine. Heavy exercise and congestive heart failure may increase red blood cell excretion in persons with no abnormalities of the kidneys or urinary tract.

White Blood Cells Two or three white blood cells per high-power field are found commonly in urine from normal men and women. Higher numbers of white cells may be found in urine from women, particularly when there is some contamination of the urine from the vulva. However, up to 20 white blood cells per high-power field occasionally are found in normal urine from persons with no urinary tract abnormalities or renal disease. Heavy exercise, congestive heart failure, and fever can increase the excretion of white blood cells.

Epithelial Cells   Large vaginal epithelial cells are found commonly in the urine sediment of women. This finding suggests contamination of the urine from the vagina, and a better clean catch urine specimen should be obtained for examination. Large, irregular epithelial cells may be seen in urine from men and women. These arise from the bladder or urethra and are of no diagnostic significance. Renal tubular epithelial cells are much smaller, rounded, and contain an eccentric nucleus. Such cells are present in only low numbers in normal sediment, usually less than one or two such cells in the entire sediment.

Casts   Tamm-Horsfall protein, a mucoprotein of very high molecular weight, is secreted by tubular cells and may gel, forming the matrix of tubular casts which are visible in the urine sediment. Hyaline casts, narrow transparent casts containing no cellular or lipid inclusions, and granular casts containing aggregates of serum protein may be seen in normal urine sediment and are increased by dehydration, exercise, and increased protein excretion.

Abnormal Urine Sediment

Increased numbers of cells in the urine usually reflect abnormalities of the urinary tract. Many red blood cells or white blood cells per high-power field are found when bleeding or inflammation occurs anywhere along the urinary tract from the glomerulus to the urethra. Abnormal urinary casts also suggest renal parenchymal disease.

Leukocyte Casts   When casts are found to contain white blood cells, one can infer that an inflammatory process is present in the renal parenchyma. Pyelonephritis and interstitial nephritis commonly result in such leukocyte casts. Acute glomerulonephritis usually is characterized by red blood cell casts (see below), but leukocyte casts occasionally may be present as well.

Erythrocyte Casts   Urinary casts containing red blood cells place the source of blood loss in the renal parenchyma. Red blood cell casts usually mean glomerulonephritis. Rarely, red blood cell casts may be seen in patients with acute tubular necrosis.

Broad Waxy Casts   Waxy casts or broad casts are found in patients with chronic renal insufficiency. They are clear and are wider than hyaline casts.

Oval Fat Bodies   Round or oval lipid-containing droplets may be found in patients with heavy proteinuria. These particles can be found by placing the urine sediment under polarized light and searching for doubly refractile bodies which have a characteristic Maltese cross appearance. They are found commonly in patients with heavy proteinuria, and no specific significance should be attached to their presence.

Patterns of these urinary sediment abnormalities may suggest different diagnoses. For example, renal insufficiency with a scant urine sediment suggests complete obstruction of one or both kidneys. Acute tubular necrosis often is characterized by sheets of renal tubular epithelial cells and increased numbers of white blood cells. In acute glomerulonephritis the sediment contains increased numbers of red blood cells, white blood cells, white blood cell casts, and red blood cell casts. This pattern is called a "nephritic" pattern. In contrast, patients with the nephrotic syndrome have oval fat bodies, but few formed elements, in the urine. Finally, patients with chronic renal failure frequently have a "telescoped sediment" with increased numbers of erythrocytes and leukocytes and elements of both a nephritic and a nephrotic sediment.

The most important thing to remember concerning the urinary sediment is that the physician should examine it personally. It has been our experience that key diagnostic findings such as erythrocyte casts or leukocyte casts are not described by standard laboratory screening, but are found when the physician carefully evaluates the sediment.

Search for Proteinuria

In normal adults the daily urine contains no more than 150 mg of protein. Most of this protein is derived from the plasma by filtration, and the rest comes from the renal tubules and lower urinary tract. Increased urinary excretion of protein may indicate renal glomerular disease, tubular disease or dysfunction, or increased production and excretion of abnormal proteins. Most types of glomerulonephritis result in damage to the filtration barrier separating the plasma from the urinary space in the glomerulus. This damage results in a more "leaky" diffusion barrier, and plasma proteins cross the barrier in higher concentrations than normal. Albumin, a protein of molecular weight 69,000, is ordinarily filtered in only small amounts. The filtered albumin is usually taken up by proximal renal tubular cells and degraded so that only 25–50 mg per day is excreted normally. In glomerulonephritis this excretion rate can increase several hundredfold to more than 4 g per day. Thus, heavy proteinuria may be a sign of glomerulonephritis.

Patients with primary renal tubular or interstitial disease likewise may have an increased renal protein excretion. In contrast to primary glomerular disease, these patients have a predominance of low-molecular-weight proteins in their urine, including molecules such as light chains and lysozyme. Normally such molecules are filtered at the glomerulus and then reabsorbed by the renal tubule. In diseases of tubular function, this reabsorptive process is impaired, and low-molecular-weight proteins are excreted in the urine in higher concentrations.

An increased production of certain proteins can result in the appearance of these proteins in the urine. When monoclonal gammopathies and myeloma result in increased production of light chains, heavy chains, and other fragments of immunoglobulins, these proteins are filtered at the glomerulus and then reabsorbed in the renal tubule. When the renal tubule's ability to reabsorb these abnormal proteins is saturated, high concentrations of these proteins may appear in the urine.

Test for Urinary Proteins

Dipstick   The most commonly used screening test for urinary proteins is a paper strip impregnated with tetra bromphenol and a buffer to maintain the pH at 3.0. If the pH is unchanged, the color of this paper changes from yellow to blue as the protein concentration rises. Although it is a good screening test, the dipstick method has two major drawbacks. First, it is definitely positive (2 + to 4 +) when the protein concentration exceeds 30 mg/dL. At lower protein concentrations, the test is equivocal (negative, trace, or 1 +). Second, the test does not detect light chains, and therefore its use would not detect the presence of abnormal proteins in the urine even in high concentrations.

Sulfosalicylic Acid Test   In the sulfosalicylic acid test, several drops of 5% sulfosalicylic acid are added to an aliquot of urine. The quantity of precipitate is roughly proportional to the protein concentration in the urine. This test takes a bit more time than the dipstick method, but is positive when albumin and abnormal proteins including light chains are present in the urine. It is the screening test which should always be used when multiple myeloma or other gammopathies are included in the differential diagnosis.

Quantitative Excretion   The best method to determine the presence of abnormal protein excretion is to measure the actual amount of protein excreted in a 24-hour period. The patient brings a 24-hour collection of urine to the laboratory, and an aliquot of this well-mixed collection is withdrawn. The protein in this aliquot is then precipitated by the addition of Esbach's picric acid-citric acid reagent or a similar reagent in a calibrated test tube. The test tube is then centrifuged, and the volume of precipitate is measured. This offers a precise concentration of urinary protein which, when multiplied by the 24-hour urine volume, results in a quantitative 24-hour urinary protein excretion rate. Excretion of more than 3–4 g of protein per 24 hours almost always means glomerular disease, although rarely, primary interstitial disease can result in this degree of protein excretion. Protein excretion of less than 3 g per day may result from glomerular or interstitial disease.

Test for Light Chains   The classic test to detect excretion of abnormal immunoglobulin is the Bence Jones test. In this test, urine is heated to 45 to 55 °C in a test tube. Light chains precipitate at these temperatures when the urine is acid (pH 4.9). Further heating of the test tube to the boiling point results in the dissolution of the precipitate. This test may be difficult to perform properly and is also somewhat insensitive. For this reason, a urine protein electrophoresis and immunoelectrophoresis should be performed when light-chain proteinuria is suspected.

Clinical Presentation of Proteinuria

Patients with fixed structural lesions of the renal parenchyma causing proteinuria will demonstrate this abnormality at any time of the day or night and in the supine or upright position. In contrast, some patients have intermittent proteinuria or abnormal protein excretion only when they are standing. Intermittent proteinuria and postural proteinuria do not have the same prognosis as fixed persistent proteinuria.

Intermittent Proteinuria Exercise, fever, or emotional stress can result in intermittent increases of protein excretion. Some patients have intermittent proteinuria with no obvious cause. Such patients are at no greater risk of progressive renal deterioration than is the general nonproteinuric population. Therefore, in patients with a positive screening test for urinary protein but no hematuria, no hypertension, and no renal functional impairment, the urine should be tested on one or two other occasions before a full evaluation for proteinuria is justified.

Postural Proteinuria Some patients have a normal protein excretion while in the supine position, but an abnormal protein excretion in the upright position. Such patients usually excrete small amounts of protein, rarely exceeding 1 g per day. In the absence of hematuria, hypertension, or renal functional impairment, this finding is probably of no clinical significance, and this population should be separated from those with fixed proteinuria. There are two ways to test for postural proteinuria. The first, performed in the office or hospital, requires the patient to collect a 16-hour urine collection while he or she is in the upright position during the course of the usual daily activity. A separate eight-hour collection is then made at night when the patient is supine. Both collections are then analyzed for protein concentration, and the quantity of protein excreted in each is extrapolated to 24 hours. Patients with postural proteinuria will have negligible protein excretion in the eight-hour nocturnal specimen and higher concentration in the 16-hour daytime collection. A more precise test can be performed in the hospital. After an overnight sleep, the patient remains supine and urine is collected for four hours after an oral water load. The patient then stands, drinks another water load, and walks around during a four-hour urine collection. In each four-hour period, the urine is collected in separate containers and analyzed for protein content. Patients with postural proteinuria demonstrate negligible protein content in the supine collection and more than 100 mg of protein in the four-hour upright specimen.

■ Tests of Renal Function

The kidney functions normally by filtering plasma at the glomerulus and reabsorbing this filtrate in the proximal and distal tubules. The composition of the final urine depends on the amount of water and solutes reabsorbed in these tubular segments. Under normal conditions, the bulk of water and solute is reabsorbed in the proximal tubule, and the distal tubule fine tunes reabsorption to suit the body's needs. Depressed rates of glomerular filtration and disorders of proximal and distal tubular function are found in disease states affecting the kidney. Patterns of functional disturbances may allow the clinician to make specific diagnoses. For example, patients with primary glomerular disease have a reduction in the glomerular filtration rate and then later an impairment in tubular function. Patients with interstitial renal diseases first demonstrate disorders of tubular function and only later develop a reduction in the glomerular filtration rate (GFR). In chronic renal insufficiency, disorders of both glomerular and tubular function are evident whatever the original insult.

Measurement of the GFR

The best overall assessment of renal function is the measurement of the GFR. The average size adult male has a GFR of approximately 130 mL/min. This value is proportional to body size and declines with age. When a substance is filtered at the glomerulus and is neither reabsorbed nor secreted by the renal tubule, the excretion of that substance is equal to its filtration rate. Therefore, the GFR can be estimated by measuring the rate of excretion of such a substance. Inulin, a polymer of fructose, is freely filtered at the glomerulus and is neither secreted nor reabsorbed by the renal tubule. It has been used to measure the GFR with great precision for nearly 50 years. When such exact values are required, patients are first given a water load of 15 mL/kg and then a 0.4 mL/kg loading dose of 10% inulin. A maintenance intravenous infusion of approximately 30 mg/min is then given. Urine samples are collected every 30 minutes, and serum samples are drawn at the midpoint of each collection. The urine and serum are measured for concentration of inulin, and then the GFR is estimated by measuring the inulin clearance according to the formula:

$$C_{In} = U_{In}V/P_{In} \times 30 \tag{1}$$

where C_{In} is inulin clearance in milliliters per minute, V is the urinary volume in milliliters, U_{In} is the urinary concentration in inulin in milligrams per deciliter, P_{In} is the plasma concentration of inulin in milligrams per deciliter, and 30 is the time of collection in minutes.

This precise measurement of filtration rate is unnecessary in most clinical situations, since the endogenous substance creatinine may be used to estimate the GFR. The tubular secretion of creatinine is approximately equal to its tubular reabsorption, so the excretion rate is approximately equal to the filtration rate. Although measurement of creatinine clearance overestimates the true GFR by an average of approximately 7%, it is accurate enough to be of great clinical use. It should be noted, however, that when the GFR has fallen below 20 mL/min the creatinine clearance may exceed the true filtration rate by 50%.

Creatinine clearance is measured by using a 24-hour urine collection. Patients are asked to collect a 24-hour specimen of urine in the following fashion. On the day of collection, the patient arises from sleep, voids, and discards this urine. Thereafter, each void is collected in a clean container. All urine voided during that day and the following night is collected. When the patient arises on the next morning, his first voided specimen is collected in the container, and the collection is then ended. An aliquot of the well-mixed urine and a serum sample are then obtained for measurement of creatinine concentration, and the creatinine clearance is calculated according to the formula:

$$C_{Cr} = U_{Cr}V/P_{Cr} \times 1440 \tag{2}$$

where C_{Cr} is the creatinine clearance in milliliters per minute, U_{Cr} is the urinary creatinine concentration in milligrams per deciliter, V is the urinary volume in milliliters, P_{Cr} is the plasma concentration of creatinine in milligrams per deciliter, and 1440 is the time of collection in minutes.

The major error often made in this calculation is an incomplete collection of urine. The adequacy of urine collection can be assessed by noting the total creatinine excreted. Since the excretion rate of creatinine is no lower than 20 mg/kg per day, a total urinary excretion substantially less than this calculated amount suggests an incomplete collection. This would lead to an erroneously low estimate of glomerular filtration rate. When urinary creatinine is much lower than the estimated amount, the 24-hour collection should be repeated. If adequate collections cannot be made, it is sometimes useful to perform a four-hour collection in-office hydrated creatinine clearance. The patient is given an oral water load of 15 mL/kg, voids, and discards this specimen. The timed urine collection then begins for four hours. The precise time of the last void is noted, and the clearance is measured according to formula (2), with the exact collection time in minutes substituted for 1440.

When body mass and hydration remain constant, changes in serum creatinine concentration reflect accurately changes in glomerular filtration rate. Thus, in a given patient a rise of serum creatinine from 1.0 mg/dL to 2.0 mg/dL represents a 100% reduction in the glomerular filtration rate. In patients with chronic, stable renal insufficiency, the rate of fall in renal function can be estimated by plotting $1/P_{Cr}$ versus time. Such a plot can be used to predict rate of rise of serum creatinine and the rate of renal deterioration.

Another common measure of glomerular filtration rate is the blood urea nitrogen (BUN). Since urea is the end product of protein metabolism and is excreted by the kidney, the BUN usually correlates with the GFR. However, several factors other than renal function may affect the BUN. Increased dietary protein or increased protein catabolism such as when gut bacteria metabolize blood in the gastrointestinal tract may raise the BUN. Furthermore, dehydration alone can raise the BUN. Likewise, patients who are protein malnourished may have a relatively low BUN despite substantial renal insufficiency. Thus, the measurement of serum creatinine and creatinine clearance are far superior to measurement of BUN in the assessment of the GFR.

Under normal conditions, the ratio of BUN to creatinine is approximately 10:1. A ratio substantially greater than this, often more than 40:1, is found in patients with dehydration and lowered renal perfusion. When the level of azotemia (abnormally elevated BUN) is out of proportion to the rise in serum creatinine, a trial of hydration often improves the azotemia substantially.

Tests of Tubular Function

Tests of Proximal Tubular Function
The proximal tubule is the site of bulk reabsorption of sodium, chloride, and water as well as most filtered bicarbonate, amino acid, phosphate, and glucose. Diffuse disorders of proximal tubular reabsorption result in the Fanconi syndrome.

Fanconi Syndrome   In the Fanconi syndrome, the urine contains abnormal amounts of amino acid, glucose, and phosphate. In children these abnormalities often result in polyuria, dehydration, vomiting, growth retardation,

98

muscular weakness, and rickets. In adults osteoporosis and muscular weakness are found. Drugs such as acetazolamide, tetracycline, and anticonvulsants may induce the Fanconi syndrome. The laboratory tests which confirm this diagnosis include tests to measure urinary amino acids, glucose and phosphate. The Fanconi syndrome is characterized by high urine levels of alpha amino nitrogen, the presence of glycosuria despite a normal serum glucose concentration, and a decreased fractional reabsorption of phosphate in the presence of hypophosphatemia.

Cystinuria Cystinuria, transmitted with autosomal recessive genetics, is characterized by impaired transport of the dibasic amino acids cystine, ornithine, lysine, and arginine. Since cystine is insoluble in the urine when present in high concentration, patients with this disease develop cystine kidney stones. Therefore, screening for cystinuria is part of the routine evaluation for renal stone disease. A laboratory test for this disease is the sodium nitroprusside test. Five milliliters of urine are added to 2 mL of a 5% sodium cyanide solution. Ten minutes later, 5 mL of 5% sodium nitroprusside are added to this mixture. Urine containing greater than 75–125 mg of cystine per g of creatinine will develop a purple color. If this screening test is positive, a quantitative test of urinary cystine can then be performed by using ion-exchange chromatography.

Proximal Renal Tubular Acidosis (RTA) Although proximal RTA is found most frequently in association with the full-blown Fanconi syndrome, some children have been reported with a defect of only bicarbonate reabsorption in the proximal tubule. Several drugs including acetazolamide, aminoglycosides, and analgesics may result in proximal RTA. This diagnosis should be suspected when patients have hyperchloremic metabolic acidosis. In such patients, the urinary pH is high (greater than 5.4) only when the serum bicarbonate is in the normal range. As the serum bicarbonate level falls through bicarbonate wasting, the filtered load of bicarbonate falls and the impaired proximal tubule is able to reabsorb all of this reduced filtered load. Therefore, the urine pH falls to normal (5.4 or less) in the presence of steady-state hyperchloremic metabolic acidosis. Extrarenal losses of bicarbonate can sometimes masquerade as proximal RTA so in such patients a history of diarrhea or laxative abuse should be carefully sought.

Tests of Distal Tubular Function
Urinary Concentrating Ability The average man must excrete 600 mOsm of urea and electrolytes each day. If the kidney were unable to concentrate the urine, this solute load would require a daily urine volume of 2 L. The normal kidney is able to reabsorb water and concentrate the urine fourfold and the osmolality of plasma to 1200 mOsm/kg, allowing for as little as 500 mL of urine per day to maintain the body's homeostasis.
Several diseases are characterized by defects in urine concentrating ability. Reduction in the GFR as is seen in acute or chronic renal insufficiency, interstitial renal injury such as postobstructive uropathy, multiple myeloma, lithium toxicity, or hypercalcemia, and hormonal deficiencies such as Addison's disease or diabetes insipidus all cause a defect in concentrating capacity. In addition, since urea plays a major role in the concentrating

mechanism, patients on a low-protein diet may have a defect in maximal concentrating capacity. Patients with an obligatory solute load to excrete, such as diabetic patients with high plasma glucose levels, undergo a solute diuresis and are unable to concentrate the urine maximally. Tests of urinary concentrating ability are useful when the GFR is not substantially impaired, when the protein in the diet is not restricted, and when no solute diuresis is present.

Urine Osmolality The best test of urinary concentration is the urine osmolality. This is a measure of the number of particles in solution and can be measured accurately using the principle of freezing point depression. A small volume of urine is placed in an osmometer, the freezing point depression is measured, and the osmolality is then calculated. Under normal conditions the maximal urinary osmolality is more than 850 mOsm/kg, and the ratio of urine to plasma osmolality ($Uosm/P_{osm}$) is ≥ 3.5.

Urinary Specific Gravity The specific gravity of a substance measures its density with respect to distilled water. It is therefore a measure not only of the total number of particles in solution, but also of the relative size of these particles. Under most circumstances the specific gravity and osmolality correlate very well. However, when high concentrations of high-molecular-weight substances are excreted in the urine, such as proteins or radiologic contrast materials, the measured specific gravity may be higher than one would predict from the measured osmolality. The specific gravity is measured easily with a hydrometer. Care should be taken to standardize the temperature at which the urine specific gravity is measured, since this variable can affect substantially the measured specific gravity. In the absence of proteinuria or recent radiographic study, this is an excellent office measure of urine concentration.

Refractive Index One or two drops of urine placed in a refractometer can measure the refractive index of urine, an accurate measure of the urine specific gravity. This device has the advantage of temperature independence and less error induced by high-molecular-weight substances. The refractometer is a fast and easy way to measure urine concentration in the office.

Tests of Urine Concentrating Ability The kidney's ability to concentrate the urine may be tested by measuring the urine osmolality or specific gravity under conditions of hydropenia. For screening purposes, a first voided morning urine can be measured for osmolality or specific gravity. If the specific gravity is greater than or equal to 1.022 or the urinary osmolality is greater than 850 mOsm/kg, the concentrating mechanism is intact. To study urine concentrating capacity more rigorously, one can perform an overnight dehydration test. The patient is instructed to eat no food and drink no fluid after 8:00 PM. Twelve hours later, at 8:00 AM, the patient voids and discards this specimen. Fluid deprivation continues until the patient voids a second urine specimen which is then measured for osmolality. If the osmolality is greater than or equal to 900 mOsm/kg, the concentrating mechanism is normal. If at this time the urine osmolality is not greater than 900 mOsm/kg, a serum sample is obtained for measurement of osmolality. Five units of

100

aqueous pitressin is then injected intramuscularly or intravenously. One hour later the plasma and urine are again collected for measurement of osmolality. A plasma osmolality of greater than or equal to 300 mOsm/kg indicates adequate dehydration and stimulation of the concentrating mechanism. A urine concentration of less than 850–900 mOsm/kg indicates a defect in concentrating capacity under these conditions.

When the diagnosis of diabetes insipidus is entertained, great care must be taken in the performance of the water deprivation test. The urine volume of patients with complete diabetes insipidus may remain very high despite water deprivation, and clinical shock can result. In such patients, careful monitoring of body weight and blood pressure must be performed during a dehydration test. If the body weight falls more than 5% during the course of the test, the water deprivation should be discontinued. In such patients, serial measurements of the plasma osmolality will document adequate hydropenic stress, and a very brief water deprivation test of only several hours is often quite adequate to document the defect in urine concentration. In both central diabetes insipidus and incomplete diabetes insipidus, the addition of aqueous vasopressin will result in a substantial rise in the urine osmolality. In contrast, patients with nephrogenic diabetes insipidus will not concentrate the urine despite water deprivation and pitressin.

Distal Tubular Acidification The distal tubule completes acid-base homeostasis by reabsorbing the remainder of filtered bicarbonate and by secreting hydrogen ions into the tubular fluid. A defect in this mechanism results in distal RTA. Primary distal RTA, a disease of young adults, is usually an autosomal dominant transmitted hereditary disease. In addition, many systemic diseases, including alcoholic liver disease, amyloidosis, cryoglobulinemia, diabetic ketoacidosis, hyperthyroidism, hyperparathyroidism, hypothyroidism, and Sjögren's syndrome, may result in complete distal renal tubular acidosis. Furthermore, sickle cell anemia, systemic lupus erythematosis, and autoimmune liver disease can result in incomplete distal RTA. In addition, renal abnormalities including chronic interstitial nephritis and chronic obstructive uropathy can cause distal RTA. Finally, several drugs, including amphotericin B, lithium, and analgesics, can cause this tubular defect. The laboratory presentation of this syndrome includes a hyperchloremic metabolic acidosis with hypokalemia. The urine pH is always greater than 5.8 despite the severity of metabolic acidosis.

When the urine is not maximally acidified (pH less than 5.4) an acid loading test is sometimes necessary to diagnose proximal or distal renal tubular acidosis. In the acute acid loading test, ammonium chloride (100 mg/kg) is given with 200 mL of water in the morning. Urine is collected hourly for the next four to six hours. At four hours, the venous pH and serum bicarbonate are measured. When the acid load is absorbed normally (demonstrated by an acidemic venous pH and a lowered serum bicarbonate level), the urine pH should be less than 5.4. If it is greater than 5.4, a defect in the distal acidification mechanism is implied.

Sodium Conservation Under the stress of dehydration, the distal tubules should reabsorb most filtered sodium and chloride. In some diseases, such as medullary cystic disease of the kidney, this ability is impaired substantially and sodium wasting results. This obligatory loss of sodium may result in significant volume depletion and a fall in the GFR. Furthermore, patients with diffuse renal disease of any cause develop an impaired ability to reabsorb sodium and chloride. The laboratory tests to assess this function include measurement of the urine sodium concentration and calculation of the fractional excretion of sodium.

Potassium Secretion Under normal conditions, potassium balance is maintained by excretion of most ingested potassium. This is accomplished by the renal potassium-secreting cells of the distal tubule and collecting duct, in a process facilitated by the adrenal mineralocorticoid hormone aldosterone. When patients demonstrate hyperkalemia in the absence of metabolic acidosis, the ability of the kidney to secrete potassium normally must be tested. Likewise, in patients with hypokalemia but no metabolic alkalosis, an assessment of the potassium secretory mechanism must be made. Patients are placed on a known fixed-potassium diet, and then the urine is collected for 24 hours. An aliquot of this well-mixed collection is then measured for potassium concentration. If potassium excretion exceeds intake in the hypokalemic patient, or if it is less than intake in the hyperkalemic patient, an abnormality of either distal tubular function or of aldosterone production is implied.

Aldosterone production depends not only on potassium balance, but also on the volume status. Care should be taken to assure adequate hydration in patients tested for potassium balance. Also, a single spot measurement of potassium concentration in a random urine sample cannot be interpreted unless the potassium intake and the patient's level of hydration are known.

■ Use of the Laboratory in Renal Disease

Renal dysfunction and renal disease are sometimes present in several ways sometimes referred to as renal syndromes. In modern practice, proper use of the laboratory is essential for the accurate diagnosis and management of patients with renal disorders. In the remainder of this chapter, we describe the most common renal syndromes and illustrate the most important laboratory tests to obtain and follow in each clinical setting.

Acute Renal Failure

Acute renal failure is defined as a sudden deterioration in GFR. Most, but not all, causes of acute renal failure are reversible. In patients with renal failure, you must sometimes await improvement in kidney function before the diagnosis of acute renal failure can be confirmed retrospectively. Determination of kidney size, by simply obtaining renal nephrotomograms without dye, may be quite helpful in distinguishing acute from chronic renal failure. The kidneys are usually normal or large in acute renal failure, but frequently small if the disorder is chronic. Acute deterioration in renal function can occur after bilateral ureteral obstruction or thrombosis of the renal arteries or veins. However, it is most commonly due to an entity known as *acute tubular necrosis*, characterized by a sudden decrease in renal blood flow and GFR with subsequent tubular damage. This entity must be distinguished from the syndrome of *prenatal azotemia,* in which renal per-fusion and GFR are decreased, usually due to intravascular volume contrac-tion, but tubular function remains intact. Examination of the BUN and serum creatinine values along with the urinary electrolytes can help differentiate acute tubular necrosis from prerenal azotemia. In acute tubular necrosis, the normal ratio of BUN to creatinine level (10:1 to 20:1) is preserved, and the serum creatinine concentration rises by approximately 1–1.5 mg/dL per day after the initial insult. In contrast, patients with prerenal azotemia usually have an elevated ratio (BUN rises more dramatically than creatinine), and the creatinine level, if elevated at all, rises very slowly from one day to the next. An even better distinction between acute tubular necrosis and prerenal azotemia can be made by an examination of urinary indices (Table 6-1). Since tubular function is preserved in prerenal azotemia, the tubules will respond to the decrease in renal perfusion by avidly absorbing sodium and water resulting in a low urine sodium concentration (UNa) and a high urine osmolality (Uosm) and elevated ratios of urine to plasma urea and creatinine concentrations. Perhaps the best index to examine is the fractional excretion of sodium (FE_{Na}), a term which factors the amount of sodium excreted by the amount filtered to give a more pure measure of tubular function. Its deriva-tion and calculation can be seen in the following equations:

$$FE_{Na} = \frac{Na\ excreted}{Na\ filtered} \times 100$$

$$= \frac{UNa\ (V)}{PNa\ (GFR)} \times 100$$

$$= \frac{UNa\ (V)}{PNa\ (Ccr)} \times 100$$

$$= \frac{UNa\ (V)}{PNa\ \left[\dfrac{Ucr\ (V)}{Pcr}\right]} \times 100$$

$$FE_{Na} = \frac{UNa}{PNa} \times \frac{Pcr}{Ucr} \times 100$$

Ccr is the creatinine clearance; Ucr and Pcr are urine and plasma creatinine concentrations, respectively, and (V) is the volume of urine. In the final equation, the urine volumes cancel out such that FE_{Na} can be calculated from random urine and blood samples obtained simultaneously, in which the sodium and creatinine concentrations are measured in each sample. The FE_{Na} is usually less than 1% in patients with prerenal azotemia and greater than 1% in patients with acute tubular necrosis or acute obstruction. It is useful to develop the practice of calculating the FE_{Na} in patients with acute renal failure. Recent studies have shown that, of all tests available, it has the greatest diagnostic accuracy in differentiating between the main causes of acute renal failure.

Examination of the urine sediment should also be performed in any patient with acute renal failure since the presence of red cell casts, infection, or free heme pigment can be a clue to the underlying etiology of the renal failure. In most patients with renal failure due to acute tubular necrosis, the urine sediment will contain white cells, tubular epithelial cells, and multiple dark brown granular casts from tubular debris. The peripheral blood smear should also be examined since microangiopathic hemolytic anemias can occur with certain types of renal failure such as scleroderma, a hemolytic uremic syndrome, and malignant hypertension. Finally, since acute renal failure can cause derangements in electrolyte, calcium, or phosphorus values and in acid-base status, these parameters should be evaluated initially and followed closely to determine the need for specific treatment or correction.

Chronic Renal Failure

In most cases of chronic renal failure, the kidney damage progresses inexorably to end-stage renal failure over some period of time. Proper use of laboratory tests is essential to help determine, if possible, the etiology of the renal failure and the management of the patient as uremia develops.

Table 6-1
Urinary Indices to Differentiate Cause of Acute Renal Failure

	Pre-Renal Azotemia	Acute Tubular Necrosis
Uosm (mOsm/L)	> 500	< 350
U/P creatinine	> 40	< 20
U_{Na} (mEq/L)	< 20	> 40
FE_{Na} (%)	< 1	> 1

Table 6-2
Essential Tests to Obtain in Evaluating Chronic Renal Failure

Initial Evaluation
  BUN, creatinine
  BUN/creatinine ratio
  24-hour measurement of urinary creatinine and protein (to evaluate protein
    excretion and calculate creatinine clearance)
  Urine sediment examination
  Serum electrolytes, calcium, phosphorus values
  Complete blood count
  Intravenous pyelogram or renal ultrasound examination (to evaluate renal
    size and shape and to exclude obstruction)
  Others where indicated, such as serologic studies
Follow-Up Studies
  BUN, creatinine
  Creatinine clearance
  Hematocrit
  Serum electrolytes, calcium, phosphorus values
  Others where indicated

Initial Evaluation
During the initial assessment of a patient with a chronic elevation in BUN
(> 30–40 mg/dL) and creatinine (> 2 mg/dL), information as to etiology can
be obtained by a careful history and physical examination. Next, examine
the BUN/creatinine ratio, kidney size, urinary protein excretion, creatinine
clearance, urine sediment, and electrolytes—all of which should be obtained
as part of the primary workup (Table 6-2). The BUN/creatinine ratio is usually
elevated (> 30–40/L) both in prerenal azotemia and in renal failure due to
obstruction. Kidney size is frequently small in chronic renal failure, by the
time creatinine level reaches 2–4 mg/dL, except in cases due to obstruction,
polycystic kidney disease, multiple myeloma, amyloidosis, and diabetes
mellitus where the kidneys remain normal to large as renal failure progresses. Measurement of the 24-hour protein excretion, obtained with concomitant measurement of creatinine excretion, can be very useful in
distinguishing renal diseases primarily affecting the glomeruli, such as
chronic glomerulonephritis, from those primarily damaging the tubulointerstitial area, such as chronic interstitial nephritis. Glomerular diseases include
all types of glomerulonephritis, malignant hypertension, and diabetic glomerulosclerosis. Chronic interstitial diseases include chronic interstitial
nephritis, polycystic kidney disease, obstructive or reflux nephropathy, and
most forms of congenital nephropathy. In chronic glomerular diseases,
urinary protein excretion is frequently greater than 2–4 g per day, whereas
in the chronic interstitial diseases, urinary protein excretion is either negligible or < 1.5 g per day. Determination of the creatinine clearance as a
measure of glomerular filtration rate is important in establishing the degree
of renal impairment. Because of the relationship between serum creatinine
level and creatinine clearance, significant decreases in creatinine clearance
cause only minor changes in the serum concentration early in renal failure,
whereas small decrements in creatinine clearance cause much more
dramatic increases in the serum creatinine as renal failure progresses.
Therefore evaluation of the creatinine clearance should be an essential part
of the initial assessment. Examination of the urinary sediment for signs of
glomerulonephritis (red cells and red cell casts) or infection (white cells or
white cell casts) is also important, although many causes of chronic renal
failure produce nonspecific changes in the sediment. It is generally accepted, although not well demonstrated, that defects in tubular function
which cause impairments in acid and postassium excretion occur early in the
course of interstitial renal disease. Thus, the finding of a high serum
potassium or low bicarbonate level in the initial electrolytes can be a clue to
the presence of interstitial rather than glomerular disease causing the renal
impairment. A serum calcium and phosphorus value should also be obtained
to exclude hypercalcemia as a cause of renal failure and to establish baseline
levels to follow subsequently.

After the initial tests, you must then decide whether other tests are indicated to establish an etiology for the renal failure. In every patient with newly
diagnosed renal failure, obstruction must be excluded since this can be a reversible process. An intravenous pyelogram, which can also outline kidney
size and shape and the anatomy of the collecting system, is frequently performed for this purpose. In patients whose risk of dye-induced acute renal

failure is greater than normal (patients with significant renal failure, multiple myeloma, or diabetes mellitus), a renal ultrasound examination is usually sufficient to rule out obstruction. If obstruction is excluded, other laboratory tests, such as serologic evaluation in a patient with suspected collagen vascular disease or a voiding cystogram in a patient with suspected reflux, should be ordered as indicated. The indication for a renal biopsy to establish the diagnosis should be made on an individual basis. This procedure is frequently contraindicated in chronic renal failure because of the small kidney size.

Follow-up Laboratory Tests

As renal failure progresses, anemia develops as well as defects in calcium, phosphorus, and electrolyte homeostasis. Therefore, in addition to following serial creatinine clearances (every 6–12 months especially if serum creatinine level is < 3 mg/dL) or serial changes in the BUN and creatinine levels, it is also important to follow the hematocrit, calcium, phosphorus, and electrolyte levels. In early renal failure (creatinine < 3.0 mg/dL), these values can be checked every 4–6 months, but should be obtained more frequently as renal failure progresses so that specific therapy can be initiated. Clinically apparent phosphorus retention does not usually occur until the creatinine clearance drops below 30 mL/min so that the finding of a serum phosphorus of > 5.0 mg/dL can be a clue that the GFR has dropped below this value. Patients with creatinine clearances below 25–30 mL/min should be seen by a nephrologist to initiate appropriate plans for future dialysis or renal transplantation.

Nephrotic Syndrome

Nephrotic syndrome is characterized by a urinary protein excretion of > 3.5–4.0 g per day in association with hypoalbuminemia, edema, hyperlipidemia, and hyperlipiduria. Many patients can have proteinuria in the nephrotic range (> 3.5 g per day = nephrosis) without the other manifestations of the syndrome; the significance of this finding is the same. Although the degree of proteinuria is greater in patients with the complete syndrome, neither etiology nor prognosis is determined by its presence. In patients with nephrosis, the protein lost is mainly albumin. This produces a positive protein dipstick test and positive sulfasalicylic acid test for protein on the initial screening procedure. Abnormal protein excretion which is not albumin can occur in patients with multiple myeloma who excrete light chains of immunoglobulin in their urine. In these patients, the dipstick test, which measures albumin, will be negative, whereas the sulfasalicylic acid test, which detects all protein, is positive. When in doubt as to the nature of the proteinuria, a urine protein electrophoresis should be performed.

For the remainder of this section on nephrosis, we will use the terms albuminuria and proteinuria interchangeably. Heavy albuminuria (> 3.5–4 g per day) is the hallmark of glomerular kidney disease; it is rarely associated with tubulointerstitial disease. Causes of proteinuria are categorized into those primarily affecting the kidney and those occurring as a result of a systemic disease (Table 6-3). The following laboratory studies should be obtained in all patients with heavy proteinuria.

Table 6-3
Major Causes of Nephrosis (> 3.5 g proteinuria per day)

Primary Renal Disease	Renal Disease Secondary to Systemic Disease

1. Lipoid nephrosis
2. Membranous glomerulopathy
3. Proliferative glomerulonephritis
   a. Mesangiocapillary glomerulonephritis
   b. Proliferative glomerulonephritis
4. Focal and segmental glomerulopathy
	1. Systemic diseases—diabetes mellitus, systemic lupus, erythematosis, amyloidosis
	2. Infection—malaria, endocarditis, syphilis, hepatitis B
	3. Mechanical—renal vein thrombosis, right-sided heart failure
	4. Toxin—heavy metals, anti-seizure medications, nonsteroidal antiinflammatory agents
	5. Tumors—lymphoproliferative, solid tumor

Initial Evaluation

The initial evaluation is aimed at determining the amount and establishing the etiology of the proteinuria. In quantitating proteinuria, it is usually wise to obtain at least two 24-hour urine collections for protein and creatinine, since one collection may be incomplete and since daily protein excretion can vary by several grams in the same patient. Determination of creatinine clearance with the same urine collection can be performed if a serum creatinine level is obtained either during or at the end of the collection period. Heavy proteinuria in association with a decrease in GFR, unexplainable by volume contraction, makes more benign forms of nephrosis, such as lipid nephrosis, less likely.

It is extremely important to examine the urinary sediment in a patient with nephrosis. Hematuria and red cell casts are much more common in proliferative glomerulopathies compared with other glomerular diseases causing nephrosis. Oval fat bodies and lipid-laden macrophages, which are visualized as "Maltese crosses" under a polarizing lens, can be seen in the urine in patients with heavy proteinuria. These findings are very nonspecific, however, and do not provide clues to the etiology of the nephrosis. Serum levels of creatinine, albumin, and cholesterol and BUN should be measured to assess the degree of renal function and protein loss. Blood glucose determinations and careful ophthalmologic examination should be performed to exclude diabetes mellitus, which is the most common cause of nephrosis in adults. Electrolyte values help provide a clue to the patient's intravascular volume status. A mild metabolic alkalosis is frequently seen in patients with a low intravascular volume due to low oncotic pressure from urinary protein losses. Serum complement levels (total hemolytic complement, C3, and C4) are frequently depressed in patients with nephrosis due to mesangiocapillary glomerulonephritis. They can also be low in patients with lupus erythematosis and other glomerular diseases associated with immune complex formation. Since a patient with systemic lupus erythematosis rarely has nephrotic syndrome alone, it is probably not necessary to perform a battery of serologic tests for lupus in each patient with nephrosis, although this is frequently done. Decisions regarding additional laboratory tests, such as VDRL, hepatitis B surface antigen, or lip or rectal biopsies for amyloidosis, depend on the index of suspicion for a particular etiology.

An intravenous pyelogram is not an integral part of the workup for nephrosis. It is mainly useful for identifying structural abnormalities and obstruction, neither of which causes nephrosis. In practice, most patients with nephrosis will undergo a renal biopsy to verify the etiology for both prognostic and therapeutic reasons.

Follow-up Laboratory Tests

After the initial diagnosis is established, with relative or absolute certainty depending on whether a biopsy is performed, urinary protein excretion can be followed by simple dipstick testing as a rough guide. Patients receiving specific therapy, such as prednisone for lipoid nephrosis, should be trained to test their own urine to determine when remission or subsequent relapse has occurred. Serum creatinine, albumin, BUN, and, less frequently, creatinine clearance and daily protein excretion should also be determined at regular intervals. The frequency with which these studies are obtained depends on the underlying disease and the clinician's knowledge of how rapidly it leads to renal failure. If patients with severe nephrosis require diuretic therapy to control edema, serum electrolytes, BUN, and creatinine should be followed more closely, since many nephrotic patients are sensitive to the volume-depleting effects of diuretics.

Acute Glomerulonephritis

Patients with acute glomerulonephritis frequently have a sudden onset of edema, hypertension, and, in older patients, congestive heart failure. There may also be associated symptoms of fever, malaise, and arthralgias. These symptoms frequently, but not always, appear after an upper respiratory tract infection, especially in children. In most patients with acute glomerulonephritis, the edema formation results not from massive proteinuria, but from an acute decrease in the glomerular filtration rate which leads to sodium retention. The key to the diagnosis can be found in the examination of the urinary sediment where red cells, red cell casts, and white cells are frequently seen. Acute glomerulonephritis frequently follows certain infections, such as streptococcal infection, or it is found in association with vasculitis. However, acute glomerulonephritis can also occur as an isolated event. In patients with suspected glomerulonephritis, the following studies should be obtained.

Initial Evaluation

The diagnosis of glomerulonephritis is considered in a patient with an "active" urine sediment (red cells, white cells, and red cell casts). In suspected cases, it is important to examine the urine sediment on several occasions since red cell casts, which are pathognomonic of this entity, are frequently not seen on cursory examination. The best way to find red cell casts is to examine the urine sediment from a first morning specimen, when the urine is most concentrated, and to examine it within one to two hours of voiding since these casts dissolve with time. Daily protein excretion and creatinine clearance should be determined along with blood tests for BUN, creatinine, total protein and albumin, electrolytes, and complete blood counts. A chest x-ray may show evidence of vasculitis such as Wegner's granulomatosis. Throat cultures and serologic tests for recent exposure to streptococcal antigen should be obtained to determine the possibility of poststreptococcal glomerulonephritis. Serum complement levels must also be evaluated since a depression in C3 and C4 occurs commonly in postinfectious glomerulonephritis, lupus nephritis, and mesangiocapillary glomerulonephritis. Blood tests for serologic evidence of lupus erythematosis, hepatitis B surface antigen, and cryoglobulins are frequently obtained in an effort to find an etiology for the glomerulonephritis. In children with obvious poststreptococcal glomerulonephritis, the diagnosis can be made with appropriate serologic data. For adults in whom poststreptococcal glomerulonephritis is less common, it is frequently necessary to perform a kidney biopsy to define the actual type of glomerulonephritis.

Follow-up Laboratory Tests
All patients with glomerulonephritis should be followed regularly with periodic measurements of serum creatinine, albumin, and BUN and determinations of creatinine clearance with daily protein excretion. Initial serologic tests should be repeated to evaluate changes in titers. Patients with specific systemic diseases such as lupus erythematosis or vasculitis should have the activity of the disease monitored with the appropriate laboratory tests.

Acute Interstitial Nephritis

Acute interstitial nephritis is characterized by acute renal failure, often secondary to an allergic reaction in the kidney to certain drugs. It has been described in patients receiving diuretics such as furosemide and thiazides, antibiotics, especially penicillins and sulfa drugs, allopurinol, and prostaglandin inhibitors such as indomethacin. The usual interval between onset of drug exposure and symptoms is 5–25 days, after which the patient has fever, skin rash (in about 50% of cases), arthralgias (in 10% to 30% of cases), and acute renal failure. The diagnosis should be suspected in any patient with acute renal failure who is taking a drug in one of the above categories. In such patients, the following laboratory studies should be obtained.

Initial Evaluation
Blood tests for BUN and creatinine levels are obtained to estimate the degree of renal failure. Urine sediment should be examined for the presence of hematuria (present in 70% to 90% of cases) or pyuria (present in almost all cases and sometimes consisting largely of eosinophils). Since this is a tubulointerstitial disease, the 24-hour protein excretion may be greater than normal, but is usually, although not always, < 2 g per day. Serum electrolyte values should be examined for the presence of hyperkalemia or acidosis, since defects in potassium and acid excretion are commonly found in this disease, even when the renal failure is not severe. A complete blood count with differential is performed since peripheral eosinophils are increased ($> 700/\mu L$) in 60% to 100% of cases. If the diagnosis is not clear after these initial studies and/or if renal function does not improve with cessation of the offending agent, a renal biopsy should be considered.

Follow-up Laboratory Tests
Patients with acute interstitial nephritis are followed at regular intervals with serum BUN and serum creatinine levels and creatinine clearance to determine the course of their renal function. Complete or partial recovery is the rule, but patients should be followed closely until it is clear that their renal function is stable.

Hematuria

Bleeding from the urinary tract can produce gross or microscopic hematuria, the latter being visible only by dipstick testing or by examination of the urine sediment under the microscope. Remember that urine can also be dipstick positive for heme pigment in the presence of either free hemoglobin or free myoglobin pigment. Leading causes of true hematuria are divided into those which produce bleeding within the kidney and include diseases such as glomerular or interstitial renal disease, renal cystic disease, malignancy, necrosis of renal tissue as in papillary necrosis, traumatic injury, and vascular malfunctions. Hematuria can also be caused by bleeding into the urinary collecting system from stones, infection, malignancy, traumatic injury, or inflammation such as cystitis. In almost all patients being evaluated for hematuria, the following laboratory studies should be pursued.

Initial Evaluation
Perhaps the most important test is an examination of the urinary sediment searching for red cell casts or evidence for infection. The finding of red cell casts suggests a glomerular origin for the hematuria and spares the patient an unnecessary workup of the lower genitourinary tract. Similarly, in patients with an infected urinary sediment, but without other features such as unilateral flank pain, the hematuria can be reevaluated after treatment for the infection is completed. Further workup may not be required. In all patients with hematuria, a urine culture should be obtained since bacteria may not be obvious in a sediment loaded with red blood cells. In the absence of red cell casts or bacteria on the initial urinalysis, protein excretion should be quantitated and creatinine clearance should be determined on the same collection. Significant proteinuria provides evidence for glomerular pathology and makes lower urinary tract disease a less likely cause for the bleeding. Pertinent blood studies should include a complete blood count, platelet count, coagulation parameters, serum BUN, and creatinine level. If glomerulonephritis is suspected, a serum complement profile and appropriate serologies (as described above) should be obtained. Black patients should also be screened for sickle cell trait, since papillary necrosis is a common cause for hematuria in this population.

An abdominal x-ray should be obtained to look for stones or calcium deposits in the kidneys (nephrocalcinosis) and to evaluate kidney size and shape. This is an important part of the initial workup even if flank pain is not present, since renal stones can produce painless hematuria. In most patients, an intravenous pyelogram is also obtained to determine the presence of obstruction, stones, cysts, malignancy, papillary necrosis, or abnormalities in the collecting system which may explain the hematuria. In the absence of flank pain, this study need not be performed as an emergency, but can be scheduled electively, subject to cancellation if heavy proteinuria is found in the 24-hour urine collection. If the diagnosis is not obvious from the above noninvasive tests, cystoscopy should be performed in adult patients to diagnose bladder tumor, ulceration, or other anatomic abnormalities. If no pathology is observed on cystoscopy or if evidence for glomerular disease is found in the initial workup, the clinician may want to consider a renal biopsy to define possible glomerular pathology, for both prognostic and therapeutic reasons. Lastly, if there is no evidence for glomerular disease, even on renal biopsy, a renal arteriogram is performed looking for unusual causes of hematuria such as A-V malformations. The order in which these studies are pursued is not fixed, and it should be based on the signs and symptoms of the patient. If the patient has painless hematuria and no clues on initial history or physical exam, the sequence of testing could proceed as outlined above, going from the least to the most invasive studies.

Follow-up Laboratory Tests

Repeated urinalysis for red blood cells is the least expensive and easiest way to determine when the problem has resolved. In a patient with persistent hematuria, the hematocrit should be followed, although the amount of blood lost through the genitourinary tract is usually small. Additional follow-up studies might include periodic determinations of creatinine clearance in a patient with intrinsic renal disease, or repeat abdominal x-ray in a patient passing a renal stone.

■ Selected Readings

General Review

Brenner B, et al: Diseases of the kidney and urinary tract, in Isselbacher KJ, Adams RD, Braunwald E, et al: *Harrison's Principles of Internal Medicine.* ed 9. New York, McGraw-Hill Book Co, 1980, pp 283–1333.

Renal Tubular Dysfunction

Buckalew VM, Moore MA: *Renal Tubular Dysfunction.* Garden City, NY, Medical Examination Publishing Co, Inc, 1980.

Hematuria

Hendler ED, Kashgarian M, Hayslett J: Clinicopathological correlations of primary hematuria. *Lancet* 1972;I:458–463.

Acute Renal Failure

Espinel CH, Gregory AW: Differential diagnosis of acute renal failure. *Clin Nephrol* 1980;13:73–77.

Miller T, Anderson RJ, Linas SL, et al: Urinary diagnostic indices in acute renal failure. *Ann Intern Med* 1978;89:47–50.

Acute Allergic Interstitial Nephritis

Linton AL, Clark WF, Driedger AA, et al: Acute interstitial nephritis due to drugs. *Ann Intern Med* 1980;93:735–741.

Cholesterol and Triglycerides

Before obtaining serum cholesterol and triglyceride levels in clinical practice, one must first consider whether an elevated cholesterol or triglyceride value is associated with the presence or development of atherosclerosis. Such an association has been found for serum cholesterol. In several studies from different populations, the incidence and prevalence of atherosclerotic coronary artery disease are directly related to the serum cholesterol level. Furthermore, the presence of an elevated cholesterol level is correlated with an increased likelihood of developing coronary artery disease in the future. Experimental studies in animals also support the role of cholesterol in atherogenesis. However, the relationship between triglyceride level and atherosclerosis is less clear. Not all prospective studies have demonstrated a relationship. Furthermore, triglyceride deposition in atheromatous plaques is not particularly excessive. Although the risk of developing atherosclerosis is definitely related to serum cholesterol, its relation to triglyceride level is much less well established.

One should next consider whether lowering an elevated cholesterol level is beneficial. Unfortunately, benefit has not been clearly demonstrated. Data obtained by the Coronary Drug Project Research Group demonstrated that lowering of cholesterol with clofibrate was not associated with a decrease in five-year mortality. A European cooperative trial demonstrated that lowering of cholesterol with clofibrate was associated with a 25% reduction in nonfatal myocardial infarction, although clofibrate administration was associated with an increase in overall mortality rate. Several other studies have failed to show the efficacy of lipid-lowering diets in preventing or treating ischemic heart disease. Thus, it remains to be demonstrated whether lowering cholesterol or triglyceride levels is associated with an inhibition or regression of atherosclerosis.

Since definitive evidence demonstrating the efficacy of lowering serum lipid levels does not exist, one cannot recommend obtaining cholesterol and triglyceride levels as a routine for all patients. Rather, we recommend obtaining values of these lipids in patients with other risk factors for developing atherosclerotic vascular disease or in patients who have already developed evidence of atherosclerosis. Furthermore, we modify this recommendation after considering the patient's age. The Framingham study demonstrated that the relative risk for coronary artery disease associated with an elevated cholesterol level is 5.5 and 5.0, respectively, for men and women under 45, but only 1.7 and 1.3, respectively, for men and women over 54. Thus, I find lipid level determinations to be less useful in the elderly patient. Before deciding

7

The Laboratory in Cardiovascular Diseases

David L. Rutlen
Charles K. Francis

111

if your patient's cholesterol level is "normal" or "abnormal" you must adjust the criteria of "normal" for age (Table 7-1).

Consideration must be given to what conditions should be maintained at the time of serum lipid determinations. Patients should maintain ambulation and a balanced diet for at least 2 weeks, and they should fast for 14 hours before testing. Determinations should not be performed in the presence of an acute illness. In particular, cholesterol may be significantly depressed after an acute myocardial infarction.

Lipoprotein electrophoresis is no longer recommended for most patients. Phenotyping can be determined on the basis of cholesterol and triglyceride levels and whether the plasma supernatant is creamy, indicating the presence of chylomicrons. Electrophoretic phenotyping provides no additional information as to risk of heart disease.

Cardiac Enzymes

Creatine phosphokinase (CPK), serum glutamic-oxalacetic transaminase (SGOT), and lactic dehydrogenase (LDH) levels are the three serum enzyme concentrations usually ascertained to determine whether a patient has had an acute myocardial infarction. For a patient with an acute infarction, CPK is usually elevated within six to eight hours, peaks at a level 2 to 10 times normal within 24 hours, and returns to a normal level within three to four days. The normal CPK value for men is approximately 1.5 times the normal value for women. SGOT is usually elevated within 8 to 12 hours of myocardial infarction, peaks at a level 2 to 10 times normal within 18 to 36 hours, and returns to normal within three to four days. LDH is usually elevated within 24 to 48 hours, peaks at a level 2 to 10 times normal within three to six days, and returns to normal within 8 to 14 days. Determinations should be performed every 8 to 12 hours for 48 hours after a patient has experienced what is thought to be a myocardial infarction. If all values are normal after 48 hours, the physician can safely exclude the diagnosis of acute infarction. Indeed, the sensitivity for each of the tests alone is in excess of 90%. Of greater concern is the possibility that enzyme levels may be elevated in the absence of acute infarction. CPK may be elevated in association with muscular dystrophy, myositis, diabetes mellitus, intramuscular injections, irradiation of the heart, myocarditis, pulmonary embolism, electrical cardioversion, severe exercise, skeletal muscle trauma, hypothermia, malignant hyperpyrexia, and Reye's syndrome. SGOT may be elevated in association with hepatic congestion due to right ventricular dysfunction, myocarditis, skeletal muscle trauma, liver disease, pulmonary embolism, electrical cardioversion, oral contraceptive use, and myositis. LDH may be elevated in association with hepatic congestion due to right ventricular dysfunction, myocarditis, electrical cardioversion, muscle trauma, Reye's syndrome, myxedema, severe exercise, renal infarction, pulmonary embolism, hemolysis, megaloblastic anemia, anemia due to ineffective erythropoiesis, neoplastic disease, and liver disease. Enzyme elevations can be reasonably attributed to acute myocardial infarction only if these conditions are absent.

For more specific assessment of cardiac enzyme release, many laboratories now perform isoenzyme determinations. Only myocardial tissue has significant amounts of CPK-MB. If CPK-MB is greater than 4% of total CPK, myo-

Table 7-1
"Normal" Values for Serum Cholesterol and
Fasting Triglyceride Levels on a Western Diet

Age (yr)	Chol (mg/dL ± SD)	Triglyceride (mg/dL ± SD)
0–19	170 ± 30	60 ± 35
20–29	180 ± 40	70 ± 30
30–39	210 ± 35	80 ± 40
40–49	230 ± 55	90 ± 40
50–59	240 ± 50	100 ± 50

cardial injury has usually occurred. CPK-MB peaks slightly earlier and disappears slightly more rapidly than total CPK. A reasonable correlation exists between peak CPK-MB and the extent of acute myocardial infarction. LDH may also be fractionated. LDH 1 > LDH 2 has been found to be a very specific indicator of infarction. Thus, fractionation of CPK or LDH may be helpful if other conditions are present which might elevate total CPK or LDH.

Most of the drugs used in the management of patients with cardiovascular diseases are potentially toxic. Measurements of serum concentrations of these drugs are widely available and, when used appropriately, can be helpful (see Chapter 4).

Hypertension

Hypertension remains one of the most significant risk factors for the development of cardiovascular disease, specifically congestive heart failure, coronary disease, and stroke, as well as renal failure. Since approximately 90% of hypertensive patients have primary or essential hypertension (high blood pressure with no demonstrable etiology), it is seldom necessary to undertake an exhaustive and expensive search for secondary causes of hypertension. Rather, a careful clinical and laboratory assessment of hematologic, renal, metabolic, and vascular status should be performed. In evaluating the hypertensive patient, the objectives of the laboratory procedures are to assess any organ damage, exclude possible secondary causes of hypertension, and establish baseline laboratory data. These baseline measurements should be established to assess the extent and severity of systemic involvement and to provide a basis for comparison with future alterations of laboratory values. Measurement of specific baseline parameters are crucial, particularly when patients are first seen, and they should be assessed serially throughout therapy. Initial therapeutic choices should be based upon objective assessment of current physiologic functioning, and future decisions should be aimed at specific therapeutic and functional goals. An outline of the minimum laboratory evaluation of a patient with high blood pressure is given in Table 7-2.

Hematologic Testing
A complete blood count is the minimum laboratory evaluation of hematologic status. Simple measurement of hemoglobin, hematocrit, white

114

Table 7-2
Minimum Laboratory Evaluation of Patient with
High Blood Pressure

Test	Reason for Test
I. Hematologic	
A. Complete blood count	General hematologic status
Hemoglobin	Anemia
Hematocrit	Plasma and red cell change
White cell count	Drug side effect
Coombs test	Drug side effect
II. Renal	
A. Blood urea nitrogen	Plasma volume change, renal disease
B. Creatinine	Parenchymal renal disease
C. Urine analysis	General renal status
Specific gravity	Plasma volume, renal concentration
pH	Drug effect
Glucose	Diabetes mellitus, drug effect
Red cells	Glomerular function
White cells	Urinary tract infection
Casts	Renal tubular function
Crystals	Kidney stone formation
III. Metabolic	
A. Blood glucose	Diabetes mellitus, drug effect
B. Electrolytes	Renal status, drug effect
Sodium	Plasma volume, drug effect
Potassium	Adrenal tumor
Chloride	Drug effect
Bicarbonate	Metabolic status
C. Uric acid	Kidney stone formation
IV. Cardiovascular Risk Assessment	
A. Lipids	Cardiovascular risk
Cholesterol	Coronary disease risk
B. Electrocardiogram	Coronary disease risk
C. Echocardiogram	Cardiac hypertrophy or dilatation
D. Chest x-ray	Lung disease, cardiac enlargement
V. Special Studies for Secondary Causes of Hypertension	

blood cell count, and differential will provide fundamental baseline information. Since hematologic side effects of drug therapy are common, careful monitoring of hematologic status allows early detection of drug-related abnormalities, including anemia, leukopenia, hemolysis, and toxic changes. Hematocrit may indicate a diuretic-induced change in plasma volume, since the hematocrit increases as intravascular volume decreases. Alpha methyl dopa has been associated with Coombs-positive hemolytic anemia which is dose related and subsides with cessation of therapy. Preexisting anemia, perhaps due to gastrointestinal blood loss or previous medications, should be established before beginning therapy. A clue to secondary causes of hypertension may also be derived from basic hematologic studies. Polycythemia sometimes occurs in adrenal forms of hypertension, including primary hyperaldosteronism, pheochromocytoma, and Cushing's disease. A low red cell count can be a marker for chronic renal failure, which is sometimes drug related.

Renal Status

Assessment of renal function with standard laboratory determinations may provide information helpful in establishing the etiology of hypertension, estimating the degree and extent of renal involvement, and detecting drug effects. The simple urinalysis, including dipstick measurement of protein, glucose, and bilirubin as well as measurement of specific gravity, pH, and microscopic examination may be surprisingly informative. Glycosuria in the hypertensive patient may suggest the need for more extensive investigation. Diabetic nephropathy or simple glucose intolerance with low renal threshold for glucose may be an early clue to diabetic glomerular disease. The loss of significant amounts of protein in the urine may have even greater importance for abnormal glomerular functioning. When abnormal amounts of protein and/or glucose in the urine are found, they should be quantitated with 24-hour urine collections, and more sophisticated tests of renal function should be done. Microscopic examination of the urinary sediment which reveals pyuria suggests urinary tract infection or tuberculosis, whereas red cells or casts suggest glomerulonephritis. Occasionally microscopic examination reveals uric acid or oxylate crystals, providing a clue to renal lithiasis. This is particularly important in patients receiving those diuretics which may increase uric acid excretion and increase the likelihood of stone formation. Blood urea nitrogen (BUN) and serum creatinine determinations are the most important biochemical tests of renal function. The BUN may be abnormally elevated in prerenal as well as renal disease and therefore may also reflect spontaneous or diuretic-related changes in intravascular volume. BUN determination, along with estimates of volume provided by hematocrit and urine specific gravity, may help in following shifts in plasma volume during diuretic therapy. The creatinine level, however, more accurately reflects intrinsic renal dysfunction and should be determined when patients are first seen and periodically during treatment with antihypertensive medication. Elevations in serum creatinine suggest the need for estimates of creatinine clearance and quantification of 24-hour creatinine excretion.

Serum Electrolytes

The electrolytes sodium, potassium, chloride, and bicarbonate should be measured in all hypertensive patients. Perhaps the most significant measurement is the serum potassium. Hypokalemia occurring in the absence of diuretic therapy is considered a hallmark of primary hyperaldosteronism. Low serum potassium may occur with other mineralocorticoid-producing tumors, but is not found uniformly in all patients with tumors. Extensive chronic licorice ingestion is a less common cause of low serum potassium, but does not cause hypertension. When abnormally low potassium levels (less than 3.5 mEq/L) are detected, 24-hour urinary excretion should be measured. When urinary excretion is high with simultaneous low serum potassium levels, more sophisticated tests for mineralocorticoid-producing tumors should be considered. The definitive diagnosis of adrenal tumors is made by computerized tomographic scanning, renal arteriography, and measurement of plasma and/or renal vein renin activity. Hypokalemia in patients with diuretic therapy has little pathologic implication, since potassium loss is a common side effect of many diuretics. With the growing use of drugs causing potassium retention, additional concern arises for the potential for drug-induced hyperkalemia. Because excess as well as deficient potassium may lead to dangerous cardiac arrhythmias, monitoring of serum potassium intermittently is necessary throughout antihypertension therapy. This is particularly important for patients receiving digitalis preparations in whom hypokalemia may lead to digitalis toxicity.

Serum sodium determinations also provide important etiologic and therapeutic information. Since sodium intake is directly related to potassium loss, a careful assessment of both is crucial. Salt intake has been related to the prevalence of hypertension, but does not directly determine serum sodium. The kidneys have the prime role in the management of salt and water excretion. Rarely, a salt-losing nephropathy may lead to hyponatremia, but generally hypertension is not a major component of salt-losing renal disease. Excess loss of free water as well as sodium may occur with diuretic therapy. Excessive sodium loss should be watched for, particularly in elderly patients. Rarely, significant dehydration may ensue. The serum sodium measurement provides additional data regarding alterations in volume status as well as renal function.

Serum Glucose
The measurement of serum glucose is valuable in the detection of occult diabetes with associated diabetic nephropathy and hypertension. In patients with known diabetes, the blood sugar is the prime marker for effective therapy. In the patient initially diagnosed as hypertensive who later becomes diabetic, clear delineation of the relative roles of diabetes and hypertension is important. This may require glucose tolerance testing or more sophisticated tests of renal function, such as creatinine clearance determinations. In the usual hypertensive patient without preexisting glucose intolerance, a simple random serum glucose determination may be helpful. If necessary, a 2-hour postprandial and/or a fasting serum glucose determination may provide more reproducible and valid assessments. Since the thiazide group of diuretics can increase blood sugar in susceptible patients, blood glucose determination should be performed before instituting diuretic therapy. If baseline measurements of blood glucose are abnormally elevated, confirmation of a true diabetic state may be aided by a glucose tolerance test before consideration of alternative types of antihypertensive treatment. With a wide choice of nonthiazide diuretics, selection of an agent not likely to raise blood sugar may be preferable.

Renovascular Hypertension

The renin angiotensin system may be deranged in renovascular hypertension and is also probably a major factor in the pathogenesis of essential hypertension. The use of renin profiling has been suggested as a valuable tool in the assessment of most hypertensive patients, particularly those suspected of having renovascular hypertension. Plasma renin activity may be clinically measured, but requires that patients be on a known intake of dietary sodium, be in an upright position for some time, and be volume depleted, usually with diuretic therapy. Because of the overlap of normal and abnormal plasma renin levels in large populations of patients with primary hypertension, the use of routine renin determinations has not been of significant benefit. Renin profiling is not indicated in the routine management of the patient with uncomplicated essential hypertension. Where secondary hypertension is extremely likely, more invasive procedures, such as renal vein renin determinations, computerized tomography, and arteriography may be more reliable in defining the precise etiology of hypertension. A useful screening test has recently been developed in which an infusion of a converting enzyme inhibitor is administered intravenously and the patient's blood pressure is monitored. Since these agents interfere with the conversion of renin to angiotensin II, a potent vasoconstrictor, patients with excessive stimulation of the renin angiotensin system due to renovascular or other forms of hypertension, should experience a fall in blood pressure. No major fall in blood pressure in response to the drug should be experienced by those patients in whom the renal angiotensin system is not a major contributor to the hypertension. This test might prove useful in identifying patients in whom more invasive measurements of the renin angiotensin system and renovascular function may be of more diagnostic value.

An additional consideration is the search for evidence of increased cardiovascular risk, since hypertension exerts its greatest detrimental effects in the pathogenesis of diseases of the heart and blood vessels. In addition to the standard evaluation of blood and urine, a chest x-ray and electrocardiogram should be obtained. Echocardiographic assessment, providing the most accurate measurement of wall thickness and chamber dimensions, may also be desirable. In patients refractory to standard therapy or in whom clinical evidence strongly points to nonprimary causes of hypertension, special studies may be considered. The rapid-sequence intravenous pyelogram may help in the diagnosis of both renal parenchymal and renovascular causes of hypertension. Other tests helpful in excluding obscure causes of hypertension include aortography with selective renal angiography, computerized tomography, and urinary or plasma aldosterone, catecholamine, or corticoid levels. In evaluating hypertensive patients who are unresponsive to appropriate medical therapy, careful attention to the role of side effects and compliance with the pharmacologic regime is crucial.

Cardiomyopathy

Whereas imaging techniques are of special help in assessing cardiomyopathy, studies of the serum and urine may be of additional benefit. A restrictive cardiomyopathy must be considered in the presence of heart failure and a normal-sized heart. Since amyloidosis is a common cause of restrictive cardiomyopathy, serum and urine protein electrophoresis and immunoelectrophoresis should be obtained in patients for whom the diagnosis of restrictive cardiomyopathy is being considered. If amyloidosis is primary, an M-component will often be identified; if amyloidosis is due to multiple myeloma, an M-component will almost always be identified. If heart failure occurs in the presence of an enlarged heart, a dilated cardiomyopathy must be considered. If the cause of the dilated cardiomyopathy is not apparent after history taking, physical examination, and electrocardiographic recording, then serum potassium, calcium, phosphate, iron, and iron-binding capacity should be determined, since a dilated cardiomyopathy may be due to hypokalemia, hypocalcemia, hypophosphatemia, or hemochromatosis.

■ Selected Readings

Ahumada G, Roberts R, Sobel BE: Evaluation of myocardial infarction with enzymatic indices. *Prog Cardiovasc Dis* 1976;18:405.

Burke MD: Cholesterol, triglyceride, and lipoprotein studies: strategies for clinical use. *Postgrad Med* 1980;67:263.

Canner PL, Forman SA, Prud'homme GJ, et al: Influence of adherence to treatment and response of cholesterol on mortality in the coronary drug project. *N Engl J Med* 1980;303:1038.

Hulley SB, Rosenman RH, Bawol RD, et al: Epidemiology as a guide to clinical decisions: The association between triglyceride and coronary heart disease. *N Engl J Med* 1980;302:1383.

Inkeles S, Eisenberg D: Hyperlipidemia and coronary atherosclerosis: A review. *Medicine (Baltimore)* 1981;60:110.

Kannel WB, Castelli WP, Gordon T, et al: Serum cholesterol, lipoproteins, and the risk of coronary heart disease. *Ann Intern Med* 1971;74:1.

Lott JA, Stang JM: Serum enzymes and isoenzymes in the diagnosis and differential diagnosis of myocardial ischemia and necrosis. *Clin Chem* 1980;26:1241.

Oliver MF, Geizerova H, Gyarfas I, et al: Co-operative trial in primary prevention of ischaemic heart disease using clofibrate. *Br Heart J* 1979;41:363.

Sobel BE, Shell WE: Serum enzyme determinations in the diagnosis and assessment of myocardial infarction. *Circulation* 1972;45:471.

Roentgenographic Examination of the Chest

The laboratory evaluation of the patient with signs or symptoms of pulmonary disease almost invariably begins with a chest roentgenograph. The presence of pulmonary disease generally is accompanied by abnormalities that are evident in the chest roentgenograph. Careful correlation of the roentgenographic abnormalities with the clinical picture will frequently allow the practitioner to arrive at a presumptive diagnosis with reasonable certainty, thereby allowing him or her to be more selective in the subsequent tests ordered in the workup of a particular patient. A complete discussion on the interpretation of the chest roentgenograph is beyond the scope of this chapter; a number of excellent texts have been written about this important area of clinical medicine. This section will focus on the different roentgenological tests available, describing the usefulness and limitations of these studies.

Plain Film

The plain film of the chest is the fundamental roentgenographic examination upon which all subsequent techniques build. Routinely two views, a *posterior-anterior* (PA) and a *lateral* projection, are obtained. While a single PA roentgenograph is an adequate screening procedure in a young (less than 40 years) asymptomatic individual, older individuals or those suspected of harboring intrathoracic disease should have both a PA and a lateral chest roentgenograph. The PA view, shot with the x-ray tube behind the patient and the beam projected through the patient from posterior to anterior, is preferable to an anterior-posterior (AP) view, since in the PA projection the heart is close to the film cassette (which is adjacent to the anterior thoracic wall), thereby minimizing its magnification and creating a sharper image. Generally the film is taken in an upright position in full inspiration (at total lung capacity) to maximize the contrast between air within the lung and intrathoracic lesions which are usually of water density. However, when an air-containing lesion, eg, a pneumothorax, is suspected, an *expiratory* film should be obtained; the crowding together of the vascular structures during expiration increases the density of the lung, thereby enhancing the contrast between the pulmonary parenchyma and air in the pleural space.

The lateral view is helpful in interpreting lesions that are visualized on the PA film, providing a three-dimensional view of the thorax and thereby allowing one to localize the lesion to a particular portion of the lung or mediastinum. It can confirm the presence of collapse of a particular bronchopulmonary segment or lobe, a frequent sign of endobronchial carcinoma. In addition, certain areas of the lung are normally difficult to

8

The Laboratory in Pulmonary Diseases

Gary T. Kinasewitz

119

visualize on a PA projection. Lesions behind the heart, in the mediastinum, or below the dome of the diaphragm which are frequently obscured by overlying structures on the PA film will be readily apparent on the lateral view.

Portable chest roentgenographs can be obtained in the seriously ill patient who cannot be moved to the radiology department without hazard. Although these films may provide much clinically useful information, technical factors dictate that caution be used in their interpretation. The portable x-ray unit is not as powerful as the unit in the radiology suite, necessitating longer exposure times and an increased likelihood of movement artifact. It is difficult to properly position the patient in a hospital bed, and the distance between the x-ray tube and the patient may vary between studies; consequently the cardiac silhoutte may appear different on consecutive films when in fact there has been no change in the patient's status. Despite these limitations the portable chest roentgenograph is a valuable aid in the management of the critically ill patient. The proper placement of endotracheal tubes and pulmonary arterial or central venous catheters should be confirmed by observing their position on a portable film. The presence of a previously unsuspected pneumothorax, the volume loss and localized density indicative of atelectasis, and the diffuse alveolar infiltrate characteristic of pulmonary edema are all readily apparent on the portable chest film.

The position of the patient, upright or supine, will change the appearance of various structures within the thorax. In the *recumbent* position the contents of the abdomen tend to displace the diaphragm higher in the chest so that the amount of air in the lungs is less than in the upright film. Unless the clinician recognizes that the film was taken with the patient in the recumbent position, a normal recumbent chest film might easily be misinterpreted as evidence of congestive heart failure. The volume of blood in the pulmonary capillaries is increased because venous return to the heart is facilitated in the recumbent position. In addition, the normal predominance of flow to the lung bases due to the effect of gravity is altered in the supine patient so that pulmonary blood flow is evenly distributed throughout all of the lung zones. The heart is further from the x-ray film so that its magnification is increased in a recumbent film; the combination of these physiological and technical factors creates the "pseudofailure" pattern typical of a recumbent chest film.

Intrathoracic fluid is easily recognized by the presence of an air fluid level on an upright chest film, but is difficult to appreciate if the patient is supine and the fluid is evenly layered over the posterior pleural space. Portable films in particular are rarely obtained with the patient completely erect; often the seriously ill patient is positioned with the head of the bed only partially raised. The resultant "upright" portable chest film would probably be better described as a "semirecumbent" film since small collections of fluid may still be layered out and the x-ray beam will not pass perpendicularly through the air-fluid interface.

Additional information about the nature and localization of intrathoracic abnormalities can be obtained through special techniques. In a *lateral decubitus film,* ie, one taken with the patient on his side, any free pleural fluid present will fall to the dependent side and be more readily visualized as an air-fluid interface abutting the chest wall. This technique is particularly useful in demonstrating small pleural effusions; less than 100 mL of pleural fluid will be evident on a decubitus film, whereas 200–300 mL of fluid may not be apparent on an upright chest film. The extent of a lung cavity or the presence of a freely moveable structure, eg, a mycetoma, within a cavity can also be demonstrated with this technique. In addition, the shifting of free fluid away from the lower lobe may allow one to visualize a parenchymal abnormality which was previously obscured by the overlying effusion.

Oblique views are useful in studying lesions that are visible on one of the routine views, but not on the other. Some of these shadows represent soft tissue abnormalities that can be detected by a careful examination of the chest wall. Frequently, however, the interparenchymal location of a lesion that is visible on only the PA or lateral roentgenograph can be ascertained by observing the rotation of the density in relation to the adjacent structures. Two objects that are in close anatomic proximity will rotate in the same direction on an oblique view, eg, a coin lesion in the anterior portion of the chest will move in the same direction as the anterior ribs, but in the opposite direction from the spine, a posterior structure. *Apical lordotic* views are useful in evaluating potential lesions in the apex of the lung. The normal overlap of shadows from the ribs, clavicle, and soft tissues in this region can sometimes make the interpretation of densities in this region difficult. To obtain an apical lordotic view the x-ray beam is angled 15° cephalad so that clearer visualization of the apices, superior mediastinum, and thoracic inlet can be obtained. Although this technique is useful in confirming the presence of disease in the apices, tomography is a better technique for studying this region.

Tomography

Tomography provides a detailed view of a particular layer of tissue. The x-ray tube and film are both reciprocally rotated about the patient so that only a thin layer of tissue is continuously in focus whereas the structures above or below this plane are blurred. The principal indication for tomography is to obtain a more detailed view of a lesion, particularly one that is obscured by superimposed images. It is an invaluable tool in studying the apices of the lungs, revealing previously unsuspected cavitary disease in some patients and in others showing that the apparent cavities on routine chest films are artifacts. Calcium can be identified in solitary pulmonary nodules; some patterns of calcification are pathognomonic of benign diseases, eg, the popcorn calcification of a hamartoma. The identification of this type of calcification spares the patient further invasive diagnostic procedures. Indistinct shadows can be clearly defined, the walls of cavities can be delineated, and the presence of satellite lesions, too small to be visualized on a conventional roentgenogram, can be discerned. The ability of tomography to discriminate fine detail when contiguous densities are superimposed is particularly helpful in evaluating the suspicious hilum. Oblique tomograms of this region are best for determining whether a prominent hilar shadow represents enlargement of the pulmonary vasculature or hilar adenopathy. Similarly, lesions in the mediastinum are often indistinct because of the contiguous soft tissue and require tomography to delineate their border.

Fluoroscopy

Fluoroscopy was once used as a routine screening procedure for intra-thoracic disease. However, fluoroscopic images are of poor quality when compared with the routine chest roentgenograph, and fluoroscopy cannot be advocated as a screening tool. Fluoroscopy is useful as an adjunct to the above static techniques; information about the dynamic activity of the structures within the chest can be obtained by observing them throughout a respiratory cycle. Diaphragmatic paralysis can be ascertained by observing paradoxical movement of one dome during a sniff test. An intrathoracic lesion which is pulsatile most likely is of vascular origin.

Contrast Studies

Contrast studies can be performed using radiodense dyes, eg, barium, to delineate the structures within the chest. The barium esophagram is a simple and inexpensive method to obtain information about mediastinal lesions. Displacement and/or invasion of the esophagus will indicate the location of a mediastinal mass and suggest potential etiologies. Bronchography has been largely replaced by fiberoptic bronchoscopy, which generally provides more information at less risk to the patient. The major indication for bron-chography at the present time is to localize bronchiectatic segments of the lung in the rare patient in whom surgical resection is contemplated.

Pulmonary angiography, the opacification of the pulmonary vasculature with water-soluble contrast media, is most commonly employed to evaluate the patient with a suspected pulmonary embolism. The visualization of an intraluminal filling defect or the abrupt cutoff of a pulmonary artery is diagnostic of an embolus; failure to demonstrate either of these abnormal-ities on a well-performed angiogram virtually excludes the diagnosis of pulmonary embolism. Not all patients suspected of having a pulmonary embolism require arteriography; in the proper clinical setting a perfusion lung scan with multiple segmental or lobar defects has an 80% to 90% likelihood of representing a pulmonary embolus; the diagnosis may be considered secure. However, those patients (1) with indeterminant lung scans, (2) in whom anticoagulant therapy is contraindicated, (3) in whom thrombolytic therapy is indicated, and (4) in whom surgical intervention, eg, caval inter-ruption, is contemplated should have the diagnosis of pulmonary embolism definitely established with a pulmonary arteriogram. Pulmonary arteri-ography is also indicated in the diagnostic workup of the patient with a suspect pulmonary arteriovenous (A-V) malformation, both to establish the diagnosis and to visualize additional unsuspected A-V malformations since in one-third of such patients there are multiple lesions, some of which may not be suspected on the plain chest roentgenogram.

Lung Scans

Radionuclide lung imaging is performed with a gamma camera that detects the intrapulmonary distribution of radioactive tracer administered either in-travenously (perfusion scan) or via inhalation (ventilation scan). When heat-treated macroaggregated human albumin labeled with technetium-99m is injected intravenously, the particles are distributed throughout the lung in proportion to regional pulmonary blood flow. The interruption of blood flow to an area of the lung by an embolus will produce a cold spot since none of the tracer is delivered beyond the occluded pulmonary artery. A normal perfusion lung scan effectively rules out the possibility of a pulmonary embolus. A defect on perfusion scanning may be due to an embolus, but other diseases can also produce regional abnormalities in pulmonary perfusion. It is important that a chest roentgenograph be obtained at the time of lung scanning, since perfusion may be decreased in areas with parenchymal infiltrates or pleural effusions. Asthma and chronic obstructive lung disease alter the regional distribution of ventilation and may produce secondary decreases in pulmonary blood flow to the poorly ventilated regions of the lung. If one performs a ventilation scan in such a patient, the region of decreased ventilation is usually greater than the area of decreased perfusion, a pattern indicating a low probability of pulmonary embolism; only 10% to 15% of patients with a low-probability ventilation-perfusion lung scan who are clinically suspected of having an embolus will have a positive arteriogram. On the other hand, if a segmental or lobar perfusion defect is larger than the defect on the ventilation lung scan, this represents a high-probability scan with a 85% to 90% likelihood of being caused by a pulmonary embolus. When the perfusion defect is approximately equal in size to the area of infiltrate on a chest x-ray or defect on a ventilation scan, this is an indeterminant ventilation-perfusion scan, which will be associated with a pulmonary embolus in approximately one-third of the patients. All patients with an indeterminant ventilation-perfusion scan should have pulmonary angiography to establish a definitive diagnosis.

Ultrasound of the Thorax
The inability of the ultrasound beam to penetrate the air-containing lung restricts the usefulness of ultrasound to delineating pulmonary lesions adjacent to the chest wall. The primary indication for thoracic ultrasound is to identify small loculated pleural effusions; frequently pleural fluid can be aspirated under ultrasonic guidance when blind attempts at thoracentesis are unsuccessful. In addition, the diaphragm can be easily visualized, and subdiaphragmatic disease, eg, abscess, can be identified.

Computerized Axial Tomography (CT)
The role of CT in the diagnosis of pulmonary disease is still being defined. Highly accurate cross-sectional slices of the thorax are produced in which differences in the density of adjacent structures can be more clearly delineated than by conventional techniques. It has already proven valuable in examining the mediastinum since many of its structures are normally outlined by fat. By precisely determining tissue density, CT scans can accurately identify a large number of benign fatty mediastinal lesions including lipomas, pericardial fat pads, and areas of focal or diffuse fat deposition, thereby sparing the patient a more invasive diagnostic procedure. Although CT scanning has proved helpful in demonstrating direct mediastinal invasion by lung cancer, oblique tomography remains the preferred technique for evaluation of the hilar lymph nodes. An aneurysm may be suspected when a mediastinal lesion is enhanced after the injection of contract media, but angiography is still required for diagnosis and to identify the site of intimal rupture. Although CT scanning is more sensitive than routine tomography for detecting parenchymal nodules in a patient with known malignancy,

many of the additional nodules discovered are benign. Therefore the main indication for CT scanning to detect metastatic disease is in the patient scheduled for resectional surgery whose primary tumor frequently metastasizes to the lung or in patients in whom resection of a "solitary" pulmonary metastasis is contemplated.

CT scanning also clearly delineates chest wall structures, allowing us to differentiate pleural from parenchymal disease and to recognize chest wall invasion by infectious or neoplastic lesions.

Pulmonary Function Tests

Pulmonary function tests are important in assessing the degree of functional impairment present in a patient with lung disease. Although the nature and extent of the disease process may be suggested by the chest roentgenograph, the correlation between the radiographic abnormalities and the severity of the functional impairment in a given patient is poor. Pulmonary function tests, on the other hand, provide an objective measure of the type and severity of the functional impairment, allow us to follow the course of the lung disease, and evaluate the response to therapy.

A variety of pulmonary function tests are available. Virtually all hospitals have a spirometer and a gas volume recorder; much useful information can be derived from the spirometry, the simplest of all tests. Other tests, eg, the determination of functional residual capacity, require more sophisticated equipment which is available in the typical well-equipped clinical pulmonary function laboratory. The patient's results are generally reported with a set of predicted values. The predicted values are derived from a large number of tests in healthy persons free of lung disease; comparing the patient's performance to the predicted value allows one to account for the normal variation in pulmonary function which occurs among patients of different body size, age, and sex.

The primary function of the respiratory system is the exchange of oxygen, necessary for aerobic metabolism, and carbon dioxide across the alveolar-capillary membrane. To accomplish this aim, mechanical work is performed as air moves in and out of the lungs each minute. Pulmonary function tests may be conveniently grouped into those that measure the mechanical properties of the lungs and those that evaluate the exchange of gas across the alveolar-capillary membrane.

Pulmonary Mechanics

Lung Volumes The quantity of gas contained within the lungs is subdivided into four primary lung volumes (Figure 8-1). Combinations of two or more of these primary lung volumes make up the four lung capacities.

The *tidal volume* (V_T) is the volume of air which enters and leaves the lungs during normal breathing. The *inspiratory capacity* (IC) is the maximal volume of air which may be inhaled from a normal resting level. The IC is composed of two lung volumes, the V_T and the *inspiratory reserve volume* (IRV).

The volume of gas within the lung at the end of a normal expiration is the *functional residual capacity* (FRC). Since the respiratory muscles are at rest

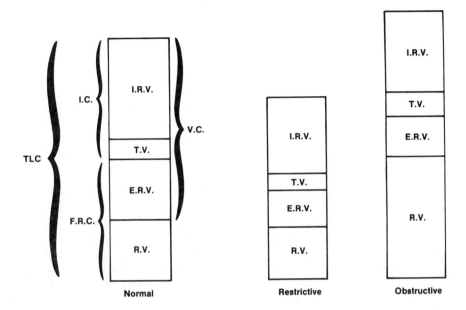

Figure 8-1 The four primary lung volumes; the four capacities are composed of combinations of two or more lung volumes. In restrictive lung disease both the VC and the TLC are reduced. In obstructive lung disease FRC and TLC may be increased because of the increased RV; the VC will be reduced if air trapping is severe.

at the end of a normal expiration, FRC is determined by the opposing recoil forces of the lung and chest wall. In a patient with a complete pneumothorax, the lung collapses and the chest wall expands; FRC is the lung volume at which the tendency of the lung to collapse is counterbalanced by the tendency of the chest wall to expand. The FRC is composed of two primary lung volumes, the *expiratory reserve volume* (ERV) and the *residual volume* (RV). The ERV is the maximal amount of gas than can be exhaled beginning from the end of a quiet expiration when the lung is at FRC. The RV is the volume of gas remaining in the lung after a maximal expiratory effort. *Total lung capacity* (TLC) is the volume of air in the lungs after a maximal inspiration, ie, the sum of all four primary lung volumes. The *vital capacity* (VC) is the maximal amount of air that can be exhaled after a maximal inspiration. While the VC and its subdivisions, V_T, IRV, and ERV, can be directly measured with a spirometer, the RV and those lung capacities which include the RV, ie, FRC and TLC, must be determined indirectly. In most pulmonary function laboratories, the FRC is measured indirectly, and RV is calculated by subtracting the ERV from the FRC.

Three techniques are commonly employed to determine the FRC. Two, the *closed-circuit helium dilution* technique and *open-circuit nitrogen washout* method, rely on the use of a tracer to measure FRC. In principle a known volume of gas with a known concentration of tracer gas is placed in communication with an unknown lung volume. After equilibration between the two compartments the final tracer concentration is measured, and by simple proportional calculation the final volume (V_f), which is the sum of both the known and unknown volumes, may be calculated as:

$$V_f = V_i \times C_i/C_f \tag{1}$$

where V_i is the initial volume and C_i and C_f are the initial and final concentrations of the tracer, respectively. In the closed-circuit helium dilution technique, beginning at end expiration (FRC), the subject breathes from a spirometer with a known volume of gas containing 10% helium. Since helium is inert and does not cross the alveolar-capillary membrane, the volume of helium within the system remains constant. After equilibration has occurred the total volume of the closed circuit, ie, the lungs and spirometer, is calculated from equation 1, and FRC is determined by subtracting the initial volume of the spirometer from that of the entire closed circuit. The open-circuit nitrogen washout technique utilizes the nitrogen present in the lung at FRC as the tracer substance. Again beginning at end expiration, the subject breathes 100% oxygen, and all of the expired gas is collected as the nitrogen is "washed out" of the lungs. The initial concentration of nitrogen in alveolar gas can be estimated, and, since all of the nitrogen in the expired air came from the lungs, when the volume and nitrogen concentration of the expired gas are measured, the initial volume of the nitrogen (FRC) can be determined by proportional calculation analogous to that used in the helium dilution method.

TLC is determined by the ability of the inspiratory muscles to expand the lungs and chest wall. Similarly, in a person free of airway disease, the RV of the lungs is determined by force which the expiratory muscles exert in compressing the chest wall, "squeezing" air from the lungs. A reduction in both the VC and the TLC is the hallmark of those disorders which produce a restrictive impairment. Infiltrative pulmonary disease, eg, pulmonary fibrosis, reduces the distensibility of the lung; the TLC and VC are therefore decreased in these disorders, primarily because of a reduction of the IC. In the massively obese person, the compliance of the chest wall is reduced, and the diaphragm is displaced high into the thorax by the abdominal contents. Both the TLC and the VC are reduced in massive obesity, primarily because of a reduction in the ERV. Other nonpulmonary conditions which may produce a pattern of restrictive impairment include skeletal deformities, ascites, pleural effusions, and pregnancy. Finally, disorders which decrease the strength of the respiratory muscles, eg, myasthenia gravis, will also reduce the amount of air which can be inspired (IC) and expired (ERV) from functional residual capacity, creating a restrictive pulmonary impairment.

In obstructive lung disease the airways are narrowed and lose some of the peribronchial support which maintains their patency. During expiration premature airway closure may occur, trapping air behind the occluded bronchioles and increasing the RV of the lung. This loss of elastic structural tissue, if widespread, may increase the distensibility of the lung, and both FRC and TLC may actually be elevated in obstructive lung disease. Nonetheless, the VC is normal or frequently reduced, typically when the air trapping and increase in residual volume are marked.

Airflow   The dynamic aspects of pulmonary function are measured by monitoring the rate of airflow from the lungs during a forceful expiration from TLC to RV. The volume of air expelled during this *forced vital capacity* (FVC) maneuver should be similar to that expired during a slow VC maneuver. However, some patients with obstructive lung disease increase their RV due to premature airway closure and air trapping during a forced expiration, and the FVC may be less than the slow VC in these individuals.

The forced expiratory spirogram is produced by having the patient inhale to TLC and then, as forcefully as possible, exhale to RV while the results are graphically recorded as a function of time (Figure 8-2). Airflow (change in volume per unit time) is usually reported as the volume exhaled over particular time intervals or over particular segments of the FVC. The *forced expired volumes* (FEVs) are measured at one-half ($FEV_{0.5}$), one (FEV_1), and three (FEV_3) seconds after the start of expiration; these timed volumes are usually expressed as absolute volumes and as percentage of the FVC, eg, the $FEV_1/FVC\%$. In addition the *forced midexpiratory flow rate* (FEF_{25-75}) is the

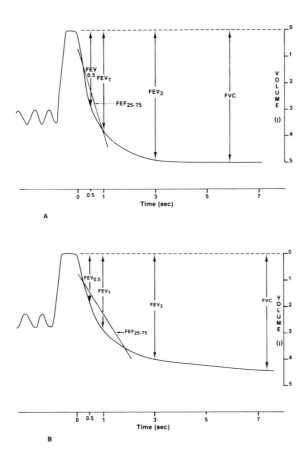

Figure 8-2 **A,** A normal forced-expiratory spirogram with the $FEV_{0.5}$, FEV_1, FEV_3, FVC, and FEF_{25-75} indicated; expiration is almost complete after three seconds. **B,** Forced expiratory spirogram in obstructive lung disease; the expiratory flow rates are lower than normal, and significant airflow is still occurring at seven seconds.

flow rate between 25% and 75% of the FVC. The FEF between 200 and 1200 mL of expired volume ($FEF_{200-1200}$) is a measure of airflow at large lung volumes.

It is important to remember that expiratory airflow over most of the VC is determined by two factors, the elastic recoil pressure of the lung and the diameter of the airways. As the length of a rubber band is progressively increased, more and more force is required per change in unit length; releasing the band at maximal stretch generates considerably more force than would be obtained if it were released when it was partially stretched. Similarly, as the volume of air within the lung increases during inspiration, progressively more negative pleural pressures must be developed by the inspiratory muscles to counterbalance the increasing elastic recoil pressure of the lung. Although airflow during the first 25% of the FVC may be influenced by the patient's effort, after this initial, effort-dependent portion of the FVC, it is the elastic recoil pressure of the lung which is the driving pressure for expiratory airflow. In addition, at high lung volumes the increased elastic recoil pressure of the lung expands and tethers the airways open. Since resistance is proportional to the fourth power of the radius, it is obvious that the resistance of the airways is decreased at high lung volumes.

This influence of lung volume on airflow can be more easily appreciated if the expiratory airflow during the FVC maneuver is plotted as a function of the volume of gas within the lungs, a maximal expiratory *flow-volume curve* (Figure 8-3). In normal persons, after the initial rapid increase in airflow at the onset of expiration, there is a gradual decline in airflow as both airway diameter and elastic recoil pressure of the lungs decrease with falling lung volumes. Obstructive airway disease is characterized by narrowing of the airways and frequently a decrease in the elastic recoil pressure of the lung. The increased TLC frequently observed in obstructive disease has the compensatory effect of increasing both airway size and the elastic recoil of the lung. Nonetheless, at any given lung volume, expiratory airflow is subnormal. In restrictive lung disease, although the absolute values for expiratory airflow may be decreased, when lung volume is considered, airflow is normal or even supranormal.

Since airflow during the initial phase of a FVC maneuver is dependent on expiratory effort, the $FEF_{200-1200}$ which is measured early during expiration may be disproportionately reduced in comparison with the other flow rates in the poorly motivated patient. On the other hand, the FEV_1, FEV_3, and FEF_{25-75} are all measured over large lung volumes, and therefore they will be relatively less influenced by a suboptimal effort. These latter tests are reliable indices of airflow obstruction. In addition to measuring expiratory airflow, it is also possible to determine the resistance of the airways.

The major sites of increased airway resistance can be identified by comparing expiratory flow volume curves breathing air and a *helium-oxygen mixture* that is less dense than air. In normal persons the major sites of airway resistance are in the large central airways where airflow is turbulent and density dependent. Breathing a helium-oxygen mixture will increase expiratory airflow at all but the lowest lung volumes. Those patients who have a significant portion of their airway obstruction in the small peripheral airways of the lung, where flow is laminar and independent of density, will have a much smaller change in airflow at 50% of the vital capacity (V_{max} 50)

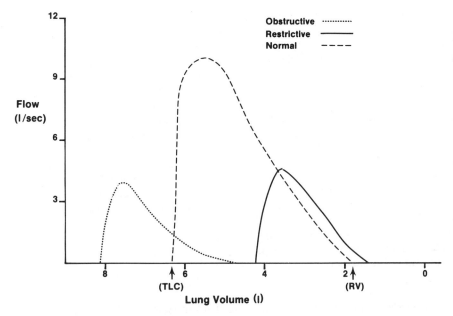

Figure 8-3 Maximal expiratory flow as a function of lung volume. Even though the volume of air in the lungs is greater than normal in obstructive disease, expiratory airflow is clearly reduced. In restrictive lung disease the low level of expiratory airflow is due to the reduced lung volume.

while breathing the helium-oxygen mixture. This test may become particularly valuable if selective pharmacological manipulation of the large and small airways becomes practical.

Diseases which produce airway obstruction, eg, asthma and chronic bronchitis, will reduce expiratory airflow in proportion to the severity of the disorder. Early or mild obstructive disease may only reduce the FEV_3 and FEF_{25-75} since these measurements include airflow at low lung volumes where the airway narrowing will have a greater effect. All the indices of expiratory airflow will fall below normal with progressively worsening obstruction. It is important when airway obstruction is detected on spirometry to administer a bronchodilator to determine whether the obstruction is reversible. A standard dose of a beta-adrenergic agonist, typically 0.5 mL of isoproterenol, is administered via a nebulizer, and the spirometry is repeated in 20 minutes when the bronchodilator response should be maximal. An improvement in FEV_1 and/or FVC of 15% or greater is considered a significant response, indicating the presence of at least partially reversible airway obstruction. In restrictive lung disorders such as pulmonary fibrosis, because the vital capacity is reduced, the FEV_1 and FEV_3 may be correspondingly decreased. Yet when the FEV_1 and FEV_3 are expressed as a percentage of the FVC, eg, $FEV_1/FVC\%$, normal or increased values will be obtained.

Inspiratory flow rates are usually not helpful in evaluating patients with pulmonary disease since inspiratory flow in most individuals is totally effort dependent. The commonest cause of a reduced maximal inspiratory flow rate is poor patient effort. Reduced inspiratory flow is also seen in patients with weakness due to neuromuscular disease, eg, myasthenia gravis, or extrathoracic airway obstruction, eg, tracheomalacia. In the latter condition, as the pressure within the trachea becomes subatmospheric during inspiration the airway is compressed by the surrounding (atmospheric) pressure, thereby reducing inspiratory flow. The *flow-volume loop* (in which inspiratory and expiratory airflow are plotted as a function of lung volume) is an important diagnostic aid. Expiratory flow may be completely normal in such cases, whereas inspiratory flow will plateau at a low rate.

The *maximal voluntary ventilation* (MVV), formerly termed the maximal breathing capacity (MBC), is another test of dynamic lung function that is highly effort dependent. The patient is instructed to breathe as hard and as fast as possible for 12 seconds, and ventilation in liters per minute is calculated. While abnormal results (MVV < 80% of predicted) are common in patients with obstructive lung disease, persons with poor strength, coordination, or motivation frequently have an abnormal MVV. In contrast the MVV is fairly well preserved in patients with pure restrictive lung disease unless their impairment is severe.

Other Tests The strength of the respiratory muscles can be tested by having the patient perform a maximal inspiratory and expiratory maneuver against a manometer or pressure gauge. These measurements are routinely included in the pulmonary function evaluation of some laboratories, whereas in others respiratory muscle testing must be specifically requested. Respiratory muscle testing is clinically indicated in all patients with neuromuscular disorders and those with an otherwise unexplained decrease in their lung volumes.

The distensibility of the lung can be quantitated by the measurement of lung compliance, ie, the change in lung volume produced by a change in pleural pressure. *Static compliance* (C_{stat}) is measured during breath holding at various lung volumes in the absence of airflow. In the acutely ill patient on a mechanical ventilator the compliance of the respiratory system (ie, the lungs and chest wall) is easily measured and can provide useful information. Since the mechanical properties of the chest wall are unlikely to change in a given patient, once baseline measurements are obtained, subsequent changes in compliance will reflect alterations in the airways and/or lungs. Most ventilators provide measurements of both airway pressure and tidal volume. Dynamic compliance at a given tidal volume can be determined from the difference between peak airway pressure and end-expiratory pressure (which is zero or atmospheric in the absence of positive end-expiratory pressure). If the expiratory line is briefly occluded at the end of inspiration, airway pressure will plateau at a value slightly less than the peak pressure; the difference between this plateau pressure and end-expiratory pressure is the pressure required to maintain the tidal volume under static conditions. Decreases in both static and dynamic compliance occur with infiltrative lung diseases, eg, pulmonary edema, and with complications of mechanical ventilation such as atelectasis, pneumothorax, and bronchial intubation. Retained secretions and bronchoconstriction of the airways, on the other hand, will decrease the dynamic compliance but not affect the static compliance.

Inhomogeneity in the distribution of ventilation (and the closing volume) can be determined via the *single breath nitrogen washout* test. After exhaling to residual volume the subject inhales 100% oxygen to total lung capacity, and the nitrogen concentration of the expired gas is continuously monitored during the ensuing exhalation to RV (Figure 8-4). The initial portion of the washout is from the anatomic dead space and contains no nitrogen (phase 1). Then, as alveolar gas begins to appear, the concentration of nitrogen rapidly rises (phase II) to a plateau. If gas enters and leaves all regions of the lung synchronously, this plateau phase (phase III) will be relatively flat, ie, the nitrogen concentration will change by less than 2.5%. However, if the distribution of ventilation is nonuniform, gas from different regions will have different nitrogen concentrations, and the expired nitrogen concentration will rise during this phase. If airway closure occurs at low lung volumes, there will be an abrupt increase in the expired nitrogen concentration (phase IV). The volume above RV at which this terminal increase in slope occurs is termed the *closing volume*. An increased closing volume is almost invariably found in those patients with chronic bronchitis and emphysema who have decreased expiratory flow rates. Many cigarette smokers will have increased closing volumes even when their spirometry is normal. In addition to airway disease however, loss of elastic recoil which occurs with aging will also increase the closing volume. Thus the demonstration of

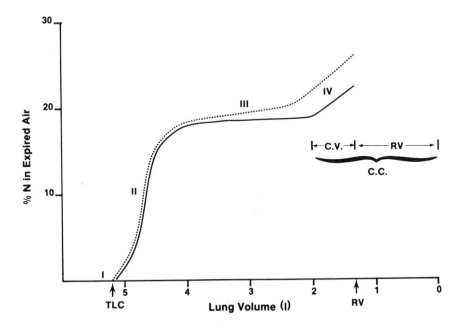

Figure 8-4   The single breath nitrogen test of a normal subject (solid line) and a patient with a small airway disease (dashed line). In the patient with airway disease the nitrogen concentration of expired air rises more steeply during the plateau phase (III), and the abrupt increase in nitrogen concentration indicating airway closure (phase IV) occurs at a higher lung volume. Abbreviations: CV, closing volume; CC, closing capacity (CV + RV).

an abnormal closing volume is nonspecific, and the potential usefulness of the closing volume test is undetermined at present.

Gas Exchange

Diffusion   The movement of oxygen in alveolar gas across the alveolar-capillary membrane into the blood and the exchange of carbon dioxide in the reverse direction occur by diffusion. Carbon dioxide is so much more soluble than O_2 that its transfer, even in severe lung disease, is relatively unaffected by an impairment in pulmonary gas diffusion. The *diffusing capacity* of the lung (D_L) is defined as the volume of gas which enters the blood per minute per millimeter of Hg partial pressure difference of the gas between alveolar air and pulmonary capillary blood. Carbon monoxide is the gas used to determine the diffusing capacity of the lung (D_{LCO}) since it is easy to measure and its diffusing characteristics are similar to those of oxygen.

The barriers which CO in alveolar gas must cross to combine with the hemoglobin in pulmonary capillary blood include the surface lining layer of the alveoli, the alveolar epithelium, interstitium, pulmonary capillary endothelium, plasma, and the red cell membrane. In essence the diffusing capacity is determined by the number of functioning alveoli in contact with red blood cells. If the number of functioning alveolar-capillary units is reduced by pneumonectomy, the D_{LCO} will be proportionately reduced. Yet when the diffusing capacity per liter alveolar volume is calculated (D_L/V_A), it will be normal, indicating that the remaining alveolar-capillary units are normal. Similarly, if the hemoglobin concentration of the pulmonary capillary blood is reduced due to anemia, the D_{LCO} will be reduced even though the alveolar capillary membrane is normal. In diseases that destroy the alveolar septa, eg, emphysema, and those which obliterate the pulmonary capillary bed such as pulmonary emboli, the D_L/V_A is markedly reduced. While increased thickness of the alveolar-capillary membrane can theoretically increase the barrier to diffusion, most of the decreased D_{LCO} observed in pulmonary fibrosis is due to the loss of alveolar volume and fibrotic obliteration of the pulmonary capillary bed.

Disorders which expand the volume of blood in the pulmonary capillaries may actually increase the D_{LCO}. Early congestive heart failure is probably the most common cause of an increased D_{LCO} encountered clinically.

Arterial Blood Gases   The ultimate purpose of the respiratory system is to provide adequate oxygen for the body's needs; the simplest way to determine how well this is accomplished is to measure the PO_2 and PCO_2 of arterial blood. Normally the P_aCO_2 of arterial blood is 40 torr (range 35–45 torr). The normal arterial PO_2 is greater than 90 torr in a young adult at sea level but, due to the increase in ventilation-perfusion mismatching that occurs with aging, the lower limit of normal for the P_aO_2 declines with age, and values of 80 torr are common in healthy 65 year olds. Far more information about the efficiency of arterial oxygenation can be obtained if one calculates the alveolar-arterial oxygen gradient (A-a dO_2). To measure the A-a dO_2 we must first calculate the partial pressure of oxygen in alveolar gas (P_AO_2) by using the simplified ideal alveolar air equation:

$$P_AO_2 = F_IO_2 \times (P_B - 47) - (P_aCO_2/R) \qquad (2)$$

where F_IO_2 is the fraction of oxygen in inspired air (0.209 for room air), P_B is the barometric pressure (760 torr at sea level), P_aCO_2 is the arterial PCO_2, and R is the respiratory exchange ratio (normally 0.8).

The simplified ideal alveolar gas equation is the mathematical expression of the concept that the alveolar pressure ("space") which both O_2 and CO_2 can occupy is limited to that not occupied by water and nitrogen. If one hypoventilates so that the P_aCO_2 rises, the P_AO_2 (and therefore the P_aO_2) must fall if the efficiency of gas exchange and therefore the A-a dO_2 remains constant. Administering supplemental oxygen (increasing the F_IO_2) increases the partial pressure that can be composed of oxygen and CO_2; if alveolar ventilation (and P_aCO_2) remains constant, the P_aO_2 must increase.

Even in normal persons gas exchange is rarely ideal. A small portion ($< 3\%$) of the arterial blood is returned to the left heart never having been exposed to alveolar air (physiologic shunt); a similar fraction, not fully oxygenated, is derived from alveolar-capillary units with low ventilation/perfusion ($\dot{V}/\dot{Q}$) ratios. Consequently, the arterial PO_2 is less than it would be if it all were fully equilibrated with alveolar gas. The A-a dO_2, which is a sensitive index of the efficiency of gas exchange, is normally less than 10 torr in a 20 year old. The normal A-a dO_2 increases with age due to the increase in closing volume and lower $\dot{V}/\dot{Q}$ ratio at the lung bases in older people, so that by age 65 a normal A-a dO_2 may be as much as 20 torr. In patients with abnormalities in gas exchange, whether due to an increase in shunt flow, worsening of $\dot{V}/\dot{Q}$ matching, or diffusion impairment, this difference in oxygen tension between alveolar gas and arterial blood, (A-a dO_2) is increased.

Clinically the A-a dO_2 is extremely useful as an indicator of the severity of respiratory disease and also in following the response to therapy. If alveolar ventilation changes and P_aCO_2 and P_ACO_2 fall, the P_AO_2 must rise and P_aO_2 will increase; determining the A-a dO_2 may enable us to diagnose an abnormality of gas exchange that is not reflected in the P_aO_2. For example, a 40-year-old patient with congestive heart failure may have the following arterial blood gas values: pH 7.50, P_aO_2 88, P_aCO_2 24. Despite the fact that the arterial PO_2 is normal, calculating the A-a dO_2 as $(150 - 24/0.8) - 88 = 32$ torr reveals a significant impairment in gas exchange.

Another patient may be in an obtunded state with the following arterial blood gas values: pH 7.21, PO_2 60, PCO_2 64. Calculation of the A-a dO_2 in this individual, $(150 - 64/0.8) - 60 = 10$ torr, reveals a normal value, indicating that there is no impairment in gas exchange due to intrinsic pulmonary parenchymal disease. The probable etiology of this patient's hypoventilation is depression of his respiratory drive secondary to his obtundation, as might be seen in a drug overdose.

An increase in the arterial PCO_2 (> 45 torr) indicates an inappropriately low level of alveolar ventilation for the patient's metabolic activity. This commonly occurs in patients with severe obstructive lung disease, but may also occur with depression of the central nervous system or neuromuscular disorders which impair the respiratory muscles and reduce the level of alveolar ventilation. An abnormally reduced arterial PCO_2 indicating alveolar hyperventilation occurs as the result of an increased respiratory drive and may be seen in a variety of disorders such as anxiety, fever, acidosis, and infiltrative diseases of the lung, eg, pulmonary fibrosis. The A-a dO_2 should be calculated in all patients with a decreased P_aCO_2 since a significant abnormality in gas exchange may be obscured by a P_aO_2 that is in the normal range due to the hyperventilation.

Arterial hypoxemia can occur for five basic reasons. At high altitudes the atmospheric pressure is decreased so that the P_AO_2 (by the ideal alveolar air equation) must fall. In Denver, where the atmospheric pressure is 690 torr, a P_aO_2 of 70 torr is normal in a 20-year-old person. Alveolar hypoventilation will produce hypoxemia as previously discussed, but again the A-a dO_2 will be normal if the patient is free of intrinsic lung disease. In patients with an abnormal A-a dO_2, hypoxemia may be produced by an increased right-to-left shunt, ventilation-perfusion mismatching, or diffusion impairment.

Most of the arterial hypoxemia associated with a increased A-a dO_2 encountered clinically is due to ventilation-perfusion mismatching. In a normal adult alveolar ventilation is about 4 L/min, and the pulmonary blood flow (cardiac output) is approximately 5 L/min, resulting in an overall $\dot{V}/\dot{Q}$ ratio of 0.8. If each individual alveolar-capillary unit had a $\dot{V}/\dot{Q}$ ratio of 0.8, the matching of ventilation and perfusion would be ideal, and, in the absence of a physiologic shunt, P_aO_2 would equal P_AO_2. However, because of the effects of gravity, relatively more blood than air goes to the bases of lungs; conversely, the ventilation of the apices of the lung is greater than their perfusion. To understand the effect of the variations in $\dot{V}/\dot{Q}$ on the arterial blood gases it is useful to first consider the extreme case of a $\dot{V}/\dot{Q}$ ratio of 0, eg, a totally unventilated but perfused alveolus. Blood coming from the capillary of this alveolus is mixed venous blood, ie, shunt, and since there is no ventilation to the alveolus, the gas within it will be equilibrated with mixed venous blood and have a $P_AO_2 = 40$ and $P_ACO_2 = 46$. If there is a small amount of ventilation relative to perfusion ($\dot{V}/\dot{Q} = 0.01$), the alveolar P_AO_2 will rise minimally while the P_ACO_2 falls only slightly with each tidal breath, and there will be only a minimal change in the gas tensions of the capillary blood from this hypothetical alveolar unit.

The opposite extreme is the alveolus that is ventilated but not perfused ($\dot{V}/\dot{Q} = \infty$), ie, alveolar dead space. The P_AO_2 and P_ACO_2 of this alveolus are 150 and 0, respectively, and any blood present in the pulmonary capillary of this unit will eventually equilibrate with the alveolar gas and have a $P_aO_2 = 150$ and $P_aCO_2 = 0$. If a small amount of perfusion is restored ($\dot{V}/\dot{Q} = 100$), then the amount of oxygen which is removed and the volume of carbon dioxide that is added to the alveolar air are small, and alveolar gas tensions change minimally, so that the P_aO_2 and P_aCO_2 of the small amount of blood which passes through this unit will still be close to those of inspired air.

The effect of an abnormal distribution of $\dot{V}/\dot{Q}$ ratios on the PO_2 and PCO_2 of expired air and arterial blood is illustrated by a hypothetical lung with three alveolar-capillary units characterized by low (1/10), intermediate (10/10), and high (10/1) $\dot{V}/\dot{Q}$ ratios. Expired gas collected in a Douglas bag will contain a total of 21 units of alveolar air; 1 unit from the low $\dot{V}/\dot{Q}$ alveolus will have a low PO_2 and high PCO_2, 10 units from the intermediate $\dot{V}/\dot{Q}$ alveolus will have normal gas tensions, whereas the 10 units from the high $\dot{V}/\dot{Q}$ alveolus will have an increased P_AO_2 and low P_ACO_2, reflecting the wasted ventilation. Arterial blood, on the other hand, will receive 10 of the 21 units of flow from the capillary with the low $\dot{V}/\dot{Q}$ ratio; blood from this alveolar-capillary unit will have a low oxygen content, producing arterial hypoxemia and increasing the A-a dO_2.

Diffusion impairment is rarely the sole cause of hypoxemia. Although a decreased diffusing capacity is common on many of the diffuse infiltrative disease of the lung, eg, pulmonary fibrosis, it is now recognized that the hypoxemia of the "alveolar-capillary block" syndromes is mainly due to $\dot{V}/\dot{Q}$ mismatching rather than to diffusion impairment.

There are two forms of shunt which reduce the oxygenation of arterial blood. The first is the anatomic shunt due to the shunting of blood from the thebesian and bronchial veins, which have no contact with alveoli. The second is the effective shunt caused by the flow of blood through areas that have a low $\dot{V}/\dot{Q}$ ratio. The combination of these two shunts is termed the venous admixture. The venous admixture at any given inspired oxygen concentration can be calculated from the shunt formula:

$$\frac{Q_s}{Q_t} = \frac{C_cO_2 - C_aO_2}{C_cO_2 - C_vO_2} \tag{3}$$

where Q_s is shunt flow, Q_t is total cardiac output, and C_cO_2, C_aO_2, and C_vO_2 are the oxygen content of end-pulmonary capillary blood, arterial blood, and mixed venous blood, respectively. End-pulmonary capillary PO_2 is assumed to be equal to alveolar PO_2 whereas either the mixed venous PO_2 can be measured or an arterial-venous content difference of 5 mL/100 mL is assumed (if the cardiac output is normal).

To understand the effect of an increased venous admixture on arterial blood gases it is important to remember the different shapes of the O_2 and CO_2 dissociation curves in blood. The relatively linear relationship between PCO_2 and CO_2 content in blood means that the content and PCO_2 of arterial blood is essentially the algebraic sum of the content and PCO_2 of pulmonary capillary and shunt blood; even if the venous admixture were to increase drastically, a modest increment in alveolar ventilation will maintain a normal P_aCO_2. The sigmoid shape of the hemoglobin dissociation curve, however, means there is little increase in the oxygen content of pulmonary capillary blood with hyperventilation since hemoglobin is almost completely saturated at a P_aO_2 of 100 torr. Therefore the P_aO_2 of arterial blood must fall as the shunt fraction increases.

When the hypoxemic patient inspires 100% oxygen for 20 minutes, thereby replacing nitrogen with oxygen and increasing the P_AO_2 in poorly ventilated lung units, hypoxemia due to $\dot{V}/\dot{Q}$ mismatching or diffusion impairment will be relieved, whereas hypoxemia due to a true right-to-left shunt, eg, an arteriovenous malformation, will persist. A reasonable approximation of the shunt fraction can be obtained from the P_aO_2 measured after 20 minutes of oxygen breathing using the formula:

$$\% \text{ shunt} \simeq (700 - P_aO_2) \times (5/100) \tag{4}$$

This estimation is relatively accurate for P_aO_2 values greater than 100 torr while breathing 100% oxygen, assuming that the patient's cardiac output is normal.

Other Tests The quantity of oxygen taken up from the alveolar gas by the blood in the pulmonary capillaries each minute is the oxygen consumption ($\dot{V}O_2$); in a normal resting person $\dot{V}O_2$ is about 4 mL/min/kg (standard temperature and pressure, dry [STPD]). Similarly the quantity of CO_2 eliminated in the expired air each minute is the carbon dioxide production

($\dot{V}CO_2$), typically 3.2 mL/min/kg (STPD). The $\dot{V}CO_2$, $\dot{V}O_2$, and respiratory exchange ratio ($\dot{V}CO_2/\dot{V}O_2$) can be determined by collecting expired gas in a bag and measuring the volume of oxygen removed or CO_2 present in the sample.

The expired air we collect in a Douglas bag is composed of air from the gas-exchanging units of the lung, the alveoli, and respiratory bronchioles and air that remains in the trachea and large airways, the anatomic dead space. The volume of gas in these conducting airways is approximately equal to a person's weight in pounds, eg, 150 mL in a 150-lb (68-kg) individual. The portion of inspired air which reaches the gas exchange area of the lung is termed the alveolar ventilation (V_A); in a 150-lb person with a tidal volume of 500 mL, the V_A is (500 − 150 =) 350 mL × the respiratory frequency. In a steady state, the $\dot{V}CO_2$ is the product of the alveolar ventilation, and the concentration of CO_2 is the expired alveolar gas. The concentration of CO_2 in alveolar air (P_ACO_2) is approximately equal to that in arterial blood (P_aCO_2) since CO_2 rapidly diffuses across the alveolar-capillary membrane and the dissociation curve for CO_2 is relatively linear in the physiologic range. (The potential error in such an assumption must be small since the difference between arterial and mixed venous PCO_2 is only a few torr.) Thus it follows that

$$\dot{V}CO_2 \times k = V_A \times P_aCO_2 \qquad (5)$$

where k is a constant (0.863) that converts liters (body temperature and pressure, saturated [BTPS]) to milliliters (STPD). Doubling the alveolar ventilation, eg, voluntary hyperventilation, will reduce the P_aCO_2 by 50% if the $\dot{V}CO_2$ remains constant. Similarly, if $\dot{V}CO_2$ increases because of fever in a patient who is unable to increase V_A, eg, a patient on control mode ventilation, the P_aCO_2 must rise.

Clinically, patients with lung disease and diminished perfusion of alveolar capillaries in some areas of the lung, eg, patients with bullous emphysema, have an increase in functional *dead space* (V_D), which means that to maintain the same level of alveolar ventilation they must increase the total volume of air moving in and out of the lung each minute ($\dot{V}_E$). This increases the work of breathing at any level of $\dot{V}O_2$ and $\dot{V}CO_2$; if the increase in V_D is large, the respiratory muscles will fatigue, and respiratory failure will ensue. However, as long as the patient is able to increase his per minute ventilation sufficiently to compensate for the rise in V_D, V_A and therefore the P_aCO_2 may be normal.

Most of the tests we have discussed measure a specific aspect of pulmonary function, eg, the volume of gas in the lungs at TLC or the oxygenation of arterial blood. Many medical centers now have the capability of assessing the performance of the entire respiratory system during *exercise*. Rapidly responding analyzers provide a breath-by-breath analysis of tidal volume, expiratory airflow, $\dot{V}CO_2$, and $\dot{V}O_2$ as well as cardiac rate for a given level of exercise. Arterial blood gas measurements obtained during exercise may reveal significant desaturation even though the resting P_aO_2 may be normal. The early onset of anaerobic metabolism which is characteristic of cardiac disorders will be detected by observing the disproportionate rise in ventilation and CO_2 production which occurs with the onset of the lactic acidemia. Exercise testing is particularly helpful in determining the etiology of breathlessness in a patient with both cardiac and pulmonary dysfunction. It is also useful in quantitating the degree of functional impairment present in a given patient and evaluating the response to therapy.

The particular pulmonary function tests ordered depend on the status of the patient. Bedside spirometry and arterial blood gases can be obtained in the acutely ill patient; daily studies are often invaluable in guiding therapy. Spirometry should be obtained as part of the routine evaluation of all patients scheduled to undergo major surgery; abnormalities on the spirogram should be thoroughly investigated with lung volume studies and arterial blood gases. The patient who has pulmonary complaints should have a determination of his or her lung volumes, expiratory airflow, diffusing capacity, and arterial blood gases performed as an initial evaluation. This represents the basic battery of tests required for an accurate physiologic assessment of the patient's impairment. Depending on the results of these initial tests further studies to test specific components of the respiratory system, eg, the respiratory muscles, may be indicated.

Clinical Laboratory Tests

The clinical laboratory is an invaluable aid to the physician evaluating a patient with pulmonary disease. The examination of bronchopulmonary secretions and/or pleural fluid will often provide a definitive diagnosis in the patient with pulmonary disease. Less frequently, the unexpected finding of an increased hematocrit or eosinophilia on a routine complete blood cell count may be the first indication of a previously unsuspected pulmonary disorder.

Sputum Examination

A properly collected sputum specimen contains the secretions and exudate from the tracheobronchial tree. The specimen must come from the lung, ie, the material must be sputum rather than saliva. Careful inspection of the collected specimen will usually verify this; if any doubt about the origin of the specimen exists, the physician should observe the patient while another sputum sample is collected. When bacteriological studies are to be obtained, the sputum specimen should be transported to the microbiology laboratory as rapidly as possible after it is obtained. Not only will the results be available sooner, but also, equally as important, the rapid processing of the sample will reduce the possibility of overgrowth by a nonpathogenic bacterial species.

A wealth of clinically useful information can be obtained simply by examining an unstained *wet preparation* of the sputum. A small drop of sputum is placed on the microscope, and the specimen is examined under low power for alveolar macrophages; their presence indicates that it is a true sputum sample from the lung. Conversely, an abundance of squamous cells indicates that the specimen originated from above the larynx and therefore is not true sputum. Eosinophils in a wet preparation of sputum can be readily identified by their bilobular nuclei and large refractile granules; polymorphonuclear leukocytes, on the other hand, have multilobular nuclei and small varigated cytoplasmic granules. (In some clinical laboratories a *Wright's stain* is preferred to distinguish eosinophils from polymorphonuclear leukocytes in sputum.) The presence of eosinophils in sputum, even in the absence of an elevated blood eosinophil count, suggests an allergic etiology for the

138

pulmonary disorder. In addition to eosinophils, the asthmatic patient's sputum frequently contains octahedral Charcot-Leyden crystals, which represent the coalescence of degenerating eosinophilic granules, and Curshmann's spirals, which are mucoid casts of small bronchioles. The presence of lipid-laden macrophages in the sputum may confirm the clinical suspicion of lipoid pneumonia in a patient with a history of mineral oil use or may support the diagnosis of fat embolism in a patient with diffuse lung disease after severe trauma.

A predominance of polymorphonuclear leukocytes in the specimen suggests that the sputum production is due to a bronchopulmonary infection. Further microbiological studies are indicated when the sputum is purulent. A *Gram stain* of the sputum provides a rapid tentative etiological diagnosis. The presence of large numbers of bacteria with a uniform appearance on Gram stain, particularly when they are observed around and within the polymorphonuclear leukocytes, indicates the probable etiology of the pneumonia and should guide the initial antibiotic selection. Neutropenic patients, and occasionally those with overwhelming pneumonia, may demonstrate sheets of organisms, but only a few polymorphonuclear leukocytes since their ability to respond to their pulmonary infection is impaired. Conversely, the presence of scant numbers of organisms with many polymorphonuclear leukocytes may indicate a nonbacterial pneumonia in the patient who has not received prior antibiotic therapy. Serial examination of the sputum is useful in monitoring the changes in bacterial flora which occur with therapy. A patient with pneumococcal pneumonia who is improving clinically may subsequently demonstrate a predominance of gram-negative organisms on smear. This merely indicates that bacteria which were not suppressed by the antibiotic therapy have overgrown and warrants no change in the patient's therapy. However, if after an initial improvement the patient's clinical course deteriorates, a superinfection must be suspected, and his antibiotic therapy should be reevaluated.

Sputum specimens which are to be submitted for culture should be transported to the laboratory as quickly as possible after they are obtained to prevent the overgrowth of nonpathogenic organisms. The predominant organism seen on Gram stain should be considered the pathogen, and an *aerobic sputum culture* should be obtained for identification and antibiotic susceptibility testing. *Anaerobic cultures* of expectorated sputum are valueless because of the likelihood of oropharyngeal contamination. Culture results from expectorated sputum must be intepreted in the context of the initial Gram stain. When the admission sputum Gram stain is loaded with gram-positive cocci and the patient is responding to penicillin, his therapy should not be modified because a few colonies of a gram-negative rod are isolated on sputum culture. *Blood cultures* should be obtained in all patients with pneumonia since any aerobic or anaerobic organism isolated would presumably be the causative agent of the pneumonia. Similarly, if pleural fluid is present in the patient with pneumonia, a specimen should be obtained for Gram stain and both aerobic and anaerobic culture.

Specimens for the demonstration of legionella, mycoplasma, and respiratory viruses require special processing that is generally available only in a sophisticated microbiology laboratory. Serological studies are often the best and most readily available method of diagnosing infection due to these agents. If serum is saved early in the diagnostic evaluation, the demonstration of a subsequent fourfold rise in specific antibody titer is good retrospective evidence that the pneumonia was due to the specific organism. (See Chapter 9 for a discussion of *Mycobacterium tuberculosis*.)

A suspected fungal infection is usually confirmed by the isolation of the organism from the sputum. The sputum should be examined as soon as possible after the specimen is obtained; to identify fungi, smears of sputum can be prepared with a *periodic acid-Schiff (PAS) stain,* Gram stain, and Giemsa stain. Culture techniques for fungi will vary depending on the type of organism suspected, so it is important that the physician indicate to the mycology laboratory his clinical impression of which fungi are potential etiologic agents.

Cytological examination of the sputum is indicated in all patients with suspected malignancy. Spontaneously expectorated or induced sputum specimens can be examined with the Papanicolaou technique, and cell blocks of the sputum sample can be prepared for histological examination. Positive cytological findings diagnostic of malignancy have been observed in up to 80% of patients with centrally located neoplasms. The positive rate is lower in those patients with peripheral lesion and metastatic disease, only 20% to 40% of such cases yielding diagnostic cytologies. False-negative results may be caused by lack of communication between the neoplasm and the bronchial lumen, or by bronchial obstruction. False-positive results are uncommon, generally about 1% in most series.

If properly instructed, most patients can produce an adequate sputum specimen. In the occasional patient who is unable to produce an adequate specimen, sputum can be induced by inhalation of a heated, aerosolized solution of hypertonic saline (10%) with or without propylene glycol. This mildly irritating solution generally induces a cough; in addition, it stimulates the mucus-producing glands of the tracheobronchial tree and increases the volume of pulmonary secretions for up to 24 hours, thereby providing additional material for pathological examination. Sputum induction has replaced gastric lavage as a means of obtaining specimens for mycobacterial culture in patients who are unable to spontaneously produce sputum.

In the comatose or obtunded patient who is unable to expectorate sputum, specimens may be obtained by transtracheal aspiration. To obtain a transtracheal aspirate, the anterior aspect of the neck is cleansed, and the skin beneath the thyroid cartilage is anesthetized. A needle is introduced through the cricothyroid membrane, and a polyethylene catheter is advanced into the trachea. In most patients the irritation of the cathether will induce coughing and permit the aspiration of a tracheal specimen. If a sample cannot be aspirated, a few milliliters of saline solution are introduced through the catheter, and the tracheal wash is aspirated and examined.

In addition to providing sputum from the obtunded patient, transtracheal aspirates are an excellent source of material for anaerobic culture since the potential contamination of expectorated sputum with anaerobic mouth flora is avoided. Transtracheal aspiration is not without risk and should not be performed on the uncooperative patient. Many patients will cough up small amounts of blood after the procedure; transtracheal aspiration is contraindicated in the patient with a bleeding disorder. Bronchopulmonary secretions can also be obtained via the bronchoscope.

Pleural Fluid

The analysis of pleural fluid is an important aid in determining the etiology of an effusion and the underlying pulmonary disorder. For a diagnostic thoracentesis, 25–50 mL of fluid is aspirated from the pleural space and divided into aliquots for bacteriological, biochemical, and cytological studies as well as the determination of its cellular content.

Pleural effusions are commonly divided into transudates or exudates depending on the mechanism underlying their formation. Transudates are commonly found in conditions characterized by an increasing venous pressure, eg, congestive heart failure, or decreased plasma oncotic pressure, eg, cirrhosis; presumably the abnormal balance of Starling forces favors the increased filtration and/or decreased reabsorption of pleural fluid in these disorders. An exudative effusion, on the other hand, is characteristic of those conditions which irritate the pleura and increase its permeability, eg, tuberculosis.

Although many methods of distinguishing between transudative and exudative pleural effusions have been proposed, the most sensitive and specific is based on the measurement of the *protein* content and lactic dehydrogenase (LDH) of the pleural fluid and serum. Biochemically there are three characteristics that determine whether a pleural effusion is an exudate: (1) a pleural fluid/serum protein ratio of greater than 0.5; (2) a pleural fluid/serum LDH ratio of greater than 0.6; and (3) a pleural fluid LDH of greater than 200 IU. If any one of these criteria is fulfilled, the effusion is classified as an exudate.

The relative numbers of erythrocytes, polymorphonuclear leukocytes, and lymphocytes in pleural fluid can provide an important clue to the etiology of an effusion. While red blood cell counts of greater than $10,000/mm^3$ are found in all types of effusions, transudative and exudative, red blood cell counts exceeding $100,000/mm^3$ are most often associated with malignancy, trauma, and pulmonary infarction. Tuberculosis and uremic pleuritis are less frequent causes of bloody pleural effusions. If a grossly bloody effusion is due to a "traumatic tap" in which a blood vessel is lacerated by the thoracentesis needle, the red blood cell count initially is high, but tends to diminish as further fluid is aspirated. Lymphocytic pleural effusions, those containing greater than 50% lymphocytes, are almost invariably due to either tuberculosis or malignancy. If the initial thoracentesis is nondiagnostic in a patient with a lymphocytic pleural effusion, repeat thoracentesis should be performed with a biopsy needle; pleural biopsy will demonstrate neoplastic tissue or granulomas in a high percentage of such cases. Bacterial pneumonia is the most common cause of a pleural effusion with greater than 50% neutrophils; high neutrophil counts are also characteristic of effusions produced by other inflammatory conditions such as lupus pleuritis and pancreatitis and are commonly observed with pulmonary infarction. A predominance of neutrophils may even be observed in an occasional malignant effusion. The presence of eosinophils in pleural fluid is nonspecific, having been observed in a variety of disorders.

Samples from all suspected malignant effusions and other undiagnosed exudative effusions should be sent for *cytological* examination. Whenever possible, a large amount of fluid (200 mL or greater) should be obtained for this purpose so that cell blocks of the centrifuged specimen can be prepared.

The initial cytological examination is positive in about 60% of the effusions eventually proven to be due to malignancy. Pleural biopsy is complementary to the cytological procedure, increasing the positive rate to 75% upon the initial thoracentesis. More than 90% of all malignant effusions will be diagnosed if, when the results of a first thoracentesis are negative, a second (and if necessary a third) thoracentesis and pleural biopsy are performed.

Whenever an infectious etiology is suspected, a Gram stain of the pleural fluid should be examined, and material should be submitted for both aerobic and anaerobic culture. Acid-fast smears are commonly negative in tuberculous effusions, and culture of the fluid is necessary to confirm the diagnosis in many cases. When a fungal infection is suspected, pleural fluid should be submitted for the appropriate smears and cultures.

In addition to the determination of protein and LDH, the *glucose* concentration of pleural fluid samples should be routinely measured. Low glucose concentrations (less than 30 mg/dL) in pleural fluid are generally due to either rheumatoid or tuberculous effusions. Occasionally however, the glucose level will be low in a large malignant effusion. The glucose concentration in an empyema is usually low, but the purulent nature of the pleural fluid renders the cause of the effusion obvious.

The determination of pleural fluid *pH* may be helpful since effusions with a pH of less than 7.28 are generally due to nonmalignant, inflammatory conditions. A parapneumonic effusion with a pH greater than 7.20 can generally be managed with antibiotics alone, whereas, if the pH is less than 7.20, a tube thoracostomy frequently is required for resolution. A pleural fluid pH of less than 7.0 is almost invariably due to either an empyema or esophageal rupture. The *amylase* level of pleural fluid is increased in pleural effusions due to pancreatitis, and also with esophageal perforation. In the latter case, the elevated amylase is of salivary origin.

When the gross appearance of pleural fluid is cloudy or milky, a chylothorax should be suspected, and *lipid levels* in the fluid should be determined. In a true chylothorax the triglyceride content will exceed 400 mg/dL. Occasionally a tuberculous or rheumatoid effusion may have a pseudochylous appearance due to an increase in cholesterol in the fluid, but the triglyceride levels will be normal. The determination of pleural fluid *complement* levels are helpful in an occasional patient with an undiagnosed exudative pleural effusion; reduced levels have been observed in patients with effusions due to rheumatoid arthritis and systemic lupus erythematosis, suggesting that immune mechanisms contribute to the development of pleuritis in these disorders.

Serological Tests (See also Chapter 10)
Serological tests are useful in diagnosing pulmonary viral or mycotic infections. Although high titers of specific antibody may strongly suggest a particular etiologic agent, rising titers in serial specimens obtained at one- to two-week intervals constitutes much stronger evidence. The self-limited nature of most viral illnesses means that these tests are of limited diagnostic value during acute viral pneumonia. Their principal value is for retrospective diagnosis or epidemiologic studies.

Serological testing is of practical value in chronic mycotic infections of the lung. The complement fixation (CF) test for histoplasmosis with both a mycelial and a yeast phase antigen is positive (titer greater than 1:16) in greater than 95% of patients with culture-proven progressive pulmonary disease. In disseminated infection, however, the CF test is less reliable; positive results have been obtained in only 56% to 80% of such cases. A latex agglutination test with histoplasmin antigen is useful in detecting acute primary infections. However 50% of patients with known chronically active histoplasmosis and positive CF sera were undetected by this test, rendering it less reliable in detecting those patients most in need of therapy. In coccidioidomycosis, precipitins may be detected within one to three weeks after the onset of the primary infection, and the CF test becomes positive shortly thereafter. The CF test remains positive in only a small percentage of cases, and a persistent high titer (greater than 1:32) should arouse suspicion of disseminated disease. In blastomycosis, the sensitivity of the CF test is so low and the incidence of cross-reactivity with other fungal antigens is so high that serological testing is of little value in diagnosing this disease. Sporotrichosis and paracoccidioidomycosis (South American blastomycosis) are uncommon mycotic infections that can be diagnosed by serological tests. Cryptococcus neoformans is generally an opportunistic pathogen; both antibody and circulating antigen may be detected in the blood of infected individuals by serological tests. Similarly, serological tests are available to detect amebiasis, toxoplasmosis, and hydatid disease, parasitic infections which are uncommon causes of pulmonary infiltrates.

Serum Chemistry

The alkaline phosphatase is frequently elevated in patients with infiltrative diseases of the liver such as sarcoidosis, miliary tuberculosis, and metastatic carcinoma. Hyperglobulinemia is common in patients with sarcoidosis. Serum electrophoresis is also useful in screening for $alpha_1$-antitrypsin deficiency since most of the $alpha_1$ globulin is $alpha_1$-antitrypsin. The young person with evidence of pulmonary emphysema can have his or her $alpha_1$-antitrypsin activity determined by more precise tests. Serum calcium levels should be determined in all patients with sarcoidosis and bronchogenic carcinoma; hypercalcemia, which is common in these conditions, is a definite indication for therapy in these disorders.

■ Selected Readings

Roentgenology

General

Felson B: *Chest Roentgenology.* Philadelphia, The W.B. Saunders Co, 1977.

Fraser RG, Paré JAP: Roentgenologic signs in the diagnosis of chest disease, in Fraser RG, Paré JAP (eds): *Diagnosis of Diseases of the Chest.* ed 2. Philadelphia, The W.B. Saunders Co, 1977, pp 341–6C1.

Specific

Dalen JE: Pulmonary angiography, in Grossman W (ed): *Cardiac Catheterization and Angiography.* Philadelphia, Lea and Febiger, 1974, pp 131–140.

Favez G, Willa C, Heinzer F: Posterior oblique tomography at an angle of 55 degrees in chest roentgenology. *Am J Roentgenol* 1974;120:907–915.

Pugatch RD, Faling LJ: Computed tomography of the thorax: A status report. *Chest* 1981;80:618–626.

Sagel SS, Evans RG, Forrest JV, et al: Efficiency of routine screening and lateral chest radiographs in a hospital based population. *New Engl J Med* 1974; 291:1001–1004.

Pulmonary Function Testing

General

Altose MD: The physiological basis of pulmonary function testing. *Clin Symp* 1979;31:1–39.

Fishman AP: *Assessment of Pulmonary Function.* New York, McGraw-Hill Book Co, 1980.

Ruppel G: *Manual of Pulmonary Function Testing.* ed 2. St. Louis, C.V. Mosby Co, 1979.

Shapiro BA, Harrison RA, Walton JR: *Clinical Application of Blood Gases.* Chicago, Year Book Medical Publishers, 1977.

West JB: *Respiratory Pathophysiology-The Essentials.* Baltimore, The Williams & Wilkins, Co, 1977.

Specific

Bone RC: Diagnosis of causes for acute respiratory distress by pressure-volume curves. *Chest* 1976;70:740–746.

Boren HG, Kory R, Syner JC: The veterans administration-army cooperative study of pulmonary function. II. The lung volume and its subdivisions in normal men. *Am J Med* 1966;41:96–114.

Buist AS: The single breath nitrogen test. *New Engl J Med* 1975;293:438–440.

Crapo RO, Morris AH, Gardner RM: Reference spirometric values using techniques and equipment that meet ATS recommendations. *Am Rev Respir Dis* 1981;123:659–664.

Darling RC, Cournand A, Richards DW Jr: Studies on the intrapulmonary mixture of gases. III. An open circuit method for measuring residual air. *J Clin Invest* 1940;19:609–619.

Dosman J, Bode F, Urbanetti J, et al: The use of a helium-oxygen mixture during maximum expiratory flow to demonstrate obstruction in small airways in smokers. *J Clin Invest* 1975;55:1090–1099.

Gibson GJ, Pride NB: Lung distensibility: The static pressure-volume curve of the lungs and its use in clinical assessment. *Br J Dis Chest* 1976;70:143–184.

Kory RC, Callahan R, Boren HG, et al: The veterans administration-army cooperative study of pulmonary function. I. Clinical spirometry in normal men. *Am J Med* 1961;30:243–258.

Kryger M, Bode F, Antic R, et al: Diagnosis of obstruction of the upper and central airways. *Am J Med* 1976;61:85–93.

Morris JF, Koski A, and Johnson LC: Spirometric standards for healthy non-smoking adults. *Am Rev Respir Dis* 1971;103:57–67.

Rodarte JR, Hyatt RE, Rehder K, et al: New tests for the detection of obstructive pulmonary disease. *Chest* 1977;72:762–768.

Sobol BJ, Park SS, Emirgil C: Relative value of various spirometric tests in the early detection of chronic obstructive pulmonary disease. *Am Rev Respir Dis* 1973;107:753–762.

Wasserman K, Whipp B: Exercise physiology in health and disease. *Am Rev Respir Dis* 1975;112:219–249.

Weinberger SE, Johnson TS, Weiss ST: Use and interpretation of the single-breath diffusing capacity. *Chest* 1980; 78:483–488.

Clinical Laboratory Tests

Barret-Connor E: The non-value of sputum culture in the diagnosis of pneumococcal pneumonia. *Am Rev Respir Dis* 1971;103:845–848.

Black LE: The pleural space and pleural fluid. *Mayo Clin Proc* 1972;47:493–506.

Buechner HA, Seabury JH, Campbell CC, et al: The current status of serologic, immunologic and skin tests in the diagnosis of pulmonary mycoses. *Chest* 1973;63:259–270.

Epstein RL: Constitutents of sputum. *Ann Intern Med* 1972;77:259–265.

Good JT, Taryle DA, Maulitz RM, et al: The diagnostic value of pleural fluid pH. *Chest* 1980;78:55–59.

144

Hahn HH, Beaty HN: Transtracheal aspiration in the evaluation of patients with pneumonia. *Ann Intern Med* 1970; 72:183–187.

Light RW, Erozan YS, Ball WC: Cells in pleural fluid. *Arch Intern Med* 1973; 132:854–860.

Light RW, MacGregor MI, Luchsinger PC, et al: Pleural effusions: The diagnostic separation of transudates and exudates. *Ann Intern Med* 1972;77: 507–513.

Oswald NC, Hinson KFW, Canti G, et al: The diagnosis of primary lung cancer with special reference to sputum cytology. *Thorax* 1971;26:623–631.

Rosa VW, Prolla JC, Da Silva Gastal E: Cytology in diagnosis of cancer affecting the lung. Results in 1000 consecutive patients. *Chest* 1973;63:203–207.

Wayne LG: Microbiology of tubercle bacilli. *Am Rev Respir Dis* 1982; 125(Suppl.):31–41.

Wimberley NW, Bass JB, Boyd BW, et al: Use of a brush protected catheter for the diagnosis of pulmonary infections. *Chest* 1982;81:556–562.

Yue WY, Cohen SS: Sputum induction by newer inhalation methods in patients with pulmonary tuberculosis. *Chest* 1967;51:614–620.

When diagnosing and treating infectious diseases some physicians limit their interaction with the microbiology laboratory to receiving culture reports and the results of antimicrobial sensitivity tests. I hope this chapter demonstrates that this is not a productive relationship to maintain between clinician and laboratory. It is also a disservice to patients, since accuracy in diagnosis and appropriate use of antibiotics can be greatly expanded by approaching the microbiologist and laboratory as one would approach any other consultant.

The Gram-Stained Specimen

Few laboratory procedures are so easily performed and have withstood the test of nearly a century of use as well as the Gram stain. Despite major advances in technology within the microbiology laboratory, the Gram-stained specimen remains a cornerstone in the evaluation of patients with suspected infectious disease. Provine and Gardner summarized its virtues and conclude:

> It is our feeling that the gram-stained smear should be considered part of the physical examination of the patient with an acute bacterial infection and belongs in the repertoire of all physicians delivering primary care to acutely ill patients. (*Hosp Pract* 1974;9:85–91)

Although physicians do not carry Gram-staining materials with them, they are generally not far from a microbiology laboratory. Yet, without a preestablished working relationship with his or her laboratory, the clinician who collected the specimen and is responsible for treating the patient often discards valuable data in the form of Gram-stained specimens without even a review. Our own laboratory initially evaluates all specimens such as sputum, urine, cerebrospinal fluid, and abscess material with a Gram-stained smear, which is then coded and saved for at least a week. The slide and its interpretation are readily available for review and consultation with a senior microbiologist. At any time, attending physicians, house staff, and medical students can work with this material in evaluating their patients with infectious processes. Often, complicated cases are initially evaluated on our service by summarizing their history, physical examination, and hospital course and then reviewing all Gram-stained specimens under a multiheaded teaching microscope *before* even considering the analysis of cultural data.

The presence of polymorphonuclear leukocytes (PMNs) is a good index of the inflammatory response to infection, and PMNs show up well with the Gram stain. The Gram-stained smear defines the adequacy of specimens such as sputum by revealing the number of PMNs and alveolar macrophages present in relation to the number of squamous epithelial cells. The more inadequate the specimen the greater the amount of oral flora contamination and numbers of epithelial cells in relation to PMNs. A good laboratory will discard an inadequate specimen rather than generate misleading data, and a good clinician will understand the reasoning behind the request for an additional specimen. House officers who leave their Gram-stained specimens and interpretations for review by laboratory personnel after their evening admissions find this an excellent teaching exercise. Frankly erroneous interpretations can be quickly corrected by more experienced laboratory personnel, and cultures that were plated the previous evening are available. Ascites, cerebrospinal fluid, pleural fluid, and pericardial fluid can be quickly evaluated for infectious etiologies on the basis of a good Gram-stained specimen. A presumptive and well-focused diagnosis often results. Additional studies such as anaerobic and fungal cultures may be suggested to a clinician simply on the basis of a Gram-stained smear that first indicates their presence and numbers.

Gram-stained specimens may be useful in unexpected circumstances. Lower intestinal secretions and stool contain largely mixed anaerobic flora, but occasionally demonstrate bacterial overgrowth, as with large gram-positive cocci, and suggest a diagnosis of staphylococcal enteritis. A stool Gram stain can be helpful in the diagnosis of *Campylobacter* infection. Staining blood by this method might seem unusual at first, but a Gram-stained buffy coat can enable the physician to make a rapid diagnosis of high-grade bacteremia in a splenectomized patient and dictate initial antibiotic coverage. Patients who have been partially treated with antibiotics before evaluation may have negative cultures of various body fluids, but a Gram-stained smear will often show the etiologic agent even if in a somewhat modified form. This can be particularly helpful in the evaluation of cerebrospinal fluid. Mixed anaerobic infections are easily recognized on Gram-stained smears and can often be diagnosed long before the isolation of the responsible pathogens.

At times what is not seen on the Gram-stained specimen can be as important as what is seen. For example, a specimen from a hemodialysis patient with pneumonia obtained by transtracheal aspiration demonstrated many PMNs and no visible bacteria when Gram stained. This was a clue that the patient might be infected by an organism which does not stain well by this procedure, such as a virus, mycoplasma, or one of the *Legionella* organisms. Legionellosis and mycoplasma infections are treatable diseases. The fact that the patient clearly had pneumonia with no visible agent dictated that coverage include erythromycin, at least until the etiology of his illness was clarified. Cultures of the transtracheal aspirate subsequently demonstrated the pathogen, *Legionella micdadei,* but performance of these specialized cultures and initial antibiotic coverage were largely dictated by what was observed on the Gram-stained smear itself.

Tissue Stains

It is beyond the scope of this chapter to discuss the many tissue stains available to surgical pathologists for the detection of microorganisms. However, along with the Gram stain, these stains may be the most underutilized clinical tools available to clinicians evaluating patients for infectious diseases. No protocol of standard stains for biopsy specimens can compensate for physicians who fail to communicate with surgical pathologists. It is simply impossible for pathologists to perform routine bacterial, fungal, parasitic, and acid-fast stains on every specimen they receive. The clinician must communicate a reasonable differential diagnosis to the pathologist, who in turn will choose the most appropriate stains for demonstrating suspected organisms in tissue. Table 9-1 lists some of the organisms which can be demonstrated by the choice of an appropriate staining technique.

Tissue stains are also helpful in evaluating the clinical significance of microbial isolates which were clinically unexpected and difficult to interpret. Infectious disease consultants are often asked to determine the clinical significance of bacterial isolates from biopsy material or excised tissue.

Example
A 68-year-old man underwent aortic valve replacement for severe aortic stenosis and received a bioprosthetic replacement. The excised valve was processed in the microbiology laboratory, and the Infectious Disease service was called several days later because broth cultures containing some valvular tissue were growing a *Bacillus* species. Since a new prosthetic valve had just been inserted, did the growth of bacteria from the excised valve indicate preexistent valvular endocarditis? Was treatment now required to prevent loss of the new bioprosthetic valve from residual infection at the valve root?

Table 9-1
Examples of Some Special Stains and Techniques for Histopathological Diagnosis of Infectious Diseases

Organisms	Typical Staining Techniques
Gram-positive and -negative bacteria	Tissue Gram stain (eg, Brown and Brenn stain)
Mycobacterium species	Hematoxylin and eosin (H&E) stains to demonstrate caseation or granuloma, and tissue acid-fast stains to demonstrate the organisms
Nocardia species	Gram stain or acid-fast stain will show the organism in an exudate, and a tissue acid-fast stain will show the organism well in tissues
Legionella species	Do not stain well on routine H&E or tissue Gram stains; request silver stain (eg, Dieterle silver stain)
Candida species	Besides the gram stain and the periodic acid-Schiff (PAS) stain, the Gomori-Grocott chromic acid methenamine silver (GMS) stain is used
Aspergillus species	PAS and GMS stains also used
Cryptococcus neoformans	PAS and GMS stains used; organisms may stain well with capsular stain such as mucicarmine
Viruses	H&E, acridine orange, and Feulgen stains may demonstrate intranuclear and intracytoplasmic inclusions which are confirmed and further characterized by electron microscopy

The question is not an unusual or a trivial one. *Bacillus* species can cause endocarditis, and residual infection could threaten survival of the new valve. The issue could be resolved by reviewing the previous clinical history and physical findings which did not suggest the presence of endocarditis. Also, three sets of blood cultures which had been drawn for a brief postoperative fever were negative. However, it was of considerable help for the pathology laboratory to review with us stains of the excised aortic valve material which had been submitted at surgery. Tissue Gram stains for bacteria were checked for the presence of large gram-positive rods within any lesions which might suggest endocarditis. Neither was found, and the *Bacillus* isolated was appropriately attributed to environmental contamination of the valve at surgery or during processing. Similar problems often arise when bone or vascular tissues are removed for insertion of prosthetic material, when suspected embolic material is submitted for culture, or when lung biopsies are processed for pathogens in immunocompromised patients. In each instance a potential pathogen may be isolated, and the data available from a complete histological evaluation of tissue are vital to the decision-making process.

Quantitation of Organisms— Interpretation of Results

When body surfaces, mucous membranes, tissues, or fluids have predictable endogenous flora or are contaminated with colonizing organisms, the quantitation of cultured bacteria taken from these areas is important. Known criteria statistically associate infection with colony counts such as those done on urine samples to delineate significant bacteriuria. Results, however, may be misleading if the basis for applying these tests is not appreciated.

Example

The microbiology laboratory has reported a urine colony count of 10^5 or greater per mL on a clean-voided midstream urine collection from your patient. Concentrating on the microbiological and not the clinical data for a moment, there are several principles and limitations on the interpretation of these data to recognize when a diagnosis of urinary tract infection or significant bacteriuria is considered.

(1) For both men and women, the distal urethra is normally colonized with a variety of organisms, both aerobic and anaerobic. It is for this reason that quantitative cultures of clean-voided midstream urine specimens are needed to determine the clinical significance of bacterial isolates.

(2) A Gram-stained smear of a drop or loopful of urine showing two or more bacteria per oil immersion field ($1000 \times$) correlates with $> 100,000$ colony-forming units per mL of urine. The presence of > 20 bacteria observed on an unstained urine sediment may also correlate with such counts.

(3) *Cultures of unrefrigerated urine that have been left standing for more than two hours cannot be interpreted by these criteria due to possible overgrowth of any bacteria present initially.*

(4) These criteria neither apply to catheterized patients nor can be arbitrarily applied to infections caused by gram-positive cocci such as staphylococci, fungi such as *Candida albicans*, anaerobic bacteria, or mycobacteria—all of which can cause significant urinary tract infections.

(5) The criteria are best applied to concentrated first-morning specimens of urine and not to urine obtained from patients who are well hydrated or undergoing a diuresis.

(6) Because even a few organisms will quickly render broth cultures turbid with large numbers of multiplying organisms, broth cultures are not used and would not be applicable to quantitation of bacteria in general.

Most important, it should be kept in mind that the original criteria for significant bacteriuria were based on the finding that 95% of cases of pyelonephritis had urine colony counts of 10^5/mL or greater, whereas contaminants had counts about 2 logs lower.

Clinical judgment and not simply statistical associations must be applied to each clinical situation as it arises. Persistent isolations of a single organism, associated with appropriate symptoms, should lead to the diagnosis of urinary tract infection even when urine colony counts are not in the range of 10^5/mL. This information must be communicated to the laboratory if the clinician expects to receive antibiotic sensitivity data on an organism present in lower numbers. The laboratory might also reasonably consider a urine culture that demonstrates polymicrobial bacteriuria as evidence for a contaminated urine specimen. The clinician may have suspected an entero-vesicle fistula secondary to tumor or regional enteritis, which is entirely compatible with polymicrobial bacteriuria. Communicate with the laboratory, or you may not receive the data you need.

With regard to surgical infections, Ellner has reviewed some simple procedures to quantitate the numbers of bacteria in wound exudates or soft tissues and distinguish "mixed saprophytic flora" from invasive microbial infection. Quantitative cultures may be performed on either wound exudate or tissue which has been ground in sterile broth and serially diluted by the laboratory to obtain colony counts in aerobic and anaerobic cultures. Plates demonstrating four or more species of organisms after 24 hours of incubation, including such organisms as viridans streptococci, enterococci, *Staphylococcus epidermidis, Micrococcus* species, diphtheroids, or non-pathogenic *Neisseria* are simply reported as "mixed saprophytic flora" and not processed further.

Studies performed on infected wounds and decubitus ulcers suggest that the number 10^5 is important when quantitating organisms infecting these areas. Regardless of the species, 10^5 organisms per g of tissue (or per mL of exudate) is associated with delays in wound healing. The presence of 10^6 organisms has been correlated with invasive infection and sepsis. Time saved by the microbiology laboratory in not processing mixed saprophytic flora more than makes up for the added efforts in dealing with those organisms likely to be responsible for invasive disease. Clinicians in turn must be aware that anaerobes assume great importance in such infections, and care must be taken to collect both tissues and exudate in a manner which will insure survival of anaerobes during transport to the microbiology laboratory.

Blood Cultures

Responsibility for the appropriate use of blood cultures lies first with the clinician who makes the decision to perform them. The method of skin preparation should be rigorous enough to reduce the risk of contamination to less than 3%. There is no advantage in doing arterial rather than venous cultures. Blood for culture must not be drawn through accessible but often colonized indwelling intravenous catheters or arterial lines. No matter how many blood culture bottles are used, each venipuncture constitutes the performance of only one blood culture. Ten milliliters of blood cultured at a 1:5 ratio of blood to broth is an effective dilution for maximum rates of isolation, although the amount of blood is more important than the ratio. Patients whose blood must be cultured while they are on antibiotic therapy such as penicillins or cephalosporins can be subjected to the same procedures. Most laboratories tend to rely on dilution rather than the addition of penicillinase (β-lactamase) to blood cultures to inactivate such antibiotics. The risk of contaminating blood cultures by the additional procedure outweighs the benefit of adding penicillinase. Commercially incorporated stable preparations of β-lactamase in culture media eliminate the need to perform an extra procedure when faced with this question.

One interesting development in the science of blood culture techniques has been in the use of antimicrobial removal devices (ARDs). They are resin mixtures which have been treated with detergents to prevent bacterial retention and then suspended in vials of saline, sealed, and autoclaved. In practice, 5–10 mL of whole blood is injected into the ARD vial and rotated to maintain contact between blood and suspended resins for about 15 minutes. This allows removal of antibiotics from blood by the resins without decreasing the concentration of bacteria which might be present. When treated blood is aseptically removed from the device for culturing, it should be substantially freed of antibiotics which might interfere with bacterial growth. This yields more positive blood cultures with less time to detection when compared with conventional blood culture techniques. If proven effective, ARDs may help recover organisms from patients who have been on antibiotics.

Any clues which the clinician has regarding the etiology of suspected bacteremia should be transmitted to the laboratory either directly or, at the very least, on an enclosed laboratory slip. All available broth media and all conditions of incubation are not equally suitable for the isolation of all bacteria and fungi. The best yields of some anaerobic species such as *Bacteroides* will occur under conditions of a low redox potential. *Pseudomonas aeruginosa* and *C. albicans* will grow better if blood culture bottles containing CO_2 are vented to the air. *P. aeruginosa* isolation rates are significantly less in thioglycollate broth than in other commercially available media. Vitamin B_6-dependent strains of viridans streptococci vary in growth from 8% to 100% depending upon the type of broth medium used for isolation. We generally suggest the use of commercially available biphasic brain heart infusion media containing agar and broth when fungal etiologies are considered.

Failure to allow the microbiologist access to clinical information suggesting the etiological agent results in a slower and decreased yield of fastidious or unusual organisms, when they could actually be detected by simple alterations in media, conditions of incubation, or subculture. The number of blood cultures required to attain maximum detection of bacteremia has been thoroughly investigated for the detection of infectious endocarditis. The following number and timing of blood cultures for suspected infective endocarditis are recommended.

(1) For acute endocarditis, obtain three blood cultures at three separate venipunctures during the first one to two hours of evaluation and begin therapy.

(2) For subacute endocarditis, obtain three blood cultures on the first day (ideally 15 or more minutes apart); if all are negative 24 hours later, obtain two more. From undiagnosed patients who have received antimicrobial agents in the week or two before admission, obtain two blood cultures on each of three successive days. Although prior antimicrobial therapy may cause blood cultures to be negative, it more often causes delayed growth. Therefore, blood cultures from partially treated patients should be incubated for at least 14 days.

With optimal culture techniques, positive blood cultures should be obtained in over 95% of cases of infective endocarditis.

Antimicrobial Sensitivity Testing

For clinicians following patients with known infectious processes, the isolation of suspected pathogens greatly increases the ability to both choose and correctly utilize appropriate antimicrobial therapy. In so doing they accept a proven concept, namely, that treating infections with agents to which in vitro sensitivity of the organism can be demonstrated will improve the chances of achieving therapeutic success. It follows that empiric therapy is avoided whenever possible to preclude situations in which infections are under inappropriate or ineffective antibiotic therapy. What appears to be a confusing array of antibiotic levels, serum bactericidal determinations, minimum inhibitory and bactericidal antibiotic concentrations, and disk diffusion assays, may so dismay physicians that they neither understand nor utilize them when their use is clearly indicated. Under these circumstances their interaction with the bacteriology laboratory is minimal, and the information obtained may be limited to reports which list the isolated organisms and their sensitivity or resistance patterns to a group of predetermined standard antibiotics by disk diffusion antibiotic assay. There is much more to be gained by an intelligent interaction between clinicians and their microbiological consultants.

Example

A 75-year-old man with an obstructed urinary tract secondary to an enlarged prostate develops gram-negative sepsis and is treated empirically with parenteral ampicillin and gentamicin after blood and urine cultures are performed. The bacteriology laboratory isolates *Escherichia coli* from the patient's blood and urine cultures which are reported as "sensitive" to ampicillin but "intermediate" to gentamicin. How are such data generated in the microbiology laboratory, and what are some of the pitfalls which might occur in the interpretation of these results?

Realize that sensitivity tests are based on a disk diffusion assay often referred to as the Kirby-Bauer test. Simply stated, the organism isolated from the patient is grown to a predetermined inoculum size and plated on standardized Muller-Hinton agar. Small disks, each containing a predetermined amount of antibiotic, are dispensed over the newly seeded lawn of bacteria. Antibiotic diffuses outward radially from each disk, and if the organism is susceptible the drug will either kill or inhibit the growth of bacteria. In either case, a clear zone with a measurable diameter surrounds the disk after overnight incubation. The diameter of the zone of inhibition is related to the ability of that drug to inhibit the growth of the test organism at the usual antibiotic levels which are achievable in blood. The interpretations of zone sizes are derived from more quantitative results obtained by the antibiotic dilution assays explained below and from known achievable serum concentrations of the antibiotics. The disk diffusion test is quite widely used since it is readily adaptable to the volume of work required in a busy microbiology laboratory. It is relatively easy to perform and quite inexpensive. The technician can read the diameter of the zone of inhibition and determine whether the organism should be classified as "sensitive," "intermediate," or "resistant" on the basis of a reference chart containing the appropriate zone diameters for each antibiotic.

There are major limitations of disk diffusion tests which could cause erroneous interpretation of results for the patient just described. Microbiologists know that variations in the size of the bacterial inoculum could give disparate results in this test and must be carefully controlled. Yet, even with the best of quality control, aminoglycoside activity against gram-negative organisms, when measured by disk diffusion, may not correlate entirely with results obtained by a dilution assay.

How does one interpret the "intermediate" result in the zone size for gentamicin versus the *E. coli* obtained from the penicillin allergic patient just described? If slightly higher doses of gentamicin were used to treat the patient, might gentamicin have been an effective single agent? Only dilution assays and measurements of antibiotic levels could satisfactorily answer this question. Had our patient been febrile but not bacteremic, with infection confined to the urinary tract, gentamicin might still have been a logical choice as single-agent therapy if use of ampicillin were precluded by allergy. Levels of gentamicin in urine far exceed those in serum. Since diffusion tests relate to achievable *serum* levels of antibiotic, experience suggests that such an organism would be readily eliminated from the urine by standard doses of gentamicin.

There are additional problems with the disk diffusion test. It does not provide a bactericidal endpoint, as can be obtained by dilution assays. For organisms which are slow growing, the procedure is difficult to standardize, since antibiotic diffusion away from the disk occurs long before the organism has been able to grow to an acceptable degree. Had our 75-year-old patient with urinary tract infection developed a new murmur associated with enterococcal bacteremia, the possibility of infectious endocarditis would have been a serious consideration. This disease requires synergistic combinations of antibiotics to achieve adequate cure rates. The disk diffusion test gives us no information regarding the effect of combination therapy on which to base our decision.

Broth or Tube Dilution Assays
A tube dilution assay answers questions unanswered by disk sensitivity tests. Gradually decreasing concentrations of the antibiotic to be tested are inoculated with a standard inoculum of bacteria (Figure 9-1). Two endpoints are examined after overnight incubation. Tubes in which bacteria are either inhibited or killed will appear clear to the eye. Turbid tubes signify bacterial

MINIMUM INHIBITORY AND BACTERICIDAL CONCENTRATIONS OF ANTIBIOTICS

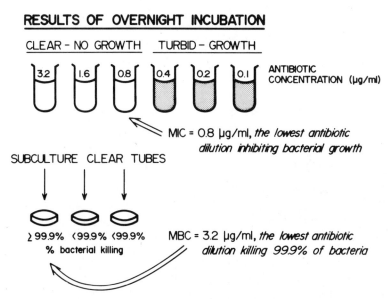

RESULTS OF OVERNIGHT INCUBATION

CLEAR - NO GROWTH   TURBID - GROWTH

| 3.2 | 1.6 | 0.8 | 0.4 | 0.2 | 0.1 | ANTIBIOTIC CONCENTRATION (µg/ml) |

MIC = 0.8 µg/ml, *the lowest antibiotic dilution inhibiting bacterial growth*

SUBCULTURE CLEAR TUBES

≥ 99.9% ‹99.9% ‹99.9%   MBC = 3.2 µg/ml, *the lowest antibiotic*
% bacterial killing   *dilution killing 99.9% of bacteria*

Figure 9-1 MIC of an antibiotic determined by tube broth dilutions after overnight incubation of antibiotic and organism to be tested. Tubes which show no turbidity are subcultured to determine the percent of bacterial killing. The lowest antibiotic dilution killing 99.9% of the bacteria initially tested is the minimum bactericidal concentration of that antibiotic for the organism tested.

growth. The lowest concentration of antibiotic which inhibits growth is referred to as the minimal inhibitory concentration (MIC) of the antibiotic for that organism under the conditions utilized by that laboratory. Subculture of clear tubes of broth to solid media free of antibiotics may demonstrate viable organisms in some of the clear tubes. The lowest dilution of antibiotic in which 99.9% of organisms were killed represents the minimal bactericidal concentration (MBC) of the antibiotic for the test organism. If all tubes which were clear after overnight incubation also show lack of growth on subculture then the MIC and the MBC are equal, as is often the case for bactericidal antibiotics. Bacteriostatic agents may be quite effective at inhibiting the growth of the test organism, but on subculture all clear tubes might still show many viable organisms. In this instance, the MIC can be determined, but there is no MBC since the antibiotic is not bactericidal for the organism at the concentrations of antibiotic tested. The range of MICs and MBCs for large numbers of bacterial isolates of various species represents one of the most important characteristic patterns of an antimicrobial agent. Pharmacokinetic studies of the agent in humans reveal the achievable serum levels for the antibiotic. The range of MICs and MBCs for an antibiotic indicate whether its achievable serum levels would be adequate for treating these various species of bacteria. It is from such data that the disk sensitivity test zone diameter criteria are extrapolated and from which the terms "sensitive," "intermediately sensitive," and "resistant" are derived.

Because bactericidal levels of antibiotics are critical for successful treatment of endocarditis, determination of MIC, MBC, and serum levels of antibiotics are routinely performed to assure the treating physician that at least the circulating levels of antibiotic exceed the MBC of the organisms causing endocarditis. Just how much greater than the MBC the serum antibiotic levels must be is not entirely clear. However, a consideration of serum inhibitory and bactericidal levels will bring the question into somewhat sharper focus.

Serum Inhibitory and Bactericidal Assays

One of the most frequently recommended tests by infectious disease consultants is the serum bactericidal concentration (SBC). It has been referred to as the Schlichter Test, based on a preliminary report of serum inhibitory effects by Schlichter in 1947. The major use of the test has been to monitor serum bactericidal levels against organisms causing endocarditis. Consider our patient with enterococcal endocarditis who requires combination therapy with penicillin and aminoglycoside in an attempt to treat the disease with a synergistic combination of bactericidal antibiotics. How is this patient's antibiotic therapy to be monitored? Individual antibiotic blood levels could be performed during treatment, but their usefulness would depend on knowing not only the MBC for penicillin and gentamicin but the results of adequate synergy studies against this patient's enterococcal isolate. The serum bactericidal level is a means of directly assaying the bactericidal activity of the patient's antibiotic-containing serum against his bacterial pathogen. Theoretically, serum which contained 16 μg of antibiotic per mL had an MBC of 1 μg/mL against a given organism would show a serum bactericidal titer of 1:16 against the organism. For example, while receiving penicillin and gentamicin a random sample of serum from a patient was obtained and tested in serial dilutions. The organism was killed at serum dilutions of 1:32 when tested accordingly. Without the need to measure individual antibiotic levels, the clinician can at least be assured that the combination of antibiotics in serum at the time the test was performed exceeded the MBC for the organism by a factor of 32.

The relative ease with which the test can be done has resulted in widespread use but lack of uniformity in methodology. Some consultants aim for an SBC of 1:8 one hour after administration of antibiotics for bacterial endocarditis. However, this level neither assures nor is required for cure. Some suggest that a sustained SBC of at least 1:8 should be maintained even when concentrations of antibiotics are at their lowest levels, ie, the trough just before the administration of the next dose of antibiotics, but there is no hard evidence to support this. Despite its shortcomings, the procedure is used rather often to obtain some evidence of efficacy during antibiotic therapy. As long as one does not look at it as an iron-clad guarantee of bacteriological cure or insist that only rigidly defined SBCs are acceptable, therapeutic regimens, then the test will not be abused. The major applications of serum bactericidal concentration are: (1) to monitor therapy during bacterial endocarditis, a disease in which effective bactericidal levels of antibiotics are important in achieving acceptable cure rates; (2) to monitor the treatment of granulocytopenic patients; (3) to monitor the synergistic effect of antibiotic combinations in vivo, when a reliable index of bactericidal effect is needed; (4) to monitor changes in antibiotic therapy, ie, when an effective parenteral regimen is replaced by oral therapy and documentation of bactericidal effect is again needed; (5) to monitor therapy of other diseases such as acute osteo-myelitis or bacterial meningitis in which bactericidal activity may also be important.

Bacterial Tolerance

The term "tolerant" as applied to bacterial isolates by a microbiology laboratory, may be a source of confusion for clinicians. Bacterial tolerance may contribute to pathogenicity by increasing the chances for survival of the organism during antibiotic therapy. The term refers to a specific phenomenon in which some bacterial isolates have MBCs which are several-fold higher than their MIC (MBC/MIC > 32) when tested against bacter-icidal antibiotics such as oxacillin. This may also be reflected during the measurement of serum bactericidal levels which are in this situation manyfold lower than the serum inhibitory level against the organism tested.

Example
A 22-year-old intravenous drug abuser had *S. aureus* endocarditis. The organism isolated from his blood was found sensitive to oxacillin by the Kirby-Bauer disk sensitivity test. However, MIC and MBC determinations were performed by the tube dilution technique and found to be 0.4 μg/mL and 50 μg/mL, respectively. The physician was informed that the patient was infected with a strain of *S. aureus* which could be interpreted as being tolerant.

This type of data is becoming increasingly common and presents some im-portant considerations for the attending physician. The basis for the phe-nomenon seems to be a deficiency in bacterial cell wall autolysin activity. This enzyme appears to increase the rate of bacterial killing when the organism is exposed to a cell wall-active agent such as penicillin. Deficien-cies in autolysin are associated with an increased MBC/MIC ratio and appar-ently increased survival of the bacteria during in vitro sensitivity tests. Whether the phenomenon is clearly associated with antibiotic failures or requires the addition of another agent such as an aminoglycoside that is not affected by the deficiency is not clear, although it has been advocated. Colonial morphology, biochemical testing of the organism, and determina-tion of MICs alone will not detect tolerant strains of bacteria.

The standard of reference for bactericidal activity is a 99.9% or greater decrease in the number of organisms over a defined time period of incuba-tion, usually 24 hours. Tolerant organisms may take 36 to 48 hours to reach this level of killing *but they do eventually reach it.* Hence, there is a bactericidal effect, but it is proceeding at a rate that is slower than expected. The phenomenon is quite common. Whereas early studies demonstrated tolerance in 36% to 63% of *S. aureus* strains tested, it is now evident that if all the organisms in a given bacterial culture are tested then all cultures con-tain some tolerant organisms with an average number of 8.6% (range 0.5% to 50%) being tolerant. Whether clinical situations in which a greater propor-tion of bacterial isolates are tolerant are associated with a worse prognosis if not treated more aggressively remains to be determined. If tolerant bacteria simply represent an in vitro phenomenon which results in slower killing of bacteria due to this associated autolysin deficiency, it is not clear to what extent tolerance will contribute to antibiotic failure, particularly if "tolerance" to some degree is always present. For now, it is suggested that the addition of an aminoglycoside antibiotic be considered for treatment of serious staphylococcal infections in which bactericidal therapy appears important.

Antibiotic Combinations— Understanding Synergy

The clinician is more likely to use combinations of antibiotics in attempts to cover multiple potential pathogens than to produce synergy. However, there are circumstances in which more than one antibiotic is used because combined effects against a single pathogen may be additive or greater, producing an increased opportunity for eradication of the pathogen, lower relapse rates, and, ultimately, cure of the infection. The treatment of enterococcal endocarditis with combinations of cell wall-active antibiotics and aminoglycosides and the therapy of *P. aeruginosa* infections in neutropenic patients with carbenicillin and aminoglycosides are well-studied examples.

To understand what synergy studies mean when reported to you from the microbiology laboratory, it is important to understand the language in which the results are summarized. Drugs act *synergistically* when their combined effects on an organism are significantly greater than the sum of their individual effects when measured separately for that organism. They act antagonistically when their combined effects are significantly less than this sum. More is known about synergy, since it is commonly sought or investigated in attempts to define regimens for clinical therapy. The term additive or indifferent is applied to two drugs when their effects on an organism are equal to the sum (or partial sum) of their separately measured effects.

The checkerboard technique and time-kill curves represent the two major methods by which such data are generated from the laboratory when these studies have been requested. The checkerboard technique is used more commonly. It requires a series of tubes or wells on a test plate which contain growth medium. The concentration of one antibiotic can be varied along the *x*-axis, and that of the other antibiotic can be varied along the *y*-axis. The resulting combinations of antibiotics are then tested against a standardized inoculum of the organism under consideration. The result is a checkerboard (Figure 9-2). It is initially set up to include concentrations of antibiotics which are both above and below the MIC of each drug for the organism being tested. After overnight incubation the turbid wells indicate viable, growing organisms at concentrations of antibiotics which are not inhibitory. The clear wells indicate antibiotic concentrations at which the organism is either inhibited or killed. By constructing a graph called an isobologram, which connects the MICs of the combinations of antibiotics in each row, a curve is generated which graphically illustrates the types of interactions just described.

In graphs A and D the results are simply additive. The MIC for each drug is 1 μg/mL. In this case a concentration of 0.5 μg/mL or 0.5 of the MIC of both drugs produces the same effect as 1.0 MIC of the single agents used alone.

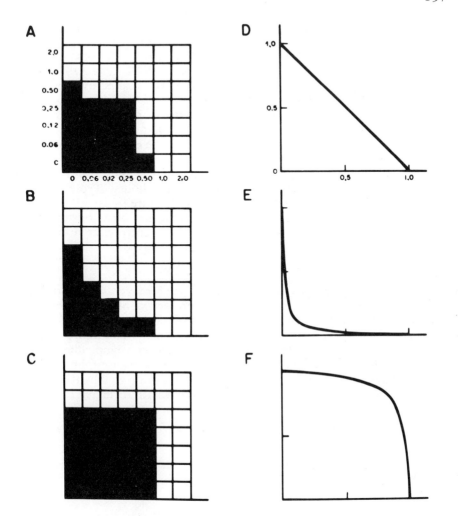

Figure 9-2 Assessment of antimicrobial combinations by the checkerboard technique. A, B, C: Arrangement of drug dilutions given as multiples of the MIC. Shading: Visible growth after incubation. D, E, F: Isobolograms plotted from results of checkerboard test to the left of each isobologram. A, D: Additive (indifferent) effect. B, E: Synergistic effect. C, F: Antagonistic effect.

Graphs B and E are the most critical for understanding synergy. In this case, 0.12 of the MIC of each drug, when used in combination, inhibits the growth of the test organism. This meets what would be considered an acceptable criterion for synergy, ie, less than 0.25 of the independently determined MIC for each drug, when used in combination, will inhibit the growth of the test organism, which would have required 1 μg of either drug per mL for growth inhibition, if used independently. The results in graphs C and F are antagonistic. One important limitation in the technique must be kept in mind. The results are given in terms of growth *inhibition* and not the bactericidal effect of the combination. However, by sampling the clear wells for subculture on agar medium, the bactericidal data can be determined.

158

To assess the actual synergistic *bactericidal* activity of antibiotic combinations by another method, the laboratory may perform and report time-kill curves. These studies involve the exposure of bacteria to one combination of antibiotics at concentrations which are in the clinically achievable range. When tubes containing bacteria and antibiotics are sampled over time and colony counts are performed at selected time intervals for 24 hours or more, decreasing colony counts will reflect the killing of bacteria in a dynamic fashion. In this context, synergy is defined as a 100-fold ($2 \log_{10}$) reduction in colony counts after 24 hours of incubation by the combination of agents as compared with the single most efficacious drug when used alone. A more convenient definition which is also acceptable would be a 10-fold colony count reduction when the test is read at eight hours. Typical curves generated by the time-kill method are shown in Figure 9-3.

The tests described above are clinically helpful, but time consuming for the laboratory. There are, however, means to obtain corroborative data with less effort, best illustrated in the following case study.

Case

A 64-year-old man was seen by his local physician for fever, weight loss, and malaise. A mitral murmur was heard, and several sets of blood cultures grew what were identified as "enterococci" by the microbiology laboratory. No additional data was generated or requested from the laboratory and the physician felt it appropriate to treat his patient with ampicillin and an aminoglycoside parenterally for six weeks. He chose to use tobramycin as the aminoglycoside. The patient appeared to have done well by the time he was discharged, but returned within a few weeks with recurrent symptoms

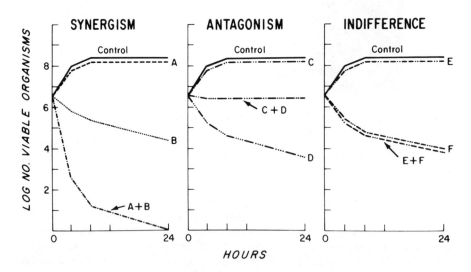

Figure 9-3 Effects of antimicrobial combinations as determined by the killing curve (time-kill curve) method. (Reproduced with permission from Krogstad DG, Moellering RC Jr: Combinations of antibiotics, mechanisms of interaction against bacteria, in Lorian V: *Antibiotics in Laboratory Medicine*. Baltimore, MD, The Williams & Wilkins Co, 1980.)

and blood cultures again positive for enterococci. This patient had a well-documented case of relapsed enterococcal endocarditis which ultimately required mitral valve surgery for cure. It might have been avoided had the laboratory been requested to provide additional data.

The enterococci are group D streptococci and include several species, among which are *Streptococcus faecalis* and *Streptococcus faecium*. Although *S. faecalis* is a more common cause of endocarditis, the organism isolated in this case proved to be *S. faecium* when ultimately speciated in our laboratory and at the Centers for Disease Control. The distinction is fairly important because in vitro studies indicate that *S. faecium* is consistently resistant to combinations of penicillins and several aminoglycosides, one of which is tobramycin. *S. faecium* produces an enzyme (6'-acetyltransferase) that inactivates tobramycin. In vitro investigations and in vivo studies using the rabbit model of endocarditis suggest that this would not be an effective combination to use for serious infections caused by *S. faecium*. The problem might have been avoided in a number of ways. Speciation of any organism for which one is planning a long and expensive course of therapy is generally indicated. This might have alerted the clinician or microbiologist to check the recent literature for problems in therapy of this uncommon isolate. Also, without actually performing synergy studies, even a small laboratory with limited personnel can perform a screening test for synergy based on demonstrating the presence or absence of high-level resistance of the organism to the aminoglycoside chosen for therapy.

For example, penicillin-streptomycin synergy against *S. faecalis* can be predicted by testing for high-level resistance of the organism to streptomycin (MIC > 2,000 µg/mL). Strains with high-level resistance or for which streptomycin has MICs greater than 2000 µg/mL do not demonstrate synergistic killing by the penicillin-streptomycin combination. The assessment of high-level resistance should be within the range of available procedures in any microbiology laboratory. It is a reasonable screening method upon which to base initial therapy. In the interest of saving time and increasing the efficiency of microbiology laboratories, it has occasionally been suggested that microorganisms not be identified as to species by the laboratory and simply be reported as they were in this case as "enterococci" with their sensitivity patterns.

Mycobacteria

Physicians must take special care to closely correlate the diagnosis and treatment of patients infected with classical *Mycobacterium tuberculosis* and other mycobacteria with data from the laboratory responsible for performing smears, cultures, and antibiotic sensitivity tests on these organisms. The responsibility begins with the collection and submission of adequate specimens. In sputum samples endogenous mouth flora outnumber and can overgrow mycobacteria because the growth rate of mycobacteria is so much slower. For this reason I strongly recommend that the physician assure that specimens are fresh, collected in sterile containers, contain a minimum of nasal secretions or saliva, and are refrigerated if not delivered immediately to the laboratory.

There is no significant increase in culture yields for *M. tuberculosis* using 24- or 72-hour pooled sputum samples over that of a single specimen;

however, in their study the rate of contamination increased from 1.6% for single specimens to 14.8% for pooled specimens. With properly collected samples there is no advantage to collecting more than five per patient, since beyond that point there is no increase in the cumulative percent positive cultures.

Gastric washings also have a place in the collection of samples from young children and others who have difficulty cooperating with sputum collection. After attempted aerosol induction of sputum, the yield of positive cultures from gastric lavage may be increased during the subsequent one-half hour. However, mycobacteria survive poorly in gastric fluid, and these cultures require processing within four hours or neutralization of acid during transport.

The laboratory performing smears for tuberculosis will use one of the standard stains that take advantage of the acid-fast properties of mycobacteria. Sputum smears for acid-fast organisms are becoming the mainstay of outpatient care, and their use will increase rather than decrease in the near future, as reliance on time-consuming cultures for monitoring bacillary numbers in response to therapy wanes. The staining procedure for "fluorescence microscopy" utilizes a yellow fluorescing dye. It is also an "acid-fast stain." With condensers and high-intensity lamps, acid-fast bacilli can be seen to fluoresce against a contrasting background. The principal advantage of this method is that large areas of a smear can be examined under a lower power far more quickly than by conventional techniques. Smears can be screened by this technique and confirmed as positive by overstaining with carbol fuchsin stain.

Positive acid-fast smears do not make a diagnosis of infection with *M. tuberculosis;* culture results are necessary to identify this species and distinguish it from other mycobacteria. The question of disease versus infection, the choice of therapy, and the epidemiology of acquisition are all dependent upon this information. For isolations of atypical mycobacteria the questions are those of disease versus colonization and the appropriate choice of an antibiotic regimen consisting of several drugs for those who have disease. Hence, the species identification of mycobacteria is of paramount importance.

There is a mistaken impression that "six weeks" is required to get answers to these questions. This is not so, provided the lines of communication with the laboratory are open. For example, mycobacteria which appear on primary isolation media after a week or less of incubation (rapid growers) are almost certainly not *M. tuberculosis,* nor are species which produce bright yellow or orange pigmented colonies whether in a light or dark environment (scotochromogen). In addition, when exposure to light causes pigment production (photochromogen), the organism is not *M. tuberculosis.* Examination of very young colonies growing on agar media may demonstrate "cording" or grouping of organisms, a property which is characteristic of *M. tuberculosis* but not unique for this species. Although occasionally other strains of mycobacteria have a positive niacin test, the positive niacin reaction strongly suggests *M. tuberculosis* and can be performed when cultures are about three weeks old if enough colonies (> 100) are present. It is at least possible to have a reasonable idea of the type of mycobacterial infection one is dealing with before a final laboratory report is issued. A slow-growing, nonpigmented, niacin-positive *Mycobacterium* may be presumed to be *M. tuberculosis,* unless proven otherwise by subsequent testing.

Sensitivity testing for mycobacteria can be confusing, particularly since patients may be well into a course of therapy before results are available. Besides the public health importance of monitoring drug-resistant strains of mycobacteria in the community or in patients undergoing retreatment, these tests are important in planning therapy for the individual patients.

When 1% of a population of *M. tuberculosis* becomes resistant to an antibiotic, that drug may not, or soon will not, be useful for chemotherapy because resistant organisms can quickly become the predominant form of the organism. If the laboratory reports the amount of growth on drug-containing media as compared with growth on drug-free controls with inocula at various dilutions, it is possible to learn the percentage of the population which is resistant to a specified level of drug in vitro.

The most important message for practicing physicians is: *Do not allow your interaction with the laboratory to be limited to submission of specimens and the reception of computerized laboratory reports.* Clinicians must individualize and evaluate the results of diagnostic tests in consultation with the clinical microbiologist. Each has much to learn by intelligent interaction with the other.

Acknowledgments

I sincerely thank Mary Murray and Deborah Beauvais for manuscript preparation and Ms Gertrude Barden MT (ASCP) MHS and Dr Jean E. Hawkins for their careful review of this manuscript.

■ Selected Readings

Coleman DL, Horwitz RI, Andriole VT: A review of the association between serum inhibitory and bactericidal concentrations and therapeutic outcome in bacterial endocarditis. *Am J Med* 1982; 73:260–267.

Douglas RG, Hall CB: Significance of virus isolation and identification and virus serology in the care of patients, in Lorian V (ed): *Significance of Medical Microbiology in the Care of Patients.* ed 1. Baltimore, The Williams & Wilkins Co, 1977, pp 159–169.

Hawkins JE: Drug susceptibility testing, in Kubica GP, Wayne LG (eds): *The Mycobacteria: A Sourcebook.* New York, Marcel Dekker Inc, 1983, (in press).

Hsiung GD: Laboratory diagnoses of viral infections: General principles and recent developments. *Mt Sinai J Med (NY)* 1977;44:1–26.

Jawetz E: The doctor's dilemma: Have I chosen the right drug? An adequate dose regimen? Can laboratory tests help in my decision? in Remington JS, Schwartz MS (eds): *Current Clinical Topics in Infectious Disease,* vol 2. New York, McGraw-Hill Book Co, 1980, pp 109–120.

Kaye DS: The clinical significance of tolerance of *Staphylococcus aureus. Ann Intern Med* 1980;93:924–925.

Kestle DG, Kubica GP: Sputum collection for cultivation of mycobacteria. An early morning specimen or the 24- to 72-hour pool? *Am J Clin Pathol* 1967;48: 347–349.

Krogstad DG, Moellering RC Jr: Combinations of antibiotics, mechanisms of interaction against bacteria, in Lorian V (ed): *Antibiotics in Laboratory Medicine.* Baltimore, The Williams & Wilkins Co, 1980, pp 298–341.

162

Kubica GP, Gross WM, Hawkins JE, et al: Laboratory services for mycobacterial diseases. *Am Rev Respir Dis* 1975; 112:773–787.

Kunin C: Principles of urinary bacteriology and immunology, in *Detection, Prevention and Management of Urinary Tract Infections.* ed 3. Philadelphia, Lea and Febiger, 1979, pp 91–150.

Reller RB: Laboratory procedures in the management of infective endocarditis, in Bisno A (ed): *Treatment of Infective Endocarditis.* New York, Grune and Stratton, 1981, pp 235–268.

Roberts GD, Washington JA II: Detection of fungi in blood cultures. *J Clin Microbiol* 1975;1:309–310.

Roberts RB, Krieger AG, Schiller NL, et al: Viridans streptococcal endocarditis: The role of various species, including pyridoxal-dependent streptococci. *Rev Infect Dis* 1979;1:955–965.

Saunders WE Jr, Saunders CC: Significance of *in vitro* antimicrobial susceptibility tests in care of the infected patient, in Lorian V (ed): *Significance of Medical Microbiology in the Care of Patients.* ed 1. Baltimore, The Williams & Wilkins Co, 1977, pp 186–197.

Sazie EM, Titus AE: Rapid diagnosis of *Campylobacter enteritis. Ann Intern Med* 1982;96:62–63.

Washington JA II: Blood cultures: Principles and techniques. *Mayo Clin Proc* 1975;50:91–98.

Wolinsky E: Mycobacteria: Significance of speciation and sensitivity tests, in Lorian V (ed): *Significance of Medical Microbiology in the Care of Patients.* ed 1. Baltimore, The Williams & Wilkins Co, 1977, pp 115–121.

This section views the humoral immune response as well as the products of this response as a means of diagnosing infectious disease. I describe briefly those pertinent aspects of the human immune system as well as the methodologies involved which help us diagnose specific infections.

Why Use the Serology Laboratory

Quite simply, properly used serological data can confirm clinical suspicions or diagnosis. In some situations the data provide the only laboratory evidence for a specific infection. Serological tests are the most easily accessible diagnostic aids for viral, parasitic, rickettsial, and chlamydial infections. Often they are the only means to diagnose one of these infections when the causative agent cannot be or is not easily isolated by existing methods.

Unfortunately, the impression has often been conveyed that much of the data generated by serology laboratories is at best only of academic interest. Useful data can be obtained *if active communication between physician and laboratory is pursued*. This communication provides the laboratory with information as to the appropriate methodology for the particular clinical setting. An understanding by the requesting physician of the methods used in the laboratory will then permit accurate interpretation of test results.

The various methodologies for measurement of antibody to *Toxoplasma gondii* serve as appropriate examples. A request received by a laboratory for an evaluation of immune status to this organism (ie, has this person ever been exposed to this agent?) permits the laboratory to use a single specimen and detection of immunoglobulin G (IgG) class of antibody. On the other hand if it is necessary to rule out a primary infection during pregnancy, then other more elaborate procedures are necessary.

Some Basic Principles for Obtaining Useful Serological Data

The first practical step is *save the sera*. Nearly all serological testing requires comparison of antibody titers (a titer is a semi-quantitative measure of levels of specific antibody).

Test results which allow us to draw some conclusions will be strengthened if serial specimens can be examined. This requires that either the laboratory or the physician have facilities for the storage of specimens, so that they may be held until the patient has been seen again and additional samples have been obtained.

Regardless of who stores these specimens it is important that serum be removed from the clot. Hemolyzed red cells and

T.J. Tinghitella

other products of cell death interfere with many assays. Sera should then be stored below 0 °C (most laboratories store sera at – 20 °C for short-term storage and – 70 °C for long-term storage).

Freezing and thawing of sera should be avoided since this may result in loss of specific immunoglobulin or may interfere with some serological techniques.

The "save the sera" principle makes possible the examination of acute- and convalescent-phase sera. The diagnosis of a recent infection requires the comparison of antibody levels during different phases of an infectious disease process. The physician must realize that the results obtained from a single specimen permit only evaluation of immune status or generation of epidemiological data from the surrounding "normal population." Laboratory "normal" ranges for single specimens or those obtained from the literature are of value if the patient falls within the parameters of the popula- tion from which the levels of specific antibody were drawn. A given patient may not fall into that population for one reason or another (socioeconomic background, past medical history, present medical problems, etc). Interpreta- tions based on the examination of a single specimen are fraught with danger and are to be discouraged. A case has often been made for interpreting an ex- tremely high titer as suggestive of a recent infection. The emphasis here is that these results only suggest a recent infection. A high titer may actually be a heterotypic rise due to infection by an agent that is a polyclonal activator of immunoglobulin synthesis. This nonspecific rise may also be observed in patients with autoimmune disease, chronic immunologic stimulation, or liver disease. All of these situations make it imperative that antibody to a number of closely related and other microorganisms be sought and that anti- body levels in acute-phase and convalescent-phase sera be compared.

Only when a seroconversion from negative to positive or a minimum of a fourfold increase in titer is obtained can a diagnosis of a recent infection be confirmed. The physician should make certain that sera from different phases of the disease process are tested in parallel and repeated by the laboratory for final confirmation of a rise in titer.

It is often difficult to obtain serum from a patient during the acute phase simply because of the delay from onset of symptoms to presentation to a physician. Nevertheless, it is still more suitable to obtain two specimens spaced two weeks apart than to interpret results from a single specimen.

Diagnosis of a Recent Infection by Class-Specific Antibody

IgM antibody has several features that distinguish it from IgG antibody. Some of these aspects have already been discussed in other chapters. Serologists are most interested in those characteristics which bear a par- ticular relationship to their ability to make diagnostic decisions concerning the etiology of infectious diseases.

Generally IgM antibody is produced during the initial or primary infection and is detectable for a limited period only. Since IgM-specific antibody often, but not invariably, appears before IgG-specific antibody, a useful rule of thumb is the presence or absence of this antibody class. In adults, low levels of specific IgM have been observed to persist after infection with some agents, making the sorting out of a recent and past infection more difficult.

Nonetheless, the detection of specific IgM raises the level of clinical suspicion and strongly supports a diagnosis of a primary infection.

There is some evidence to suggest that a rise in the specific IgM titer may also occur with recurrent infection or reinfection with the same or a closely related agent, so that serial determinations of specific IgM are useful in the diagnosis of reactivation of latent viral agents.

Specific antibody of the IgG class clearly persists for a long period of time, if not for life, although it may be seen to fluctuate somewhat with time as the immune status or health of the individual also changes. Detection of specific IgG antibody in a single specimen indicates only that antigenic exposure has occurred. As with acute- and convalescent-phase sera, only a significantly rising titer of specific IgG is evidence for a primary or reactivated infection.

One of the most interesting and useful contrasts, however, between IgG and IgM is that only IgG freely crosses the placenta; hence, in the neonate the IgG present is solely of maternal origin. It is not for some months later that the IgG is predominantly that of the child. If one uses methodologies which do not distinguish antibody class (as discussed below), then examination of the serum of newborns is simply looking at maternal antibody. IgM, on the other hand, does not cross the placenta; hence any IgM which is detected has been synthesized by the child. The concentrations of this immunoglobulin in infants are relatively low, less than 30 mg/dL, and do not reach adult levels until nearly the end of the first year of life. This fact provides the clinician with supportive evidence for the infectious etiology of congenital or neonatal disease. Elevated quantities of this immunoglobulin increase the level of suspicion and should be pursued by studies of specific IgM antibody to infectious agents. Table 10-1 provides a scheme of interpretation of IgM- and IgG-specific antibody in both the adult and neonate.

Serological Examination of Cerebrospinal Fluid

In normal persons the immunoglobulins are present in the cerebrospinal fluid by passive transfer. The levels of specific antibody there are much too low to be detected by the routine methods found in a serology laboratory.

Table 10-1
Generalized Scheme of Antibody Response in Patients with Primary or Recurrent Viral Infections

	Acute Serum		Convalescent Serum		
	IgG	IgM	IgG	IgM	Interpretation
Adults	+	+	+	+	No evidence of recent infection
	−	−	+	+	Primary infection
	+	−	+	+	Recurrent infection
Neonates	+	−	Not done		No evidence for infection
	+	+	Not done		Probable congenital infection
	+	−	+	+	Primary neonatal infection

166

During the course of meningeal or encephalitic disease, cells recruited to the site of infection may produce specific immunoglobulin. Under these circumstances, the levels of antibody may be measurable by routine methods and surely would be measurable by sensitive techniques such as radioimmune assay and enzyme-linked assay (see methods of detection below).

An ideal situation would be to examine the cerebrospinal fluid serially for a change in specific antibody titer. If this cannot be accomplished for humane or ethical reasons then comparative examination of serum and cerebrospinal fluid may be useful. Recent publications have suggested that the levels of specific antibody in cerebrospinal fluid should be 1/20 or less of that observed in serum. This consideration, then, is needed particularly in cases where the levels of specific antibody in serum are elevated and hence elevated nonspecifically in the cerebrospinal fluid.

Routine Methods of Antibody Measurement

Agglutination Tests

The earliest serological tests for the detection of antibody were those that either caused agglutination of particulate antigens or resulted in the formation of precipitates from soluble antigen matrixes. These methods are still used in most clinical laboratories for the detection of antibody to the well-studied bacteria which cause acute febrile illnesses. Generally these tests utilize whole, killed bacteria and are performed in an aqueous phase (generally a buffer at a particular pH, in tubes or on glass slides). Patient serum is generally diluted serially and mixed with the antigen. Observation of an agglutination pattern is then made after an appropriate incubation period. The agglutination produced is the result of the cross-linking of the particulate or soluble antigen by IgM and IgG specific for that antigen. The efficiency of IgM in this matrix is much greater due to its larger number of binding sites.

A qualitative determination of class-specific antibody can be made by chemicals that decrease the efficiency of agglutination, notably, 2-mercapthoethanol or dithiotreitol. Primary infections with *Brucella* can often be demonstrated by running in parallel untreated patient sera and patient sera treated with one of the above-mentioned reducing agents. The presence of IgM antibody and hence evidence for a recent infection is circumstantially obtained by significant reduction in the agglutination titer of the treated sera as compared with the untreated sera. Most clinical laboratories, however, do not deal with such reagents that are noxious and toxic. Only specimens with high titers of antibody should be examined by this method.

Agglutination reactions have been extended beyond particulate antigens by their chemical attachment to red blood cells or to small latex particles. An excellent example of this type of methodology is the indirect hemoagglutination assay for the detection of antibody to *T. gondii*. Various types of blood cells are used by different commercial companies, but the technology is basically the same. Antigen extracts from *T. gondii* are bound to red blood cells. In the presence of antibody these red cells now agglutinate and in so doing form a mat-like appearance at the bottom of a tube or a microtiter plate. The appropriate controls are required, one of which is to determine whether there is agglutination of red cells by nonspecific or non-antigen detecting antibody.

CF Assays

Complement fixation (CF) assays—at best cumbersome and tedious—have been the backbone of serological testing for viral antigens as well as some other microorganisms. Recently it has been streamlined for performance in microtiter plates or read spectrophotometrically. The basic principles, however, are the same and can be found in any serology or immunology manual. Briefly, the assay system can be used for detection of either antigen or antibody. In the clinical serology laboratory it is used to detect antibody, whereas in the clinical virology laboratory it is used to detect or to type viral antigens. The assay is simply a competition for complement (added exogenously) by the antigen-antibody system being detected and the binding of anti-red blood cell antibody and red cells. If complement is bound by the antibody being sought, none remains to be bound by the red blood cell–anti-red blood cell complex and the cells remain intact. Results are generally reported as a titer. Unfortunately, in this assay the freezing and thawing of specimens, bacterial contamination, or high levels of lipoprotein also bind complement. Hence, specimens submitted for analysis should be freshly drawn, separated from the clot, and frozen only once before testing. Sera in which hemolysis has occurred are unsuitable for testing.

Most important, it is essential for the clinician to interpret results obtained by this method as previously outlined. CF tests as generally performed do not inform us as to the class of antibody, hence the requirements for an acute and convalescent specimen. In addition, many viral antigens tested by CF demonstrate heterotypic rises. Antibody to a number of closely related viral agents should be requested. Only those with the most significant rises (fourfold) should be considered as supporting evidence for a recent infection.

IFA and EIA

More recently, indirect immunofluorescence assays (IFA) have found their place in the clinical laboratory routine. A significant modification of this basic methodology known as the enzyme-linked immunospecific or immunosorbent assay (EIA) is becoming increasingly popular, but has not yet replaced more well-known techniques for many popular tests. Either methodology used is characterized as a sandwich technique and follows the sequence outlined below. The antigen, whether viral, bacterial, or fungal, is passively adsorbed to either a solid support or a glass slide. The antigen can be either the entire microorganism itself, as in most IFA for bacterial and fungal antigens, or cell cultures infected with a particular virus. EIA technology generally uses an extract or a soluble antigen that is either passively adsorbed to tubes, beads, or disks of paper or covalently attached to these same solid supports. The serum in which antibody is to be detected is then incubated with these attached antigens. Unattached or nonspecific antibody is then removed by successive washings. This is then followed by incubating a tagged antibody; that is, anti-human immunoglobulin which is conjugated or covalently linked to a fluorescent molecule such as fluorescein or rhodamine (for use in indirect fluorescent assays) or attached to an enzyme such as horseradish peroxidase or alkaline phosphatase (for use in EIA methods). A positive result is either the last dilution of patient serum that is fluorescent as compared with the negative sera or the color change of an enzyme substrate. Indirect fluorescent assays, of course, require the use of microscopes equipped with a wavelength of light which will cause excitation of the fluorescent molecule. EIA can often be read visually, although most laboratories prefer to use a spectrophotometer to measure the extent of the color change.

These assays are faster and more efficient than CF and agglutination tests and more importantly, they permit the determination of class-specific antibody.

Unfortunately, they have their own disadvantages. IFA and EIA tests when read visually are subject to a great deal of reader variation, making it imperative that only results from the same laboratory be compared. Both methods are subject to false-negatives and -positives. Generally these problems are due to interferences by rheumatoid factor of high levels of IgG antibody competing for antigenic sites. Competent laboratories, however, can provide technical services which (with careful interpretation) can provide significant evidence for primary or recent infections.

The State of the Art

The clinician should be aware that not all serological tests are done by the same technology. Different organisms require different levels of technical sophistication. It is also important to keep in mind that different methodologies may not only give different types of information but may also provide more sensitive or more specific information for that particular disease. *Only by discussion with the laboratorian will this information be available to the physician.*

Miscellaneous Methods

Detection of antibody to some agents is best accomplished by methods tailored to a particular characteristic of the organism. A striking example is detection of antibody to streptococcus. The antigens detected are to the enzymes produced by the organism: streptolysin, hyaluronidase, and DNase B. Antibody is measured by the inhibition of the activity of these enzymes. Regardless of this, the general rules of serology of a need for a rising titer or the cautious interpretation of elevated titers apply. Unfortunately, these assays as done in clinical laboratories do not allow for antibody class determination. More recently, latex particles or red blood cells coated with extracts of these enzymes have become popular, altering the method of an agglutination assay. As would be expected, titers obtained by this method do not correlate very well with those obtained by the more classical methods of enzyme inhibition. In addition these tests are susceptible to all of the problems associated with particle agglutination.

Methods of Antigen Detection

Although the above discussions have emphasized the detection of antibody, all of the above techniques can be altered to detect antigen. Antisera prepared in animals replaces the human sera in which previously antibody was being detected. The best example of this is the direct fluorescent antibody technique. Fluorescence indicates the presence of viral or bacterial antigens in smears, aspirates, sedimented urine, or biopsy material.

Latex agglutination has also been used to detect antigen. Again, the methodology used is similar to that described above. The surface of the latex particle is coated with antiserum, with agglutination occurring in the presence of antigen. False-positives do occur if rheumatoid factor is present, but this is easily controlled by using latex particles coated with nonspecific immunoglobulin from the same animal species. Many commercial kits are now available for the detection of cryptococcal antigen, *Haemophilus influenzae* type b as well as streptococci. The methods work best when the body fluid examined is cerebrospinal fluid but serum and urine can also be tested. The principle advantages are increased sensitivity over other methods (see counterimmunoelectrophoresis, below), speed (generally requires no more than 30 minutes [total time] for results), and the ability to detect antigen even when antibiotic therapy has begun.

A similar method is coagglutination; a particular strain of *Staphylococcus aureus* possesses a protein (called protein A) which binds to the Fc portion of immunoglobulin (notably IgG). The surface of the organism can easily be coated with specific antiserum. In the presence of antigen the staphylococcus aureus is observed to agglutinate. This technique has the same advantages as latex agglutination, but theoretically is not as susceptible to the number of false-positives due to the presence of rheumatoid factor. Most often, microbiology laboratories employ this technique for typing cultured organisms rather than for detection of antigen in body fluids.

Countercurrent immunoelectrophoresis or counterimmunoelectrophoresis (CIE) has been used for rapid detection of antigen for the past decade. CIE employs the force of an electric current to drive antigen and specific antibody together with the formation of a visible precipitin line in a solid support such as agarose. Its advantages are similar to latex and coagglutination, although it generally requires more time than latex or coagglutination. It is somewhat less sensitive than either of these, although this depends on the antisera used. Its major disadvantage appears to be that some antigens do not move in an electric field.

It is important for the clinician to remember that, although all of these rapid tests provide answers in a short period of time, they are no substitute for culturing the organism when possible. The need for determining antibiotic sensitivity still remains. *Hence, the clinician should remember that a specimen sent to a laboratory for antigen detection must also be sent for culture.*

Update on Some Clinically Important Infections

Streptococcal Disease
Serological evidence for streptococcal disease is often more useful than throat culture because of the high carriage rate in the normal population. Most physicians are familiar with the antistreptolysin O (ASLO) test (see miscellaneous methods, above) with results often expressed in Todd units (based on the standardization of streptolysine used). An elevated result may be a useful indicator in adults with pyoderma or streptococcal complications such as in acute glomerulonephritis.

A number of other tests measuring antibody to streptococcal enzymes have been developed in recent years, notably anti-DNase B and anti-hyaluronidase tests. Although the performance of all these tests would be ideal for diagnosis of streptococcal disease, the best single test appears to be the anti-DNase B test. It is reproducible by competent laboratory technologists and extremely sensitive. In addition, it is subject to fewer false-positives than the ASLO. It is now the test of choice for streptococcal pyoderma and useful in the diagnosis of acute rheumatic fever and Syndenham's chorea.

Antigen detection is easily accomplished by the latex agglutination test with a commercially available kit and is useful in the diagnosis of streptococcal meningitis in neonates.

Streptococcus Pneumoniae

Until recently there was little need for antibody measurements in patients with pneumococcal pneumonia. The advent of the polyvalent pneumococcal vaccine for "at risk" populations makes it more than an academic exercise. The assays developed for measurement of antibody to *S. pneumoniae* are not readily available in most laboratories because of the need to assay each one of the serotypes by radioimmune assay. Measurements of an antibody response to the vaccine should not be undertaken until two to three weeks after inoculation. The antibody appears to be long lasting, but reaches a peak response at about one month postvaccination.

Although culture is still the most valuable tool for the diagnosis of bronchial pneumonia, counterimmunoelectrophoresis for detection of antigen is useful. Serum and urine appear to be good specimens for counterimmunoelectrophoresis detection with true-positive results occurring more frequently in urine.

Legionella

The laboratory diagnosis of legionellosis relies primarily on culturing the organisms (presently six serotypes as well as numerous legionella-like organisms). Detection of legionella organisms can also be accomplished by direct fluorescent antibody testing of appropriate body tissue using specific antisera. Sputum examinations in this disorder are unreliable. Transtracheal aspirates or lung biopsy are the specimens of choice for detection of these organisms.

Epidemiological or retrospective studies can be accomplished by indirect fluorescence tests using cultured organisms. The general rules of serology apply here, particularly since little or no work regarding class-specific antibody has been accomplished.

Mycoplasma Pneumoniae

The culturing of mycoplasma organisms is still not easily accomplished in routine bacteriology laboratories; hence, the diagnosis of this disease still relies heavily on serological methods. The most specific and sensitive test for antibody to this organism is the metabolic inhibition test, which prevents growth of a stock culture of mycoplasma. This test is not generally available to most physicians. What is available is the CF or IFA test. Again, the general rules of serology apply. Cold agglutinins, although useful when they appear (particularly when a rise is observed) are nonspecific and occur, at best, in only 50% of patients with primary atypical pneumonia.

Cryptococcus Neoformans

Rapid detection of *C. neoformans* has been accomplished by a widely available latex agglutination assay. Semiquantitative levels of this antigen can be measured by this method, making it a suitable test for following the efficacy of the intensive therapy that is often needed for treatment of this disease.

Herpes Simplex

Herpes simplex infection is generally indicated by typical vesicular lesions from which the virus is readily cultured. In the absence of these lesions (during the periods of quiescence) or if a clinical virology laboratory is not readily available, serological investigations become important. In addition, diagnosis of encephalitis may also be accomplished serologically, particularly if both cerebrospinal fluid and serum are examined. In theory, if both fluids are positive, it may not be necessary to perform a brain biopsy.

CF has been the mainstay of serological testing for herpes virus infection or recurrences. While it still has its place, it suffers from the usual disadvantages of CF tests and in addition cannot distinguish infections of herpes simplex type 1 from type 2. The use of immunofluorescence can determine the serotype or type of each virus as well as detect the presence of class specific IgM antibody in neonates or immunocompromised patients (see Table 10-1).

CMV

Essentially the same type of assays and interpretations made with herpes simplex virus apply to the diagnosis of cytomegalovirus (CMV) infection. Although a number of antigenic and genetic variants of CMV do exist and cause disease, they generally are not significant problems in serological diagnosis. Detection of class specific antibody to CMV is useful for diagnosis of infection in infants and for detection of recurrent infection in renal transplant patients.

Rubella

Determination of immune status to rubella can be accomplished by either the standard HIA or more recently by a commercially available EIA. When the need for determining a recent infection with rubella does arise during pregnancy, the presence of IgM with a rising IgG titer by IFA or EIA can provide this information.

Infectious Mononucleosis

Nonspecific agglutination tests for the detection of the heterophile antibody which arises during the course of infectious mononucleosis is still the most useful serological indicator. A number of commercially available kits of easily performed agglutination assays are available, but they require a significant amount of technical skill in interpretation. Those assays which utilize adsorptions to remove other agglutinins are the most reliable for use as spot tests. A number of laboratories today will screen patient sera with a spot test and then employ some other method for confirmation. Commonly used is the ox cell hemolysin test. It is very important for the clinician to discuss with the laboratory the tests performed to determine the sequence of events that occur in establishing a diagnosis of infectious mononucleosis.

The physician should also be aware that while nearly all serum from patients with mononucleosis will become heterophile positive, a single determination in the face of the clinical symptoms of the disease or other laboratory findings (lymphocytosis, increased number of atypical lymphocytes) is not sufficient. A second examination of the serum should be undertaken a few days later.

If the serum of a patient continues to remain negative, a laboratory should be sought which performs the specific tests for antibody toward Epstein-Barr virus.

Toxoplasma Gondii

Infection with *T. gondii* as a significant cause of adult and neonatal disease has only been recognized within the past few years. As with many of the other agents discussed in which congenital disease can be serious, it is important for the clinician to communicate the purpose for which the assay is being sought. If one is interested in immune status, then the standard hemagglutination test (similar rubella screening described above) is sufficient. However, if the diagnosis of a recent maternal infection or congenital infection is necessary, then methods identifying IgM specific antibody are essential for correct interpretation.

Conclusion

Communication between the physician and laboratory about the purpose for which a test is being requested and the methods by which these tests are accomplished can provide significant confirming or supporting evidence for the etiology of an infectious disease process. Measurment of IgM- or IgG-specific antibody, because of their different biological properties, can help distinguish recent infections.

Immunodiagnosis of infectious disease antigens can also be accomplished rapidly with such techniques as CIE, latex, or coagglutination.

These newer techniques, coupled with a philosophy of communication between laboratory and physician, can make serology a useful tool in diagnosis.

■ Selected Readings

Cappel R, de Cuyper F, de Braekaleer J: Rapid detection of IgG and IgM antibodies for cytomegalovirus by the enzyme-linked immunosorbent assay (Elisa). *Arch Virol* 1978;58: 253–258.

Carroll JF, Booss J: Cerebrospinal fluid IgG level in herpes simplex encephalitis. *JAMA* 1976;236:2092–2093.

Cradock-Watson JE, Bourne MS, Vandervelde EM: IgG, IgA and IgM responses in acute rubella determined by the immunofluorescent technique. *J Hyg (London)* 1972;70:473–483.

Gardner PS, McQuillin J: Detection of virus-specific IgM by immunofluorescence, in *Rapid Virus Diagnosis*. London, Butterworths, 1980, p 259.

Groedbolk-DeGroot LE, Michel-Bensing N, Vanes-Boon MM, et al: Comparison of the titers of ASO, anti-DNase, and antibodies against the group polysaccharide of Group A streptococci in children with streptococcal infections. *J Clin Pathol* 1974;27:891–896.

Grant S, Edward E, Syme J: A prospective study of cytomegalovirus infection in pregnancy. 1. Laboratory evidence of congenital infection following maternal primary and reactivated infection. *J Infect* 1981;3:24–31.

Reimer CB, Black CM, Philips DJ, et al: The specificity of fetal IgM: Antibody or anti-antibody. *NY Acad Sci* 1975; 254:77.

Thirumorrthi MC, Dajani AS: Comparison of staphylococcal coagglutinations, latex agglutination and counterimmunoelectrophoresis for bacterial antigen detection. *J Clin Microbiol* 1979;9:28–32.

Voller A, Bidwell DE: Enzyme immunoassays for antibodies in measles, cytomegalovirus infections and after rubella vaccination. *Br J Exp Pathol* 1976;57:243–247.

Cells and Antibodies of the Immune System: Testing for Immunodeficiency

Lymphocytes located throughout the body comprise the essential cells of the immune system. Lymphocytes can be divided into B cells (Bursa equivalent or bone marrow derived) and T cells (thymus derived). B lymphocytes differentiate into plasma cells, which produce antibodies that play a major role in humoral immune defenses for fighting bacterial infections. In contrast, cellular immune responses are mediated by T cells and function primarily in fighting infections due to viruses, fungi, and facultative intracellular bacteria such as mycobacteria. The division of the immune system into humoral and cellular compartments is useful as long as it is kept in mind that together they form a functional unit and interact in many and often complicated ways. T and B lymphocytes cannot be distinguished by light or electron microscopy. Both are small mononuclear cells with a large nuclear/cytoplasm ratio. Differences can be determined by examining surface markers and functional properties.

T Lymphocytes (SRBC Rosetting Cells)

In most laboratories T cells are quantitated by mixing sheep red blood cells (SRBC) with a mononuclear fraction of blood leukocytes (polymorphs are removed). The mixture is centrifuged together and carefully resuspended. The SRBC adhere selectively to the cell membrane of T cells forming cellular aggregations that are called E rosettes (E for erythrocyte). The percentage of E rosettes is the percentage of the total mononuclear cells that are T cells. They can be purified from B cells by separating the rosetting cells and lysing the SRBC, leaving a pure population of T cells.

Some congenital immunodeficiency diseases (such as DiGeorge's syndrome, in which the thymus is absent) feature low numbers of T lymphocytes, and some viral infections have been shown to reduce T-cell numbers. In some autoimmune diseases the suppressor subset is decreased, and this may be one reason for overactive B-cell responses leading to autoantibodies and hypergammaglobulinemia. Evaluation of the in vivo functional capacity of the T-cell system is most easily accomplished by delayed-type hypersensitivity (DTH) skin testing. Skin testing with commonly encountered antigens such as *Candida,* purified protein derivative of tuberculin, trichophyton, streptokinase/streptodornase, and tetanus toxoid serves as a simple and valuable screening test. Nearly all patients react to one of these antigens in 24–48 hours with erythema and induration of more than 5 mm. A normal response to intradermal skin testing requires intact T-cell and

P. W. Askenase
T. J. Swartz
K. Erlendsson
T. J. Tinghitella

175

macrophage function. In small children that have not had sufficient experience with these antigens, T-cell function can be evaluated in vivo simply by skin testing with the T-cell mitogen phytohemagglutinin (PHA). This substance activates T cells non-specifically and they produce a skin test response similar to activation by specific antigen. Thus, DTH skin tests with antigens can be negative if the T cells have not been exposed to the antigen before, but the PHA skin test should be positive if the cells are present and normal.

In vitro assays of T-cell function are restricted to specialized laboratories of large referral centers and are only necessary in unusual cases.

B Lymphocytes

B cells do not form spontaneous rosettes with SRBC. In contrast to T cells, B cells have on their surface easily detectable immunoglobulins. These are similar to serum antibodies that are secreted when B cells are introduced by antigen and T cells to differentiate into plasma cells. B cells are enumerated by staining their surface immunoglobulin with fluorescein-conjugated, anti-human immunoglobulin. The distribution of B cells in the body is different from that of T cells. They are shorter-lived cells (7–10 days versus 30 years) and usually not as common in the circulation. They differentiate in the bone marrow and reside there, in peripheral lymph nodes, and in the spleen. Within a lymph node the B cells reside in the cortical areas, forming germinal centers that become very pronounced when cellular proliferation, caused by antigen exposure, takes place. In contrast, T cells reside closer to the hilus in the paracortical area in a more uniform distribution. Immunoglobulin levels (quantitative serum immunoglobulins) are a simple and highly reliable screening test of B cell function in vivo. With normal quantitative immunoglobulin levels, B-cell abnormalities can virtually be ruled out. In rare cases with low immunoglobulin levels (congenital and acquired hypogammaglobulinemias), quantitation of immunoglobulin surface-positive B cells is helpful.

In Bruton's congenital, sex-linked agammaglobulinemia, B cells are totally absent. In acquired cases of hypogammaglobulinemia, B cells can be present, but do not differentiate into antibody-forming plasma cells because of intrinsic defects, insufficient T cell help, or overactive suppressor cell function.

Immunoglobulins

Immunoglobulins are a diverse group of plasma proteins produced when B cells are induced by antigen and helper T cells to differentiate into antibody-producing plasma cells. Normal serum contains a mixture of antibodies. Levels can become very high when the humoral immune system is stimulated, accounting for the polyclonal hypergammaglobulinemia seen in inflammation and infections.

Five classes (isotypes) of immunoglobulins have been identified on the basis of structure and function. Immunoglobulin G (IgG) is the most abundant group with the basic structure of immunoglobulins: two heavy chains and two light chains. IgG binds antigen very avidly and can activate complement to promote phagocytosis and induce cytolysis. Absent IgG severely damages the body's defense against bacteria and viruses, although many viruses are resisted by T cell-dependent mechanisms.

IgA is the second most abundant class of immunoglobulin in serum. However, its best known function is in secretions of the gastrointestinal and respiratory tracts. It exists there in a dimer form connected by a J-chain and secretory piece made by surface epithelial cells. Approximately one person per 400 has an IgA deficiency, the most common immunodeficiency. Most persons with IgA deficiency are asymptomatic, but some have an increased incidence of infections, especially upper respiratory tract infections and otitis media. Coincident deficiences of IgG subclasses (IgG_1, IgG_2, IgG_3, or IgG_4) may contribute to the predisposition to infection in some of these patients. Low IgA is often associated with infantile diarrhea. There is an increased incidence of Giardia infestation in the gut and of Crohn's disease in patients with low IgA.

IgM is a large molecule composed of five basic immunoglobulin units joined by a J-chain. It is the class that appears first after antigen stimulation and has good antigen-binding capacity and superb complement-binding activity. Isolated IgM deficiency is very rare.

Serum IgD is present in low concentrations, and its function is unknown. IgE antibody is associated with atopic allergic diseases. The level in serum is often high in such instances, especially in atopic dermatitis.

Normal immunoglobulin levels in serum vary from one laboratory to another and with age (Table 11-1).

Workup of Immunodeficiency

Frequent and persistent infections are the problem that most often makes a physician consider an immune deficiency. Other well-known and less well explained problems such as infantile diarrhea, atopic eczema, and autoimmune diseases can also be associated with abnormalities of the immune system.

After history and physical examination, simple screening tests can be undertaken. A complete blood cell count with differential counts gives the number of neutrophils, eosinophils, and lymphocytes. A total lymphocyte count of $< 1500/mm^3$ may indicate that an immunodeficiency is present. Quantitative immunoglobulins in serum and IgA level and secretory piece in saliva are good screening tests for the integrity of the humoral immune system. DTH skin tests with common antigens or PHA will grossly evaluate the cellular immune system. Low immunoglobulin levels or no response to skin testing require further investigations, usually in research laboratories. A

Table 11-1
Variations of Immunoglobulins with Age*

Age	IgG (mg/dL)	IgM (mg/dL)	IgA (mg/dL)
Newborn	1000 ± 200	10 ± 5	2 ± 3
1–12 mo	600 ± 250	40 ± 5	30 ± 20
13–24 mo	750 ± 200	60 ± 20	50 ± 20
3–16 yr	900 ± 200	60 ± 20	130 ± 60
Adult	1100 ± 300	100 ± 30	200 ± 50

*These values are adapted from Stiehm ER, and Fudenberg HH, *Pediatrics* 1966;37:715. They are not the result of any particular statistical study, but rather represent the accumulated data and experience of the author.

simple and convenient method to differentiate congenital from acquired hypogammaglobulinemia is to look at iso-hemagglutinins or to follow anti-viral titers after routine childhood immunizations. Iso-hemagglutinins are IgM antibodies to blood group antigens present on the red cells of other individuals. They probably are found in response to cross-reacting antigens of microorganisms that stimulate the immune system. Viral titers after vaccination are largely due to IgG antibodies. Thus, the presence of iso-hemagglutinins and antiviral titers after routine immunizations suggests that normal IgM and IgG responses have occurred. This favors the diagnosis of acquired rather than congenital hypogammaglobulinemia.

The importance of understanding each patient's immune defect becomes clear when we look at the progress that has been made in treatment and reconstitution of immunodeficiencies. It is also very important to know about immune defects in a particular patient. Even though the defect may not be corrected, such patients require a different approach when dealing with an infection that would be considered minor in a normal host.

Immediate Versus Delayed Hypersensitivity

Immediate Wheal and Flare Skin Tests

Immediate wheal and flare skin tests are useful in evaluation of atopic allergic diseases. They are the simplest, quickest, most sensitive, and most useful tests for detecting IgE antibody-mediated sensitivity to allergens, as occurs in allergic rhinitis, asthma, and stinging insect sensititivity. By injecting intradermally extracts containing allergens from pollens, animal danders, fungi, and dust, the presence of allergen-specific IgE antibodies on skin mast cells is detected because IgE-sensitized mast cells release histamine and other vasoactive substances. This gives rise to a wheal and flare skin reaction that can be interpreted semiquantitatively depending upon the size of the wheal and presence of pseudopods. A negative reaction shows no wheal and flare or at least less than the control injection of saline diluent. A 3–4 mm wheal with erythema is considered +; a 4–8 mm wheal and erythema + +; over 8 mm wheal with erythema but without pseudopods + + +; and a wheal, erythema and pseudopods should be considered + + + +. Pseudopods are important because their presence indicates a strong reaction with leakage of large amounts of fluid from the vessels filling the interstitial space and dissecting around vessels and nerves to form pseudopods. A positive reaction develops within 20 minutes and is designated immediate-type hypersensitivity.

In many instances there is a good correlation between positive wheal and flare skin tests and clinical symptoms (eg, ragweed-induced allergic rhinitis). Skin testing for immediate hypersensitivity to stinging insects gives the most accurate results of all skin tests. It may be that these skin tests with actual venom proteins simulate the natural stimulus and, therefore, are more reliable. There are other instances where correlation is not as good, but the test is useful in documenting definite IgE-dependent allergic sensitivity, as in patients who are resistant to parting with an offending cat or dog. One possible explanation for a poor correlation between skin test results and clinical symptoms is that IgE antibody may be lacking on mast cells at the skin test site (giving a negative reaction), but may be present on cells in the organ(s) giving symptoms. Another possibility is that IgE is necessary, but may not be sufficient, to give rise to clinical symptoms, a suggestion that seems to gain support when looking at radioallergosorbent test results (see below).

Skin tests are far less useful in detecting food allergy. There are false-negatives and -positives, some food extracts give irritative reactions, and the relevant antigen, modified by digestion, may be lacking in the usual extracts used for skin testing.

Sometimes allergens are introduced into the skin by prick or scratch tests instead of intradermal testing. Scratch tests are particularly useful in children who abhor injections. Also, less antigen is introduced, and irritative reactions are less likely.

Total IgE Levels

Measurement of total IgE in serum does not identify the cause for an allergic reaction. Atopic patients, that is, those with a familial tendency to form IgE antibody in response to environmental allergens, usually have higher total IgE levels than normal persons. In addition to the classical atopic diseases, ie, asthma, hay fever, infantile eczema, and acute urticaria, IgE has been found elevated in other instances such as parasitic infestations, IgE myeloma, certain disorders of immunoregulation, acute graft versus host reactions, mononucleosis, sarcoid, coccidioidomycosis, some cases of pulmonary hemosiderosis and rheumatoid arthritis.

The concentration of IgE in the serum of nonatopic healthy persons is much less than that of all the other immunoglobulins. Therefore, quantitative methods are of necessity different from those used for the other immunoglobulins. Routine measurements are made by either solid-phase radio immunoassay (RIA) or by an enzyme-linked immunosorbent assay (ELISA). Concentrations are generally reported in international units (1 IU = 10 ng). Many laboratories today utilize commercially available kits which are well standardized. Nonetheless, if serial determinations are to be made it is wise to compare results from the same laboratory.

There are few clinical indications for the measurement of total IgE in serum. Essentially, it is a means of differentiating some IgE-mediated from non-IgE-mediated disorders. Hence, a workup for diseases such as rhinitis, asthma, dermatitis, chronic urticaria, and food intolerance may benefit from quantitation of IgE. Unfortunately, IgE levels can be within established normal ranges even in IgE-mediated diseases, and nonatopic disorders such as parasitic infestations can elevate total IgE, but are usually diagnosed by other means.

Present data suggest that serum IgE levels are useful in confirming clinical diagnoses and provide supportive evidence when differential diagnosis of allergic disease is difficult. One must not discount allergy when levels are low or normal and must not automatically diagnose allergy when the level is high.

Tests for Allergen-Specific IgE Antibodies (RAST)

In RAST (radioallergosorbent tests), particles coated with a particular allergen are mixed with the patient's serum. IgE antibodies to the allergen will bind to the particle. The IgE is then detected by the addition of radiolabeled anti-IgE antibodies and compared with particles incubated with normal sera. Attempts to correlate the diagnostic value of a positive RAST (which measures antigen-specific IgE antibodies) with in vivo allergen challenge tests such as skin tests or nasal or bronchial provocation tests (which are more sensitive and measure IgE-triggered release of mediators and subsequent tissue responses) have yielded correlations from 40% to 90% depending on the allergen. Correlation with severity of clinical symptoms is even less. Skin testing is more sensitive, and results are available immediately. RAST is most useful in suggesting specific allergens in a situation when skin tests cannot be performed.

Thus, RAST should be reserved for those patients who, for either physical or emotional reasons, cannot tolerate skin testing. In addition it should be used in only those situations in which IgE-mediated disease has been implicated. For example, while some laboratories may offer RAST for "allergy" to codeine, or contrast media, there is no evidence to implicate an IgE-mediated response in these reactions.

In evaluating an atopic patient, the history is of paramount importance, whereas skin tests and, to a lesser extent, RAST serve most often as confirmatory tools that are useful when their limitations are kept in mind.

DTH Skin Tests
DTH skin tests are used to evaluate T cell competence in vivo. In contrast to immediate-type hypersensitivity, these delayed-onset reactions begin 6 to 8 hours after intradermal injection of antigen and are read at 24, 48, or 72 hours. In these reactions, T cells, rather than mast cells, are of primary importance, and IgE plays no role. DTH responses are characterized by *prolonged* erythema and induration. No reaction takes place unless normal T cells that were sensitized by prior exposure to the antigen are present. Challenge by intradermal injection of antigens such as streptokinase/streptodornase, tetanus toxoid, or *Candida* results in presentation of antigen by skin macrophages to specific T cells. The T cells then release lymphokines locally, leading to a cellular infiltrate. Normal DTH skin reactions (erythema and induration >5 mm in diameter) suggest grossly intact cellular immune responsiveness. Anergy (inability to mount DTH response to previously encountered antigens) is seen in primary T-cell immune deficiencies and also transiently in many infectious diseases (tuberculosis, certain viral infections), malignancies, connective tissue disorders, and sarcoidosis. Further evaluation of T-cell function in such instances requires specialized in vitro studies, usually in research laboratories.

Quantitation of Immunoglobulins and Complement in Serum and Cerebrospinal Fluid
Introduction
The quantitative assessment of the major immunoglobulins as well as complement components found to be most useful clinically is accomplished by similar techniques. Hence most laboratories can measure serum IgG, IgA, IgM, C3, and C4. IgE requires more sensitive assays.

Methodological Considerations
Quantitation of these serum proteins is most often performed by one of the

following methods: (1) radial immunodiffusion, (2) nephelometry, or (3) rocket or Laurell electrophoresis.

Radial immunodiffusion quantitates a specific serum protein such as C3 by including specific antibody to that protein in an agarose support medium. Patients' sera are added in defined volumes to wells cut into the agarose, and the serum component diffuses out from the well radially until a critical concentration is reached and a precipitate is formed with the antibody in the agar. Since agarose is clear, precipitation of antigen (C3) and antibody (anti-C3) complex can be observed. This precipitation of an insoluble antigen-antibody complex takes the form of a circle whose diameter squared is directly proportional to the concentration of the protein (C3) being measured. Quantitative results are obtained by comparison of these circles to those obtained with known standards. This technique has become the standard procedure in most laboratories, principally because it is inexpensive and gives reproducible results. However, it has a number of disadvantages. Since it is dependent on diffusion it generally requires 24 to 72 hours to give results. This time is extended further if the specimen has abnormally high or low values, since these samples usually need to be rerun after dilution (when values are high) or with substitute gels with greater sensitivity (when values are low). *Thus, if high or low values are anticipated you should warn the laboratory when submitting the sample.*

Recently, nephelometric techniques have been popularized. These have become fully automated, making it the technique of choice. Nephelometry measures by light scatter the rate of formation of antigen-antibody complexes. Results are obtained in a matter of minutes, as compared with hours or days, and there is little variability. Its major disadvantage is that it consumes more antiserum, resulting in higher reagent costs. It is also less suitable for quantitation of immunoglobulins in those sera which are highly lipemic and in those with cytoglobulin activity, because these produce light scatter.

Regardless of the technique for quantitative measurement of proteins, discrepancies in results both within and between laboratories arise from the use of different anti-serum preparations as well as different standards. The World Health Organization provides reference standards for many of these proteins, and we recommend that laboratories be sought which utilize these standards.

Clinical Usefulness

Patients suspected of having an inherited or acquired deficiency of immunoglobulins can only be assessed accurately by quantitation of these proteins in serum. In addition, a thorough investigation requires an assessment of IgA in external body secretions such as saliva or intestinal juice. Although it is not necessary or technically easy to quantitate IgA in these fluids, one should have the laboratory examine in a qualitative manner not only the presence of IgA but also its secretory component. The absence of both these proteins would indicate that IgA is either not synthesized or not transported into the environment in which it does its work.

The clinician should also keep in mind that normal total immunoglobulin concentrations do not exclude the possibility of deficiencies of particular subclasses (ie, IgG_1, IgG_2, IgG_3, IgG_4) or *specific* antibody deficiency or immune unresponsiveness. Patients with immunoglobulin deficiencies who receive gamma globulin therapy should be monitored serially for the effectiveness of treatment. Ideally this should be accomplished by using the same method of quantitation.

Measurements of serum immunoglobulins are also useful in distinguishing the so-called benign monoclonal gammopathies. In multiple myeloma there is a progressive rise in the monoclonal component and a decrease in serum polyclonal immunoglobulins, whereas in more benign disease the monoclonal component is not as elevated (< 2 g/dL) and the (polyclonal) immunoglobulins remain within the normal range.

In contrast to normal or polyclonal immunoglobulins, many monoclonal immunoglobulins are difficult to measure by immunochemical means. Radial immunodiffusion often underestimates their concentration, as the antibody used to measure them is prepared against "normal" immunoglobulins. The avidity or tightness of the antigen-antibody interaction is generally reduced. These reactions make it more accurate to monitor changes in the quantity of a monoclonal protein by some other means. Generally, this is done by measuring the area under a monoclonal "spike" as obtained by serum electrophoresis (see below). If immunochemical means must be used, then care must be taken to use the same preparation of antibody in the assay.

Radial immunodiffusion and nephelometry provide information on the concentration of some of the individual components of the complement system. Although the complement system (both classical and alternative pathways) has over 15 components, it is generally only useful to measure two or three of these in most clinical situations. It should be emphasized that these measurements do not directly inform us of the functional nature of complement or the components, but rather of the concentration of antigenic determinants of the components. Although measurements of complement components by immunochemical means are not as sensitive to changes induced by handling and storage, compared with assays for functional complement activity, a serum specimen should be delivered to a laboratory within a few hours after being drawn. If not, it should be separated from the clot and frozen for delivery to the laboratory. In contrast, any functional studies require processing within one hour and freezing the serum at $-70\,°C$ or lower.

Quantitation of C3 and C4 together provides the bulk of clinically useful information, although many laboratories today are able to provide measurements of C1q, properdin, factor B, and C1 esterase inhibitor. The need to measure other complement components is generally less appropriate to a routine clinical setting.

Many of the complement components act as acute-phase reactants. Levels of C3 and C4 often rise in serum when increased synthesis occurs after inflammation or trauma or during the course of many autoimmune diseases. Decreased levels may be due to decreased synthesis in genetically deficient persons but usually it is the result of utilization, ie, activation of the complement sequence with a transient decrease of circulating components. Quantitation of C3 and C4 is used to monitor patients with glomerulonephritis, immune complex diseases like systemic lupus erythematosus, forms of vasculitis, and certain viral and bacterial infections. C3 and C4 levels are usually parallel in the pathological states in which they are likely to be determined. Both C3 and C4 levels are decreased in autoimmune hemolytic anemia, acute viral hepatitis, gram-negative septicemia, subacute bacterial endocarditis and the synovial fluid of rheumatoid arthritis. In SLE C3 will be decreased while the C4 may be decreased or normal. In streptococcal glomerulonephritis C3 will be decreased while C4 is expected to be normal. In the serum of patients with rheumatoid arthritis, C3 may be decreased or normal whereas C4 is expected to be normal. In mixed cryoglobulinemia C3 is decreased or normal and C4 is decreased. Effective use of the values obtained requires that serial determinations be made.

The complement cascade may follow either the classical or alternative pathway. The classical pathway is activated by the interaction of IgG or IgM antibody with antigen. The alternative pathway is activated by a different set of substrates and is initiated by a different set of components (properdin, etc). These interact with the classical pathway, from C3 to the terminal components. In general, C4 measurements are an earlier and more sensitive indicator of complement consumption than C3, but measuring the two complement components in the same specimen also allows for an interpretation as to which of the pathways is being utilized. A depression in C3 *and* C4 indicates activation of the classical pathway, whereas depression of C3 with a normal C4 implicates the alternative pathway.

Hemolytic Complement Assays
Many laboratories offer an assay which assesses the functional capacity of the complement system. This is generally called CH50 or total hemolytic complement. This method assesses the ability of a serum to lyse a standard suspension of SRBC coated with anti-SRBC antibody. Results are generally reported as CH50 units and are derived from a dilution of the serum which results in 50% hemolysis. Principally, it is an assay of the functional integrity of the classical pathway, since it is activated by an antigen-antibody complex. A few laboratories will, in addition, use a standardized suspension of rabbit red cells, which activate the alternative pathway. Both tests are technically difficult and subject to a number of variables. Unless properly collected and stored (serum separated from the clot within one hour and frozen at $-70\,^\circ$C), specimens may give falsely low values. In clinical practice, this assay analyzes those complement components not generally measured routinely in laboratories (ie, C2, C5 through C9, factor D, properdin). Unfortunately, a significant reduction in these components is unnecesary for detection of an abnormality. Measurements of total hemolytic complement are made if complement consumption or a genetic defect in complement is suspected.

C1 EI
The C1 esterase inhibitor (C1 EI), a plasma protein, is a nonspecific esterase inhibitor. In addition to blocking the activation of C4 by C1s in the early portion of the classical pathway of complement, it also inhibits activated Hageman factor, plasmin, and kallikrein. Hereditary angioneurotic edema (HAE), caused by a lack of functional C1 esterase inhibitor, is an autosomal dominant disease characterized by recurrent episodes of brawny, non-pruritic, and nonerythematous angioedema that can include laryngeal edema

and abdominal visceral edema causing abdominal pain, vomiting, and/or diarrhea. Eighty percent of persons with this disorder lack C1 EI as measured by immunodiffusion techniques. The remaining 20% have immunologically detectable but nonfunctional C1 EI. In addition to absent or nonfunctional C1 EI, these persons often have a low C4 level, especially during attacks. This is due to activation of the early components of the complement cascade.

There also appears to be an acquired form of angioneurotic edema associated with absent or nonfunctional C1 EI. In these cases, depletion of C1 is more pronounced than depletion of C4, C2, or C3. An underlying lymphoproliferative or connective tissue disease has often been found in patients with acquired C1 EI deficiency.

C1 esterase inhibitor measurement is not a useful test in the routine evaluation of urticaria or angioedema. It should be reserved for patients with recurrent noninflammatory angioedema and a family history compatible with HAE.

Analysis of Immunoglobulins by IEP

Standard electrophoresis of serum conducted on paper, cellulose acetate strips, or agarose resolves all of the components into five major fractions (albumin, alpha-1, alpha-2, beta, and gamma). Except for the albumin fraction, all are heterogeneous mixtures of proteins with similar electrophoretic mobilities. This simple protein fractionation should be used as a screening test, not a diagnostic test for any disease. The presence of a "monoclonal spike" or a paraprotein in this assay is the only diagnosis that can be made. This method does not provide any identification of the protein involved. It is here that immunoelectrophoresis (IEP) comes into play. IEP allows for the ready identification of the major immunoglobulin classes as well as an accurate assessment of whether or not a monoclonal protein is present.

IEP can be used to study the immunoglobulins in any body fluid, but its greatest clinical value is in the assessment of those proteins found in serum, urine, and intestinal juice. Principally, the methodology combines electrophoresis in agarose with the precipitation properties of specific antisera. It is the use of monospecific antisera in this assay which allows ready identification. In general, the procedure is the following. Agarose is prepared with a buffer which will easily conduct an electric current. This preparation is liquified and then poured onto a glass slide and allowed to cool and gel. The agarose provides solid support for initial separation of proteins by electrophoresis as well as a medium for specific precipitation of protein by the antisera. Holes are punched in the agrose gel so that control sera and patient sera are placed side by side. This is usually done in triplicate. The appropriate specimens are added to the punched holes, and the agarose is electrophoresed for one to two hours. Then a trough, the length of the electrophoresis path, is cut between the holes. Monospecific antiserum is placed in each of the troughs, and diffusion of this antibody is allowed to take place overnight. Most laboratories will put into the first trough antisera to IgG, IgA, and IgM. The second and third trough will have monospecific antisera to the light chains, one for kappa and the other for lambda.

Normally a delicate precipitin arc line is formed by the interaction of the antisera and the protein. Each point on the line represents the secretion of a single clone of plasma cells. With proliferation of a single clone the cell product at the corresponding point is increased, leading to bulging and an abnormal shape of the line in that region. Other changes may be differences in mobility, shape, or size and in addition may be reflected by only one of the light-chain types. The criterion for being monoclonal is filled if the abnormal precipitin arc is observed with only one of the light chains. The identification of the light-chain type is also necessary for the diagnosis of Bence-Jones proteins in urine (excreted light chains) and is thought to have prognostic significance in myeloma. Use of antisera to each of the light chains also allows for the detection of monoclonal components present only in small amounts and, therefore, not very prominent against a background of normal polyclonal gamma globulins.

The identification of some monoclonal IgM proteins may require additional laboratory procedures. Generally initial separation of IgM from IgG by size will then permit identification of the light-chain type associated with the monoclonal IgM.

Clinical Usefulness
IEP of serum and urine are the tests of choice when there is a clinical suspicion of myeloma, Waldenstrom's macroglobulinemia, heavy chain disease, amyloidosis, or immunoglobulin deposition disease. A pathological finding such as a spike on protein electrophoresis, the presence of a cryoglobulin, increased serum viscosity, or an appreciable discrepancy between an immunochemical quantitation of immunoglobulins and more direct methods, indicates the need for further study by IEP.

Detection of Circulating Immune Complexes

A significant body of evidence indicates that antigen-antibody complexes can be measured in many disease states. These "immune complexes" appear to be involved in the pathogenesis of some diseases; hence, their detection is helpful in assessing and monitoring disease activity.

Circulating immune complexes can be detected by more than 30 methods. Two different interactions of these complexes form the basis of their detection by the assays used most frequently: (1) aggregated or complexed immunoglobulin will bind a portion of the first component of the complement system (C1q), and (2) many cell surfaces have receptors for the Fc portion of IgG or various complement components. The standard methods for detecting immune complexes are, therefore, binding of radiolabeled C1q, binding to Raji cell surface receptors, and inhibition of Fc binding by monoclonal rheumatoid factor. Studies by the World Health Organization have found these to be the most readily reproducible of all of the proposed assays.

The collection and storage of samples for immune complex detection should be done with great care. Bacterial contamination or repeated freeze-thawing of specimens results in the formation of immune complex-like aggregates producing false-positives. Hence, specimens sent to reference laboratories should be freshly drawn and, after clot separation, frozen at $-70\,°C$ or lower (dry ice).

The Raji cell binding assay can present problems. This cell is a human lymphoblastoid cell line which has high affinity receptors for C3; hence, immune complexes that have bound complement components will adhere to the cell. Radiolabeled anti-IgG which reacts with the bound complexes is then used to measure the amount of immune complexes present. Unfortunately, false-positives may occur if the patient has antilymphocyte antibody that binds to antigenic determinants of the lymphoblastoid line. This can occur in systemic lupus erythematosis (SLE) and other connective tissue disease. In addition, the results obtained by this assay are often discordant with those obtained by the C1q binding assay. Different methods appear to measure different sizes and types of complexes, so that comparisons between tests, patients, and disease entities are difficult to make. However, serial determinations can be useful in any given patient using the same method from the same laboratory. Levels often fluctuate with clinical exacerbation or improvement in some disease states (SLE, subacute bacterial endocarditis).

Clinical Indications

The detection of immune complexes does not now appear to be essential in the diagnosis of any clinical condition. Lesions induced by deposited immune complexes can exist without detectable levels of circulating immune complexes. Similarly, their presence in serum does not provide evidence for, or the necessity of, immune complex-associated lesions. In all conditions where immune complex deposition is suspected, only analysis of tissue samples by biopsy is confirmatory. Because discordant results are often obtained with various assays, the clinician should obtain results by two or three methods. Once a method has been found to give positive results it may be used serially to monitor the rise and fall of the circulating complexes.

Cryoproteins/Cryoglobulins

Cryoproteins are plasma proteins that precipitate in the cold and resolubilize when rewarmed. These proteins are usually immunoglobulins, and thus the term cryoglobulins is often used, although other proteins such as fibrinogen can also have this property.

To detect cryoglobulins, blood is drawn into a warmed tube without anticoagulants and allowed to clot at 37 °C. An insulated disposable coffee cup containing 37 °C tap water is a simple and convenient temporary incubator for bedside use until the tube can be placed in a regulated incubator. The tube is centrifuged subsequently at 37 °C and then cooled in a conical centrifuge tube at 4 °C. Formation of the precipitate usually occurs in 24–48 hours, but may take up to seven days. It is useful to demonstrate resolubilization of the precipitate upon rewarming to establish that it is a true cryoglobulin. Once the precipitate has formed, it is measured either as a cryocrit (percentage of total volume) or the mass of protein per volume of original serum. Greater than 0.2 mg/mL is definitely significant. It is important to identify and to quantitate the components of the precipitate because the clinical manifestations and etiologies differ according to the type of cryoglobulin. The components are determined and quantitated by radial immunodiffusion of the resolubilized proteins.

The classification of cryoglobulinemia is based on the types of immunoglobulins involved and whether they are monoclonal or polyclonal. Table 11-2 is a summary of types of cryoglobulinemia. It is important to determine

Table 11-2
Cryoglobulins and Cryoglobulinemias

Type	Frequency	Component	Amount of Cryoglobulin	Diseases	Symptoms (Frequency)
I	25%	Monoclonal IgM > IgG > IgA	+ + +	Lymphoproliferative	Hyperviscosity (50%)
II	25%	Monoclonal IgM (IgG, IgA < 10%) and polyclonal IgG	+ +	Lymphoproliferative, rheumatic, inflammatory, infectious	Vasculitis (> 50%)
III	50%	Polyclonal IgM (IgA rare) and polyclonal IgG	+	Infectious, rheumatic, inflammatory, "essential"	Vasculitis (> 70%)

the amount and nature of the cryoglobulin because symptoms and associated diseases vary among the types.

Thus, type I cryoglobulinemia, which consists entirely of a monoclonal immunoglobulin (single light chain, single heavy chain subclass, single idiotype), is marked by large amounts of cryoglobulins, symptoms of hyperviscosity (Raynaud's phenomenon, thrombosis, hemorrhage, and distal extremity cyanosis, necrosis, and ulceration) and is usually associated with an underlying lymphoproliferative disease of B cells (multiple myeloma, chronic lymphocytic leukemia, lymphoma, or Waldenstrom's macroglobulinemia). Types II and III cryoglobulinemia usually have less cryoglobulin, symptoms of vasculitis (purpura, arthralgias, peripheral neuropathy, and glomerulonephritis) and are less often associated with a lymphoproliferative disorder. Most cases of essential cryoglobulinemia (cryoglobulinemia without evidence of another disease present) are type III. As many as two-thirds of the patients with essential cryoglobulinemia have hepatitis B antigen or antibody in either their serum or cryoprecipitate. Presumably a hepatitis B virus infection is the basis of their "essential" cryoglobulinemia.

Because cryoglobulinemia is usually secondary to an underlying disease, the discovery of cryoglobulins requires a search for the primary lymphoproliferative, rheumatic, inflammatory, or infectious disease.

Antibodies to Tissue Antigens

Antibodies to tissue antigens are widely used in the diagnosis of many autoimmune diseases. These antibodies include organ-specific antibodies (eg, thyroid or parietal cell antibodies), non-organ-specific antibodies (eg, antinuclear and anti-smooth muscle antibodies), and antibodies against formed blood elements (eg, erythrocytes and platelets). The presence of these antibodies is not in itself diagnostic of a disease since they are present in healthy persons and increase in frequency with aging. The presence of these antibodies is, in many cases, secondary and not directly pathogenic. Some of these antibodies are also found in relatives of affected patients, suggesting a genetic link. High titers are usually diagnostic of specific diseases, but do not correlate with severity of disease and are not useful in following the course of the disease. Despite these shortcomings they are useful markers of particular diseases because of their high incidence.

Thyroid Antibodies
The most commonly measured thyroid antibodies are antithyroglobulin and antimicrosomal antibodies. These are most useful in the diagnosis of Hashimoto's thyroiditis in which there is a 100% incidence when measured by radioimmunoassays. They are also present in 50% to 60% of patients with Grave's disease and primary myxedema. High titers are frequent in Hashimoto's thyroditis and Grave's disease. They are present in lower titer in 10% to 20% of the patients with adenomatous goiter, thyroid carcinoma, and normal, elderly females. These antibodies are also present in some cases of autoimmune diseases that fall into a group called the thyrogastric cluster. In addition to Hashimoto's thyroiditis and Grave's disease, these include pernicious anemia, Addison's disease, insulin-dependent diabetes mellitus, myasthenia gravis, and some cases of rheumatoid arthritis and Sjögren's syndrome. The presence of these antibodies correlates with the presence of lymphocytic infiltrates in the affected organs.

Antibodies in Pernicious Anemia
Among patients with pernicious anemia, 80% have antibodies to parietal cells and 30% have antibodies to intrinsic factor. These are usually measured by indirect immunofluorescence. Parietal cell antibodies are present in up to 30% of elderly normal persons and patients with other diseases of the thyrogastric autoimmune cluster and so are not specific for pernicious anemia. Additionally, up to 60% of patients with atrophic gastritis have parietal cell antibodies. Intrinsic factor antibodies are more specific for pernicious anemia, but may be present without vitamin B_{12} malabsorption.

Other Organ-Specific Antibodies
Other organ-specific antibodies are present in diseases with a postulated autoimmune basis, but assays for these antibodies are not routinely available. These include adrenal antibodies in idiopathic adrenal insufficiency, basement membrane antibodies in Goodpasture's syndrome, islet cell antibodies in insulin-dependent diabetes mellitus, melanocyte antibodies in vitiligo, and antibodies to proteins that link epidermal cells in pemphigus. These are usually measured by indirect immunofluorescence methods. The same constraints about their interpretation apply as for other tissue antigen antibodies.

Non-Organ-Specific Antibodies
The most widely used of the non-organ-specific antibodies is the antinuclear antibody. The other commonly used tests are antimitochondrial and anti-smooth muscle antibodies, which are frequently present in some types of chronic liver disease.

Antimitochondrial Antibodies
Antimitochondrial antibodies appear to be directed against a lipoprotein on inner mitochondrial membranes and can be of IgG, IgM, or IgA class. They are measured by indirect immunofluorescence on kidney tubule cells and are present in 85% to 90% of primary biliary cirrhosis cases (generally in high titer; $> 1:200$ in 50% of the patients). They are useful in excluding biliary duct obstruction, but they have been reported in up to 7% of patients with

chronic large duct obstruction. They are present infrequently in normal persons (< 5%), but occur in up to 30% of patients with chronic active hepatitis or cryptogenic cirrhosis. Low titers are sometimes seen in Sjögren's syndrome, adrenalitis, thyroiditis, idiopathic hemolytic anemia, and myasthenia gravis.

Anti-Smooth Muscle Antibodies

Anti-smooth muscle antibodies are directed against an actomyosin component of smooth muscle and are usually detected by indirect immunofluorescence on thin sections of rodent stomach. They are present in the highest titer (usually > 1:80) and highest frequency (65% to 86% of patients) in chronic active hepatitis. They are also seen in 40% to 50% of patients with primary biliary cirrhosis and up to 30% of those with cryptogenic cirrhosis. Patients with other diseases such as acute viral hepatitis, infectious mononucleosis, extrahepatic biliary cirrhosis, drug-induced hepatitis, ovarian tumors, and malignant melanoma may have low titers (< 1:80) of anti-smooth muscle antibodies. Less than 5% of a normal population will have low titers.

Table 11-3 is a summary of the disease for which tissue antibodies are used diagnostically.

ANAs

Antinuclear antibodies (ANAs) are a group of immunoglobulins directed against various molecular components of mammalian nuclei. The diagnosis and definition of various forms of systemic connective tissue diseases, especially systemic lupus erythematosis (SLE), rely on the detection of ANAs. Measurement of ANAs leads to a better understanding of pathogenic mechanisms in these diseases and is important in monitoring disease activity.

The lupus erythematosis cell factor (LE cell factor) was the first antinuclear antibody described. When sera containing this factor are incubated with phagocytic polymorphonuclear cells and leukocytes that have been slightly damaged to expose previously hidden nuclear antigens, the antibody binds to the nuclear antigen, leading to phagocytosis of nuclear material by the polymorphs. Thus, LE cells are polymorphs containing homogenous

Table 11-3
Antibodies to Tissue Antigens and Associated Diseases

Antibody	Disease	% Incidence
Antithyroglobulin	Hashimoto's thyroiditis	100
	Grave's disease	50–60
Antimicrosomal	Hashimoto's thyroiditis	100
	Grave's disease	50–60
Anti-parietal cell	Pernicious anemia	80
	Atrophic gastritis	60
Anti-intrinsic factor	Pernicious anemia	30
Antimitochondrial	Primary biliary cirrhosis	85–90
	Chronic active hepatitis	30
Anti-smooth muscle	Chronic active hepatitis	65–85
	Primary biliary cirrhosis	40–50

cytoplasmic inclusions that stain like nuclei. The LE cell phenomenon occurs most often in SLE, but is also present in drug-induced lupus erythematosis and other connective tissue diseases such as scleroderma. ANA determinations have generally replaced the LE cell test because they are simpler, more quantitative, and more sensitive.

The best method to screen for ANAs is an indirect immunofluorescence technique that relies on the binding of these antibodies to nuclear antigens exposed in sections of rodent tissues such as liver and kidney. Other tissues such as leukocytes, thymus, spleen, thyroid, tissue culture lines, and tumor cells have also been used. Dilutions of the patient's serum are applied to the sections or smears, which are then washed. Antibodies binding to nuclear constituents are then detected by the addition of fluorescein-conjugated antibodies to human immunoglobulin. The slides are then examined with a fluorscence microscope for the presence and pattern of nuclear fluorescence.

In interpreting ANA results it is important to consider the incidence of a positive result for a given disease, the titer of the antibody, and the pattern of fluorescence. Table 11-4 lists the incidence of a positive ANA for several diseases. A negative ANA in SLE is very unlikely, although a small proportion of patients produce antibody against cytoplasmic rather than nuclear ribonucleoproteins (the Ro antigen). Higher titers of ANA in a patient's serum make SLE a more likely diagnosis. With diseases other than the connective tissue diseases the ANA titer is usually low. A weakly positive and transient ANA can occur in benign conditions such as infectious mononucleosis.

Four well-recognized patterns of fluorescence correlate with various antigens related to subsets of the connective tissue diseases. A homogeneous pattern with total nuclear fluorescence is the most common. It is due to antibodies against deoxyribonuclear proteins and correlates with the antigen for the LE cell factor. In low titer, it is found in normal persons and in patients with chronic infectious processes, drug-induced lupus, and many connective tissue diseases and is, therefore, nonspecific. In high titer ($> 1:160$), it is fairly specific for SLE. The peripheral or rim pattern shows fluorescence localized to the edge of the nucleus and is due to antibodies against DNA. This pattern is unusual in diseases other than SLE. The speckled pattern is caused by antibodies against ribonuclear proteins. It is seen in SLE, scleroderma, and Sjögren's syndrome. When present in high titer, it is a marker for mixed connective tissue disease. Finally, the nucleolar pattern is characteristic of scleroderma and appears to be due to antibodies against nucleolar RNA.

If a screening test for ANAs is positive in sufficient titer, further characterization of the antibody is worthwhile. This is usually done by radioimmunoassay or hemagglutination techniques. Among the ever-increasing numbers of specific antinuclear antibodies, those that are most available and useful are against DNA and extractable nuclear antigens.

There are three types of anti-DNA antibodies. Antibodies to double-stranded DNA are found exclusively in SLE. They appear as a peripheral pattern in the indirect immunofluorescence assay. Not only are these antibodies specific for SLE, but also the titers correlate with disease activity and the presence of renal lesions and fall with successful treatment. Eluates of the kidneys of patients with renal lesions of SLE contain high anti-DNA activity with specificity for double-stranded DNA. The presence of these antibodies

191

Table 11-4
ANA Positivity in Various Diseases

Disease	Percent with a Positive ANA
SLE	95
Scleroderma	50–80
Rheumatoid arthritis	20–60
Felty's syndrome	100
Sjögren's syndrome	40–75
Dermatomyositis/polymyositis	10–30
Polyarteritis nodosa	15–25
Mixed connective tissue disease	80
Cirrhosis	10–20
Ulcerative colitis	60–80
Chronic lymphocytic leukemia	10–20
Waldenstrom's macroglobulinemia	10–20
Infectious mononucleosis	50–65
Drug-induced lupus	50
Normal (< 60 years old)	0–4
Normal (> 60 years old)	Up to 20

should initiate a search for renal disease even in the presence of seemingly normal renal function. Some patients have antibodies against single-stranded DNA. These are much less specific and are present in other connective tissue and rheumatic diseases as well as SLE. The third type of anti-DNA antibody reacts against both single- and double-stranded DNA. These are also less specific, being present in low titer in several connective tissue diseases besides SLE.

Among the extractable nuclear antigens, the Sm (Smith) and ribonucleoprotein antigens are the most discussed. Both are saline extracts, usually from thymic cells, and are ribonucleoproteins. The Sm antigen is an RNase-resistant, acidic component. It is present exclusively in SLE. It appears as a speckled immunofluorescence pattern. The ribonucleoprotein antigen is RNase sensitive and also appears as a speckled pattern by immunofluorescence. It is less specific and is present in SLE, discoid lupus, and scleroderma. When present in high titers, however, it is indicative of mixed connective tissue disease, an overlap syndrome with clinical features of SLE, polymyositis, and scleroderma. Table 11-5 lists these and some other less frequently used, antinuclear antibodies.

Antibodies to Peripheral Blood Components
Whereas antibodies directed against some of the tissues already mentioned are associated with, but not necessarily causally related to, certain diseases, antibodies directed against peripheral blood components (eg, erythrocytes, platelets, and neutrophils) often appear to be the etiology of anemia, thrombocytopenia, and neutropenia, respectively. Because tests for antiplatelet and antineutrophil antibodies are not readily available, only antierythrocyte antibodies will be discussed here.

The classical test for detecting antibodies against red cells is the Coomb's test. The direct Coomb's test detects antibodies that are attached to red

Table 11-5
Various ANAs

Name	Antigen	Disease Association
dsDNA*	DNA	SLE
ssDNA†	DNA	SLE, other connective tissue diseases
ds + ssDNA	DNA	SLE, other connective tissue diseases
Sm	Nuclear ribonucleoproteins	SLE
RNP	Nuclear ribonucleoproteins	Mixed connective tissue disease, SLE, scleroderma
La‡	Nuclear ribonucleoproteins	Sjögren's syndrome
Ro	Cytoplasmic ribonucleoproteins	SLE (ANA negative)
RANA§	Epstein-Barr virus-induced protein	Rheumatoid arthritis

*dsDNA, Double-stranded DNA.
†ssDNA, Single-stranded DNA.
‡Also called Ha or SS-B.
§RANA, Rheumatoid ANA.

blood cells, whereas the indirect Coomb's test detects erythrocyte antibodies free in the serum. Up to 8% of hospitalized patients show a positive direct Coomb's test with no evidence of hemolytic anemia. Thus, a positive test must be interpreted in light of other clinical findings. A positive indirect Coomb's test with a negative direct test is weak evidence of a hemolytic anemia.

In the direct Coomb's test, antihuman globulin is added to a saline suspension of the patient's erythrocytes. This mixture is then examined for agglutination. Initially, a polyspecific antiglobulin is used. If the test is positive with this serum, monospecific antiglobulin reagents are then used that will detect either IgG or C3 bound to the erythrocytes. IgM is difficult to detect, but readily fixes complement. Complement-specific reagents are therefore used to detect IgM. In addition to characterizing a hemolytic anemia by whether it is IgG (gamma) or IgM (nongamma) mediated, it is also useful to characterize it as warm or cold reactive. The antibodies combine with erythrocytes at 37°C in the former and at 4°C in the latter. Warm-reactive antibodies may be directed against the Rh group, whereas cold-agglutinating antibodies are usually against the I antigen (another red blood cell membrane structure). Since certain drugs and diseases give a characteristic type of direct Coomb's test, characterization allows better definition of the etiology of the hemolytic anemia. Table 11-6 gives a brief summary of the different types of immune hemolytic anemias and their associated diseases or drugs.

Biological False-Positive VDRL
The VDRL (venereal disease research laboratory) is a test that has been widely used in screening for syphilis. It is read qualitatively as nonreactive, weakly reactive, and reactive. Serial dilutions of sera are usually done to give a titer. Up to 30% of positive VDRLs are biological false-positives. These are usually weakly reactive, of low titer (< 1:8), and associated with negative specific antitreponemal antibody tests (fluorescent treponemal antibody-absorbed

[FTA-Abs] and *Treponema pallidum* immobilization [TPI] test). The acute biological false-positive test is seen in both viral and bacterial diseases and reverts to negative within six months. The chronic biological false-positive remains positive for greater than six months and is most often seen in connective tissue diseases, especially SLE. About 10% of chronic biological false-positive VDRLs are due to SLE. Heroin use and diseases such as lepromatous leprosy may also cause a chronic biological false-positive. On occasion a false-positive FTA-Abs test may be seen in SLE and other autoimmune diseases. These are usually atypical in appearance and are accompanied by a negative TPI test. The titer of the VDRL is not useful in following the course of diseases with a chronic biological false-positive. A biological false-positive VDRL in SLE is often associated with the presence of a circulating anticoagulant.

Acute-Phase Reactants
Acute-phase reactants are glycoproteins whose concentrations rise within hours to days after acute tissue injury or an inflammatory reaction. If the stimulus is self-limited, the values of these proteins return to normal, but if the stimulus is chronic the concentration of acute-phase reactants remains elevated. Among the proteins that act as acute-phase reactants are complement components, ceruloplasmin, alpha-1-antitrypsin, haptoglobin, fibrinogen, and C-reactive protein (CRP). Of these only the CRP and the

Table 11-6
Immune Hemolytic Anemias

Disease or Drug	Antibody	Direct Coomb's Gamma	Coomb's Nongamma	Indirect Coomb's
Penicillin	IgG	+	–	+
Quinidine	IgM	–	+	±
Cephalothin	IgG	+	+	+
Alpha methyldopa	IgG	+	–	+
Autoimmune hemolytic anemia SLE Chronic lymphocytic leukemia lymphomas Granulomatous diseases Idiopathic	IgG (warm)	+	–	+
Cold agglutinin hemolytic anemia *Mycoplasma pneumoniae* Viral infections Waldenstrom's macroglobulinemia	IgM (cold)	–	+	–
Paroxysmal cold hemaglobinuria Syphilis Viral infections	IgG (cold)	–	+	±

erythrocyte sedimentation rate (ESR), which reflects primarily elevation of fibrinogen, are widely used.

An elevated acute-phase reactant has no diagnostic specificity, but does reflect the presence of inflammation or tissue injury. Acute-phase reactants are also of value in following the course of some inflammatory diseases. A persistant elevation suggests ongoing inflammation. The level of the elevation only weakly correlates with the degree of tissue injury.

The CRP is a glygoprotein complex with a molecular weight of approximately 105,000. It is detectable in low concentrations in all subjects. After tissue injury or an inflammatory stimulus the CRP becomes elevated within hours, reaches peak elevation in two to three days, and falls within eight to ten days. In chronic inflammatory diseases the CRP will remain elevated. Most infections, solid tumors, tissue destruction, and connective tissue diseases will cause an elevated CRP. Although it has not been well described as a method of following the course of disease, the development of better techniques to quantify the amount of CRP may lead to wider use. Since elevations of CRP begin within hours, it is useful in the early diagnosis of inflammatory diseases. As with most acute-phase reactants, serial levels are more reliable than a single level.

The ESR has been used clinically for over 50 years and is the most widely used measurement of acute-phase reactants. The ESR measures the rate of settling of anticoagulated red blood cells. It is an indirect reflection of increased fibrogen. In addition to increased amounts of fibrogen, the ESR can be elevated by microcytosis, anemia, and the presence of other globulins. It is decreased by high plasma viscosity, spherocytosis, sickle cell disease, and polycythemia.

The two methods most commonly used to measure the ESR are the Westergren and Wintrobe methods. In the Westergren method a sodium citrate diluent is added to the blood. The cells are allowed to settle for one hour in a 200-mm long tube, and the ESR is read as the volume of plasma above the red cell column. The Wintrobe method is similar, but no diluent is added to the anticoagulated blood and the tube is 100 mm long. It is simpler but less accurate at high ESRs because of red blood cell packing. Normal values for both are shown in Table 11-7.

The ESR is a nonspecific but fairly sensitive measure of an inflammatory process. In addition to infectious, neoplastic, and lymphoproliferative diseases, it is elevated in vasculitis and most connective tissue diseases. In the vasculitis, especially Wegener's granulomatosis, giant cell arteritis, and polymyalgia rheumatica, the ESR is markedly elevated and returns to normal as the disease is treated. An elevated ESR in these diseases may be evidence

Table 11-7
Erythrocyte Sedimentation Rate

Sex	Age (yr)	Normal Value (mm/h)
Male	< 50	15
Male	> 50	20
Female	< 50	20
Female	> 50	30

of smoldering activity. The ESR is less useful in diseases with more specific organ injury indices (eg, cardiac enzymes in myocardial infarction, anti-DNA antibodies in SLE). In addition to being useful in the diagnosis and treatment of the vasculitides, the ESR is used to follow the course of acute rheumatic fever, to differentiate rheumatoid arthritis from osteoarthritis, and to diagnose urticaria with an underlying vasculitis.

■ Selected Readings

Gell PGH, Coombs RRA, Lachmann PJ: *Clinical Aspects of Immunology.* ed 3. Oxford, Blackwell Scientific Publications, 1975.

Middleton E Jr, Reed CE, Ellis EF: *Allergy: Principles and Practice.* St. Louis, C.V. Mosby Co, 1978.

Parker CW: *Clinical Immunology.* Philadelphia, W.B. Saunders Co, 1980.

Samter M: *Immunological Diseases.* ed 3. Boston, Little, Brown and Co, 1978.

Stites DP, Stobo JD, Fudenberg HH, et al: *Basic and Clinical Immunology.* ed 3. Los Altos, Calif, Lange Medical Publications, 1982.

The use of the laboratory in the differential diagnosis of rheumatic diseases is extremely important. Many illnesses in this class have well-defined but overlapping clinical criteria. When used to strengthen the case for one diagnosis over another, the laboratory has a direct impact on treatment. In some situations the clinician must use the laboratory to make a definitive diagnosis. Two such examples are the finding of crystals in synovial fluid to diagnose gout or pseudogout and the finding of a positive culture in infectious arthritis. I have chosen to include a broad spectrum of rheumatic diseases under the heading of rheumatic diseases—not only joint disease but also the so-called collagen vascular diseases: vasculitis and amyloidosis.

The clinician sees two broad categories of joint disease— chronic and acute arthritis. The former problem usually allows leisure for a careful diagnostic workup, but an acute arthritis demands a more immediate approach, often with the laboratory playing a prominent role in assessing the picture. The differentiation of inflammatory from noninflammatory arthritis when clinical grounds may suggest one or the other requires a synovial fluid analysis for confirmation. This is also often needed for differentiation of which specific type of inflammation is causing the problem. Synovial analysis revealing cell counts over 50,000, low sugars, and positive Gram stains strongly suggests infection. Culture is requisite for a definitive diagnosis and approach to treatment.

Synovial Fluid Examination

Probably the most important laboratory test in differentiating rheumatic diseases is the synovial fluid analysis. The indications for examination of the synovial fluid are its presence in a patient with joint symptoms, the ease of obtaining fluid from most joints and the safety of aspiration (Table 12-1).

The clinician must handle the aspirated fluid properly. Fluid utilized for cell counts and crystal analysis should be heparinized either in a heparinized test tube or in a syringe rinsed with dilute heparin. The use of other anticoagulants may introduce extraneous crystals which can be misinterpreted during examination under polarized light. Fluid for culture should be kept in a sterile container (without any bacteriostatic substance) and transported *immediately* to a laboratory. If this is not possible, transport medium should be added to the fluid in an attempt to keep organisms alive (this is less ideal than prompt transport). Specimens for chemical analysis and immunologic study are usually not anticoagulated, but transported in a plain tube to the laboratory. Certain special requirements may be needed as per instruction from your particular service facility. Samples

Eric P. Gall

197

for complement studies must be frozen (preferably at − 80 °C) until studied. Heparin should not be added as it inhibits complement activity.

Synovial fluid is first observed for its viscosity and clarity so that the fluid may be classified as belonging to one of four basic groups: noninflammatory, inflammatory, septic, and hemorrhagic (Table 12-2). The table highlights the basic groups of synovial fluids and a number of illnesses falling in each group. Noninflammatory fluid is seen in normal joints, degenerative arthrosis, and mild trauma. It is viscous because of hyaluronic acid, a mucopolysaccharide secreted by synovial lining cells. The fluid is transparent, and newspaper print may be read through a test tube containing it. The clarity reflects a low cell count.

Viscosity is tested by placing a drop of fluid on your fingertips or by letting a few drops drip from the needle. Noninflammatory fluid will string out several centimeters resembling egg albumin due to its viscosity. These basic observations suggest a benign or at least noninflammatory disorder. In contrast to this, inflammatory synovial fluid is turbid due to the elevated cell count. Print cannot be read through it. The viscosity is decreased due to destruction of the hyaluronic acid molecule by neutrophil hyaluronidase. The viscosity is more like that of water.

Septic fluid is similar to inflammatory fluid. However, because cell counts are higher, the turbidity is higher; when cell counts approach 100,000 or more, pus is obvious. This, of course, may be viscous because of the density of cells present. Hemorrhagic fluid connotes trauma, a bleeding disorder such as hemophilia, or tumor.

Thus, the four basic synovial fluid categories are separated by observation and by cell count. The older mucin clot test (Ropes test) is not advocated because it gives information that is similar to, but less reliable than, that already discussed.

The microscopic examination is divided into wet preparation examination, crystal examination, and examination of a Wright-stained smear. The most important observations under wet preparation examination include finding cartilaginous fragments suggesting degenerative disease, blood cells suggesting trauma, tumor, or hemorrhagic arthropathy, and fat and/or marrow fragments suggesting an intraarticular fracture. The last finding may be missed if not looked for and provides an important clue requiring orthopedic intervention. Examination of neutrophils in the wet preparation may show small refractable dots in the cytoplasm. These have been shown to contain immunoglobulin and complement and are particularly common in rheumatoid arthritis. Such cells have been called RA cells or ragocytes. They are not pathognomonic, however, for rheumatoid arthritis.

Examination for crystals is performed under compensated polarized light. This should be done on all patients with inflammatory arthritis, since gout and pseudogout may often masquerade as rheumatoid, septic, or degenerative arthritis. Many primary care physicians now use a polarizing microscope in their office since the finding of crystals is often easy, and the instant diagnosis made is both important and gratifying. A plain microscope can be rapidly converted into a polarizing scope with two pieces of Polaroid (one in the ocular and one in the condenser) (Figure 12-1). Polaroid microscope pieces can be bought or improvised from a pair of inexpensive Polaroid sunglasses. A relatively inexpensive, first-order red compensator may also be

Table 12-1
Indications for Joint Aspiration

1. Any collection of joint fluid of unknown etiology
2. Unexplained flare of arthritis in a patient with otherwise diagnosed joint disease
3. Fever in any patient with a joint effusion. (part of a culture workup)
4. Persistence of joint inflammation despite what is thought to be proper medical therapy
5. Removal of excess joint fluid for reasons of comfort
6. When injecting medications (steroids) into the joint to make sure there is no infection and that the needle is in the joint space

purchased or may be made from a glass slide covered with plain (not frosted) cellophane tape. For details of the crystal examination the reader is referred to a reference source.

The synovial fluid is screened under low power with plain polarized light. Crystals stand out because of the birefringent characteristics and, once identified, are studied in detail with a first-order red compensator. Strong negatively birefringent (yellow parallel to the axis of a first-order red compensator) needle-shaped crystals are usually sodium urate crystals and substantiate a diagnosis of gout. Weak positively birefringent (blue parallel to the axis of a first-order red compensator) rhomboidal crystals are diagnostic of pyrophosphate arthropathy (chondrocalcinosis and pseudogout). The diagnosis of both these disorders has other implications besides the treatment of the arthritis itself. For instance, gout may be caused by a genetic enzyme disorder, rapid cell turnover from a malignancy, renal failure, lead poisoning, and other problems which need medical attention themselves. Calcium pyrophosphate arthropathy is sometimes the first manifestation of hyperparathyroidism, hemochromatosis, and a variety of other metabolic diseases.

Another crystal which may be seen in synovial fluid is cholesterol (overlapping squares with a corner missing from each). This crystal looks like uric acid seen in the urine at low pH and may be called such by an inexperienced laboratory technician. At synovial fluid pH, sodium urate (needle shaped) is always the crystal that will be seen. Cholesterol is found in chronic rheumatoid and septic effusions. Steroid crystals may look like other pathologic crystals. If corticosteroid injections have occurred in the aspirated joint this must be taken into consideration. Hydroxyapatite crystals are not birefringent and look like intracellular amorphous debris. Although they may cause inflammatory arthritis, electron microscopy is required for their definitive identification. Finally, debris on a slide may be mistaken for crystals, but is readily identifiable with experience.

The white cell count in synovial fluid is most helpful in differentiating types of arthritis (Table 12-2). This must be done using a nonacid hemolysin if the clinician does this in his or her office. HCl (0.1 N), the usual diluent to lyse red cells, will coagulate synovial fluid and cause an inaccurate cell count; 0.3 N saline is the preferred diluent for such counts.

The broad guidelines for interpretation of synovial fluid white cell counts are as follows. (1) Counts less than 2000/mm^3 are noninflammatory (class 1

Axial arthropathies	Turbid	Poor	1000–50,000 (19,000)	High	N	N–high	
SLE	Slightly turbid	Fair	1000–18,000 (2700)	Low	N	Low	LE cells
Rheumatic fever	Slightly turbid	Fair	3000–98,000 (18,000)	Moderate	N	N	
Class 3, Septic							
Pyogenic	Turbid or pus	Poor (pus may be viscous)	10,000–250,000 (75,000)	High	Low	N low with GC and SBE	Culture positive, may see cholesterol
Tuberculosis	Turbid	Poor (pus may be viscous)	2500–100,000 (19,000)	Low	Low	N	Culture positive 50%
Hemorrhagic							
Traumatic	Bloody or clear	Good	1000–12,000 (1500)	Low	N	N	Blood frequent, may see marrow fragments
Tumor	Bloody	Good	500–2000	Low	N	N	Tumor cells may be seen

*PMNs, Polymorphonuclear leukocytes.
†N, Normal.

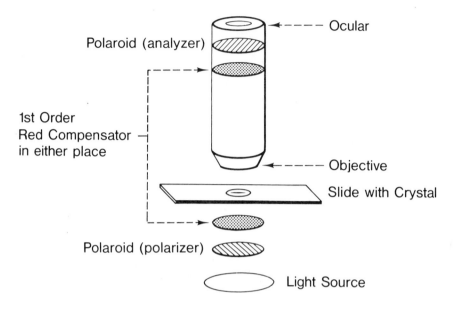

Figure 12-1 Compensating polarizing microscope.

fluid). (2) Cell counts from 2000–50,000/mm³ are inflammatory and may be benign inflammatory disease or infection. (3) Cell counts above 50,000/mm³ are assumed to be infection until proven otherwise (although patients with diseases such as rheumatoid arthritis and gout may have cell counts this high, it is not common). When interpreting red cell counts and white cell counts together, consider the ratio of white to red cells in whole blood. Thus in an otherwise normal patient with a traumatic hemorrhage (hematocrit 30% in the joint) a white cell count of 2500 would not be inflammatory and could be accounted for by the hemorrhage alone. However, a white cell count in the same synovial fluid of 25,000/mm³ would suggest something else besides trauma.

The differential analysis by stained smear of the synovial fluid may be helpful in several ways. The percentages of PMN leukocytes and lymphocytes vary in several diseases (Table 12-2). This is particularly useful in chronic infections where a large percentage of lymphocytes suggests either tuberculosis or fungal organisms as etiologic agents. More helpful, however, is finding abnormal cells. For instance, tumor cells found in synovial fluid of patients with leukemic arthritis or metastatic carcinoma to the joint are diagnostic. Similarly, the finding of a typical LE cell in stained synovial fluid strongly suggests systemic lupus erythematosus (SLE). The joint provides the requisite ingredient for an LE prep without doing the actual test. A source of cell trauma (due to joint motion), the appropriate 7S antibody for nuclear transformation, and neutrophils are all present.

Less specific would be the finding of large macrophages containing PMN leukocytes or other cellular particles. These cells (Reiter's cells) are common in that syndrome, but may also be seen in a variety of other disorders. Of course, other stains to the dry smear (Gram stain for bacteria, acid-fast

Table 12-3
Drugs Frequently Affecting Serum Uric Acid Levels

Lowers Serum Uric Acid	Raises Serum Uric Acid
Aspirin (more than 12 tablets per day)	Aspirin (low dose)
Probenecid	Diuretics
Phenylbutazone	Furosemide
Coumarin	Thiazides
Clofibrate	Ethacrynic Acid
Radiographic dyes	Acetazolamide
Telapaque	Phenytoin (Dilantin)
Cholagrafin	Levodopa
Oragrafine	Ethambutol
Hypaque	Alcohol
	Lactate
	Lead

stains, fungal stains, etc) may also provide important diagnostic information. A few comments are in order about when to order and how to interpret other synovial fluid tests performed by clinical laboratories. Chemistry tests include the protein and sugar analysis. I feel the protein analysis of synovial fluid is not warranted. Information regarding the inflammatory nature of fluid is more easily and accurately assessed by visual examination and cell counts. Synovial fluid sugars should be interpreted only with concomitant serum values. Synovial fluid values of 25 mg/dL or more below serum level thus suggest inflammation; when values are more than 40 mg/dL lower, infection is suspected. This is particularly true if the absolute synovial fluid level of glucose is less than 10 mg/dL. Rarely, however, this may occur with rheumatoid arthritis alone.

Immunologic measurements are seldom done on synovial fluid. The measurement of rheumatoid factors and antinuclear factors in synovial fluid is rarely of any more benefit than the same serum values. The complement levels in synovial fluid may occasionally influence your diagnosis. The most commonly measured complement levels are C3, C4, and CH50. The former two are preferred since there are fewer things that will interfere with an accurate determination. Complement values should only be interpreted when concomitant serum values are done. Both specimens should be obtained in a nonheparinized container since heparin inactivates complement. Although there are many ways to interpret synovial fluid complement levels, I think the easiest is to consider normal being one-third to two-thirds of the serum level. For all practical purposes anything less than one-third of serum level suggests immune complex disease, rheumatoid arthritis being the most common entity. Other common immune complex diseases include subacute bacterial endocarditis (SBE), gonococcal arthritis in the migratory phase, serum sickness, hepatitis, other types of viral arthritis, and SLE. In SLE however, serum levels of complement are often also low. More detailed discussion of serum complement levels appear in Chapter 10.

The final common laboratory procedure performed on synovial fluid is a culture. Fluid should be transported immediately to the laboratory in a syringe with a fresh needle or in a sterile tube. It is suggested that the clinician switch needles before injecting aspirated fluid into a culture tube to prevent contamination with skin bacteria. Aseptic aspiration with iodine and alcohol preparation should be done. Fluid which will take more than a few moments to transport should be placed in transport medium (check with your laboratory).

Because tuberculous and fungal agents will often (50% of the time) not grow from synovial fluid, biopsy of synovium provides a much higher yield in these infections. Obviously, special media and measures are required. The laboratory must be notified as to what you are expecting. Effusions in gonococcal arthritis often will not grow organisms, although the yield will be improved by plating in an enriched hypertonic chocolate agar media at the bedside. The culture should grow under 10% CO_2 as well as aerobic incubation. Often cultures will be positive from pharynx, rectum (with the swab not touching stool), urethral scraping, endocervix, skin lesions, and blood when the synovial fluid is negative. Such cultures should be performed before antibiotic treatment is begun.

Synovial Biopsy

Closed synovial biopsy with the Parker-Pearson needle is useful when fluid analysis and radiographic studies are not diagnostic. Diseases that may be definitively diagnosed by this method include benign neoplasms (pigmented villonodular synovitis), primary or metastatic malignancies of the joint, infections, hemochromatosis, and ochronosis. Other inflammatory arthritis may be difficult to differentiate on biopsy and may only show nonspecific synovitis. The synovial biopsy is most helpful in monarticular arthritis.

Sedimentation Rate

An extremely high sedimentation rate, no matter what kind, can be seen in 3% of normal persons. Such values should be put in proper context, and diagnostic workup should not be predicated on this value alone. If a careful history and physical examination are normal, I suggest a serum protein electrophoresis to make sure there is not a hidden immunoglobulin dyscrasia. If that is normal, just follow the patient carefully. Conversely, all serious disease is not reflected by elevated sedimentation rates. Remember that the test, while useful, is crude.

The rheumatoid factor is a misnomer. This test is not specific for rheumatoid arthritis and merely indicates the presence of an antibody to gamma globulin (an antibody to an antibody). The test is performed by affixing gamma globulin physically to a particle such as a latex bead or immunologically to a sheep red blood cell. This changes the conformation of the gamma globulin slightly and allows the particle to be agglutinated by IgM anti-gamma globulins. There are also immunoglobulin G (IgG) and IgA rheumatoid factors, but they are not readily measured in clinical laboratories.

To properly interpret a serum rheumatoid factor assay the clinician needs to know four basic facts: the type of test being done, the titer of the assay, and the sensitivity and the specificity of the procedure. All persons exposed to the environment have small amounts of anti-gamma globulin (rheumatoid factors) since circulating gamma globulin is constantly being insulted and made antigenic.

The sheep cell agglutination test (SCAT) produces lower serum titers than the latex test when tested in patients and is only about 50% sensitive in patients with active rheumatoid arthritis. The specificity, however, is about 90% if it is positive in a significant titer (1:32 or higher). Lower values are to be ignored. Thus, this assay is a poor screening test for rheumatoid arthritis, but is quite (although not completely) specific. The higher the titer the more likely the patient is to have rheumatoid arthritis.

The latex (or bentonite) rheumatoid factor test is far more sensitive (75% to 80%) than the SCAT. The significant titer of this test is 1:80 or higher, and the specificity is less than that of the SCAT, about 75%. Once again, the higher the titer, the more likely that the patient has rheumatoid arthritis.

Both tests can be positive in many other illnesses. Some of the most common include the following: (1) chronic infections such as subacute bacterial endocarditis, leprosy, tuberculosis, and osteomyelitis; (2) fibrotic diseases such as pulmonary fibrosis and cirrhosis; (3) chronic pulmonary disease; and (4) old age.

Recommendations for using the rheumatoid factor test are as follows. Do not interpret positive screening slide tests; a positive result means nothing and requires a titer anyway. Use the latex fixation test for screening; if the titer is 1:80 or higher, think about rheumatoid arthritis and the other diseases mentioned above. Titers of 1:1280 and higher are often associated with active extraarticular disease (Sjögren's syndrome, nodules, vasculitis, Felty's syndrome, etc). Since the patient presentation is more important than the laboratory test, the further specificity of the SCAT is rarely needed. Remember that rheumatoid arthritis is diagnosed by 11 criteria that are all nonspecific in and of themselves. A positive rheumatoid factor in significant titer is only one of the 11 criteria and is no more specific for the disease than any of the others. Rheumatoid factor tests of synovial fluid are rarely more helpful than serum levels. Occasionally, the rheumatoid factor test of pleural or pericardial fluid will be helpful with other tests in differentiating rheumatoid arthritis from infections.

The antinuclear factor and the LE cell test have been used frequently to diagnose lupus and other collagen diseases. The antinuclear factor may be performed by using a number of assay cell types, most often kidney and liver cells from tissue slices (less often white blood cells and tissue culture cells from a variety of sources). There are also a number of kits available for performing antinuclear factor tests by agglutination techniques. I discourage their use. Basically one must know the system he or she is dealing with and the normal values for that system.

To understand the antinuclear factor, a brief discussion of the test is in order. A frozen section of normal kidney or liver is affixed to a glass slide. The patient's serum is then layered over this tissue. If antibody to nucleus (or other tissue elements) is present it will be bound to the appropriate receptor site. After washing, fluorescein-tagged antibody to human gamma globulin is again layered on top of the preparation and will bind to the sites where patient antibody has adhered to the cell (a sandwich preparation). The specimen is once again washed and read under a fluorescent microscope. The positive assay is reported, and the pattern of the fluorescent stain in the nucleus is reported. Finally, the highest titer of serum with remaining positivity is noted. The combination of receptor cell type, pattern of staining, and titer is then used to interpret the test result.

The test is usually done at a screening dilution of 1:10 and, if positive, is then diluted further. Titers of less than 1:40 are rarely significant; the higher the titer the more significant the test.

There are four basic patterns of antinuclear staining. Each has a certain significance. The rim or peripheral pattern is the most specific. It is caused by an antibody to native DNA and is usually seen in SLE which is active, most commonly with active renal disease. Although it may be seen in other situations, the rim pattern in significant titer should alert the clinician to strongly suspect SLE.

The homogeneous pattern covers the entire nucleus and is caused by an antibody to DNA-histone complex. It is caused often by the antibody that also causes a positive LE prep. This also is seen in SLE, particularly if it is drug induced and in a variety of other autoimmune diseases, particularly in rheumatoid arthritis. Thus, it is a confirmatory, but not diagnostic, test in SLE.

The speckled pattern of nuclear staining is still less specific. It can be caused by antibodies to a variety of antigens, particularly soluble ribonucleoprotein and a RNase resistant antigen Sm (Smith). While both of these saline-soluble antigens are seen in SLE, the soluble ribonucleoprotein is also frequently cited in overlap diseases such as mixed connective tissue disease (a combination of rheumatoid arthritis, SLE, scleroderma, and polymyositis). There are a variety of ways to be more specific in identifying the antibody.

The final common antinuclear antibody (ANA) pattern is the nucleolar pattern. This is seen in scleroderma and Sjögrens' syndrome most commonly and is caused by an antibody to RNA.

Much is written about more specific assays for antibodies to nuclear antigens. I feel that these techniques are more important in research than in daily patient care and, with the possible exception of measuring specific antibodies to DNA (a test which I rarely use), are best left to the specialist.

Using immunologic tests to screen patients with suspected rheumatic disease frequently leads to confusion. The patient with mild arthralgias, a positive ANA, and no other systemic illness should not be labeled as having lupus. The patient should, of course, be followed for the development of other systemic signs and symptoms. Frequently, patients will be entirely well months and years later; thus, common sense should be used in working up such patients. Certainly, invasive procedures should be avoided in patients with only a positive laboratory test.

Conversely, the ANA in selected patients along with other tests such as serum complement assays may occasionally be helpful in predicting flares of disease before they become manifest. The clinician will learn by experience the individual patients for whom this practice will be most helpful.

The LE cell test is of historic value only. The ANA is both more sensitive and, when interpreted with titer and pattern, more specific. We have abandoned the use of the LE prep in our unit at the University of Arizona.

Serum complement levels are discussed in Chapter 10. The CH50 is a functional test which should only be used in hospitals or laboratories doing large volumes of assays and where specimens are handled promptly. The C4 and C3 assays are more readily available. These are immunologic precipitin tests which depend on the presence of a particular complement component whether or not functionally active. For practical purposes, activated complement is cleared in vivo by the reticuloendothelial system. If activation and clearance exceed the ability to synthesize new complement, serum levels drop. The early complement components in the cascade (C1, C4, C2) are usually decreased because of activation by immune complexes, the classical activation pathway. Thus, a low C4 suggests the presence of an immune complex disease such as SLE, serum sickness, SBE, and other immune complex mediated infectious syndromes (disseminated gonococcal sepsis, for instance). Lowering of the late components of the complement scheme (C3 and C5 + 9) can be due to either immune complex or alternative pathway activation. The alternative pathway is activated by materials such as the bacterial cell wall of gram-negative organisms and certain unknown factors in diseases like idiopathic immune glomerulonephritis. C3, an abundant protein, is directly affected by both classical and alternative pathways.

Thus, for practical purposes, if the C4 is low, suspect immune complex disease. If the C3 is low, either immune complex disease or disease activating the alternative pathway may be present. However, if the C3 is low and the C4 is normal, the disease process is probably due to alternative pathway mechanisms (gram-negative sepsis and idiopathic membranoproliferative glomerulonephritis). Serum for complement assays must be handled carefully and promptly frozen and stored at − 70 to − 80 °C if not studied immediately by the laboratory. Normal values depend on the particular laboratory standards used.

Immune complex testing is available to detect immune complex in a more direct fashion. The simplest screening test available is the cryoglobulin test. This test is done by drawing a clotted specimen of blood (preferably clotted at 37 °C), centrifuging (at 37 °C), and then removing the serum. Serum should then be refrigerated in ice (not frozen) for 48–72 hours. The specimen is then inspected for turbidity and centrifuged. If precipitate is present at the bottom of the tube, it is most likely cryoglobulin. It should go back into solution at 37 °C and reprecipitate at 4 °C. Material rising to the top of the tube on spinning is lipid. The cryoglobulin can be washed, and the contents can be identified. The presence of immunoglobulin and complement suggests immune complexes, and one can look for specific antigen and antibody. Other monoclonal proteins may also precipitate by this method. More sensitive and specific assays for immune complexes include C1q precipitation, monoclonal rheumatoid factor precipitation, and the Raji cell assay. Interpretations of all of these assays are discussed elsewhere.

HLA typing has received much attention, both as a diagnostic test for seronegative arthropathies and as a help in understanding the pathogenesis and epidemiology of many disorders. While the tests are somewhat useful, I would discourage the reader from ordering them except rarely when it would change clinical management. The best understood instance where HLA testing has been advocated is in the diagnosis of ankylosing spondylitis and related diseases (Reiter's syndrome, gastrointestinal related arthropathies such as Crohn's disease and psoriatic arthritis). These diseases are best diagnosed on clinical and radiologic grounds. While the HLA B-27 antigen is found in approximately 85% of patients with ankylosing spondylitis, it is seen in 6% to 8% of the normal white population; its presence is meaningless without clinical disease. Its absence also means nothing if a patient has the clinical grounds for a diagnosis.

Chemical analysis of blood and urine particularly for uric acid and muscle enzyme is helpful in the diagnosis of certain rheumatic diseases.

Gout most often affects older men, although it may affect patients of all ages, sex and races. Definitive diagnosis is made by crystal identification in the synovial fluid or tissue. The serum and urine uric acid tests are also helpful, however, in confirming the diagnosis, determining the cause of the gout, or determining proper treatment. If crystal analysis fails or is not possible, the elevation of the serum uric acid along with an acute monarticular arthritis and a response to colchicine, is accepted as a strongly suggestive triad for the diagnosis of gout.

In intrepreting serum uric acids, the clinician must know what methods and normal values his laboratory employs. The literature frequently cites lower normal uric acid levels than clinical laboratories since the research laboratories commonly use enzymatic determination of uric acid levels, rather than the more commonly used colormetric technique.

Values of serum uric acid in the high-normal range are often above the solubility product so that crystals and tophi can form even at normal levels. This is particularly important to know in treating patients since the uric acid level must be lowered enought to allow dissolution of tophi and microtophi in tissues. Thus, if the normal upper limit value of 7.8 to 8.0 mg/dL is used by your laboratory, you must lower serum values to 6.0 mg/dL or lower to reduce the uric acid pool in the body.

Up to one-third of all patients with gout have normal serum uric acid levels either between attacks or at the time of an acute attack. Because of uricosuria, the serum uric acid commonly drops 2–3 mg/dL within 24 hours of an acute attack. Conversely, elevated serum uric acid levels do not prove gout even with acute arthritis. Many patients will take aspirin when arthritis pain becomes evident. This drug may elevate the serum uric acid several milligrams per deciliter by blocking secretion in the renal tubule. Many other drugs will affect the serum uric acid levels. (Table 12-3).

Urine uric acid determinations are used to help classify the etiology of gout and to determine treatment. Levels may be measured by 24-hour urine collections. Greater than 800 mg per 24 hours suggests overproduction and overexcretion of uric acid. Levels less than 600 mg per 24 hours suggest underexcretion of the chemical. Uric acid excretion may also be estimated by measuring a spot urine uric acid/creatinine ratio and multiplying that figure by the serum creatinine. Values greater than 0.7 suggest overexcretion. This is best done on a midmorning specimen which is not as accurate as a good 24-hour specimen, but suffices for most clinical situations.

Overproducers of uric acid may have a number of underlying diseases with high cell turnover or congenital enzyme disorder (Table 12-4). They also put their kidneys at risk to stone formation and require allopurinol to decrease risk of urolithiasis.

Patients with underexcretion of uric acid either have intrinsic renal disease, competition for renal tubular secretion of uric acid, or idiopathic gout (Table 12-4). They may be treated with probenecid if clinically appropriate.

Muscle enzymes are important in the diagnosis of myopathies, and are discussed in Chapter 15.

Table 12-4
Diseases Causing Overexcretion and Underexcretion
of Urinary Uric Acid

Causes Overexcretion	Causes Underexcretion
Myeloproliferative disorders	Intrinsic renal disease
Leukemias	Renal failure
Lymphomas	Lead poisoning
Other malignancy	Competition for uric acid secretion
Psoriasis	Drugs
Glycogen storage diseases	Lactic acidosis
Cytotoxic drugs	Ketosis
Primary gout (enzyme abnormalities)	Idiopathic gout
HGPRTase deficiency	
Increased PPRP synthetase	
Other defects	

Biopsy of tissue along with special stains and histologic study are often helpful in the diagnosis of many rheumatic diseases. Examples include biopsy of skin, sural nerve, muscle, kidney, testes, and other tissue in vasculitis. Amyloid may be identified by use of Congo red stain and polarized light to give a distinctive apple-green birefringence. Patients with suspected amyloidosis should also have serum and urine protein electrophoresis and quantitative immunoglobulin performed. Muscle biopsy is requisite in the diagnosis of myopathy.

I have summarized the use of the laboratory as it is utilized in the diagnosis and treatment of rheumatic diseases. I have not, obviously, covered all possible utilization of the laboratory, nor have I covered many of the rare exceptions to the more likely explanations of laboratory results. As in all diseases, laboratory results must be interpreted in light of the clinical presentation of rheumatic patients. Abnormalities do not always indicate disease, and of course the reverse is true. The laboratory, however, is invaluable in the modern approach to patients with rheumatic diseases.

■ Selected Readings

Cohen AS: *Laboratory Diagnostic Procedures in the Rheumatic Diseases.* ed 2. Boston, Little, Brown and Co, 1975.

Dumonde DC, Steward MW: *Laboratory Tests in the Rheumatic Diseases—Standardization in Laboratory in Clinical Practice.* Baltimore, University Park Press, 1979.

Kelley WN, Harris ED Jr, Ruddy S, et al: *Textbook of Rheumatology.* Philadelphia, The W. B. Saunders Co, 1981.

McCarty DJ: *Arthritis and Allied Conditions.* ed 9. Philadelphia, Lea & Febiger, 1979.

Phelps P, Steele AD, McCarty DJ: Compensated polarized light microscopy. *JAMA* 1968;203:508–512.

Scott JT: *Copeman's Textbook of the Rheumatic Diseases.* ed 5. Edinburgh, Churchill Livingstone, 1978.

Steinbrocker O, Neustadt DT: *Aspiration and Injection Therapy in Arthritis and Musculoskeletal Disorders.* New York, Harper & Row Publishers, 1972.

Tests for gastrointestinal disorders are, like intestinal fluid, in constant flux. Some, like gastric secretory tests, may soon be superseded. Others, like gastrointestinal hormone tests, are very rapidly expanding. Still others, like stool fat tests, have retained their value despite generations of use. This chapter describes the less controversial tests in use today, which we hope will be proved the truth in years to come.

■ Diseases of the Esophagus

Laboratory tests are seldom useful for diagnosing diseases of the esophagus. There may be occult bleeding in neoplastic and inflammatory conditions (see Occult Blood Loss, below). Cytology may be useful in diagnosing carcinoma of the esophagus. Esophageal smears may help in diagnosing monilial esophagitis.

■ Diseases of the Stomach

In diseases of the stomach it may be of interest to measure gastric secretions and serum gastrin. The secretion of acid and intrinsic factor is clinically relevant. The secretion of pepsin and mucus has, until now, been mainly of research interest. Table 13-1 is a summary of the diagnosis of gastric diseases.

Gastric Secretions

Acid Secretion
Description of Tests   Quantitative analysis of acid output is performed after an overnight fast. The stomach is intubated, and gastric secretion is quantitatively collected for four 15-minute intervals. The amount of acid in the gastric aspirate is titrated to pH 7 or calculated after a precise measurement of the pH value. The initial unstimulated one-hour collection is designated as the basal acid output (BAO). Subsequently the stomach is stimulated to secrete maximally, and the collection is similarly continued for one hour. This is the maximal acid output (MAO). The two maximal quarter-hourly outputs are added and multiplied by two, the result is termed peak acid output (PAO). The most commonly used stimulant is pentagastrin (6 μg/kg of body weight [BW]) given subcutaneously. Betazole (Histalog) given subcutaneously (1–1.5 mg/kg of BW) or histamine phosphate (0.04 mg/kg of BW) given subcutaneously (with the obligatory addition of an antihistaminic such as diphenhydramine hydrochloride [Benadryl] intramuscularly) are now rarely used. Insulin-induced hypoglycemia (Hollander test) can be used as a test for evaluating the

Tuvia Gilat
Yochanan Peled
Yoram Bujanover

212

completeness of a vagotomy. Regular insulin (0.1-0.2 U/kg of BW) is given intravenously. Gastric secretion is collected as before for one hour before and two hours after stimulation.

To establish the presence of achlorhydria, pentagastrin is given as above, and aliquots of gastric contents are sampled for one hour. Achlorhydria is diagnosed if the pH does not drop below 6 in any of the aliquots. Tubeless gastric analysis is performed by giving orally a resin-bound dye (ie, Diagnex Blue) that is released by the action of gastric acid. The appearance of the dye in the urine indicates the presence of gastric acid. The test can be repeated by using a stimulant of gastric secretion.

Acid Secretion: Values   The normal range for BAO is 0-5 mEq/h; higher values are found in duodenal ulcer. Values above 15 mEq/h are highly suggestive of gastrinoma. The normal range for MAO is 12-40.0 (mean, 22) mEq/h; values below 12 mEq/h usually exclude the diagnosis of duodenal ulcer. Low values are found in atrophic gastritis, gastric carcinoma and Menetrier's disease, but are not diagnostic. High values above 45 mEq/h are suggestive, but not diagnostic, of duodenal ulcer. A BAO/MAO ratio of more than 0.6 is suggestive of gastrinoma. In the presence of gastroenteroanastomosis (after surgery), an MAO of > 15 mEq/h is suggestive of anastomotic ulcer.

In the Hollander test, basal acid concentrations above 10 mEq/L or a rise of 20 mEq/L above the basal value after insulin hypoglycemia indicate incomplete vagotomy.

Achlorhydria is mandatory for the diagnosis of pernicious anemia, and its presence with gastric ulcer is highly suggestive of malignancy.

Limitations and Indications   Tests using a nasogastric tube are unpleasant for the patient and time consuming. Most of the stimulants have side effects. The tests can be used in screening for gastrinoma (BAO) and in the diagnosis of achlorhydria. The Hollander test helps to evaluate the completeness of vagotomy. Its accuracy is limited, and the test may be hazardous. Where endoscopy is available, these tests are rarely used for the diagnosis of ulcers. The tubeless tests are qualitative and imprecise.

Secretion of Pepsin and Mucus
The secretion of pepsin is low in atrophic gastritis. Before the introduction of pepsin inhibitors its analysis had not been useful in clinical practice. The analysis of blood pepsinogen is used in research. The protein content of gastric mucus is 1.8 mg/mL. It may be greatly increased in Menetrier's disease (over 9 mg/mL).

Secretion of IF
Intrinsic factor (IF) is essential for vitamin B_{12} absorption. In its absence the absorption of B_{12} will be impaired. The secretion of IF is evaluated by the vitamin B_{12} absorption test (Schilling test—see Vitamin B_{12} malabsorption, below).

In the process of gastric mucosal atrophy, acid and pepsin secretion disappear first and IF disappears last; thus, inadequate secretion of IF is diagnostic of atrophic gastritis (gastric atrophy).

Table 13-1
Diagnosis of Gastric Diseases

Disease	Recommended Tests	Less Specific Tests
Duodenal ulcer	X-rays, endoscopy	MAO
Gastric ulcer	X-rays, endoscopy, biopsy	Test for achlorhydria
Recurrent ulcer after surgery	Endoscopy	MAO, Hollander test
Pernicious anemia	Schilling test, test for achlorhydria	
Menetrier's disease	X-rays, endoscopy, tests for GI protein loss	Protein content of gastric mucus
Gastrinoma (ZE)	BAO, serum gastrin	Gastrin provocative tests

Tests for Gastrin

Serum Gastrin
The gut hormone gastrin is produced by G cells mainly in the gastric antrum and duodenum and by gastrin-producing tumors. It is released into the blood, where it is present in several molecular forms, which are, however, detected by most available commercial kits. The radioimmunoassay is the commonly used method of measurement.

Normal values (fasting) are 20–160 pg/mL, depending upon the method, kit, and laboratory. High values with low gastric acid secretion are found in atrophic gastritis. High values associated with gastric acid hypersecretion are mainly found in gastrinoma (Zollinger-Ellison syndrome), isolated retained gastric antrum (after surgery), and also in renal failure and the short bowel syndrome.

Indications A serum gastrin test is indicated whenever gastrinoma is suspected. Screening for gastrinoma is recommended in all cases of familial, complicated, and atypical duodenal ulcer disease. It is reasonable to check serum gastrin at least once in any patient with duodenal ulcer.

Gastrin Provocative Tests
To differentiate between gastrinoma and other above-mentioned conditions associated with hypergastrinemia and gastric acid hypersecretion, the following methods may be used.

Secretin Test After an intravenous bolus injection of secretin (1 clinical unit per kg) the serum gastrin level in gastrinoma rises within 5–15 minutes by more than 50% and more than 100 pg/mL above the basal level. This rise does not occur in other conditions and is diagnostic of gastrinoma.

Calcium Infusion Test Ca^{2+} is infused intravenously at a rate of 5 mg/kg per h for three hours. In gastrinoma, serum gastrin level rises by more than 50% or by more than 500 pg/mL. The maximal gastrin level is usually achieved during the final hour of the infusion.

■ Diseases of the Pancreas

The main diseases of the pancreas in which laboratory tests are useful are acute pancreatitis, chronic pancreatitis, and, less frequently, pancreatic tumors.

In acute pancreatitis blood and urine levels of various elements may be abnormal. In chronic pancreatitis pancreatic secretion may be diminished with resultant malabsorption. This may also happen with pancreatic tumors. Pancreatic insufficiency is also present in cystic fibrosis. Gastrinoma has been discussed with diseases of the stomach. Table 13-2 is a summary of the diagnosis of pancreatic diseases.

Diagnosis of Acute Pancreatitis

Amylase

Serum Amylase   Serum amylase is raised in most cases (80% to 90%) of acute pancreatitis. The rise occurs within a few and up to 24 hours. The levels return to normal within several days, except in cases with persistent activity of the disease and especially pseudocyst. Normal values are 80–180 Somogyi units per dL or 14.7–33.1 IU/dL. (1 Somogyi unit per dL = 1.85 IU/L).

High values are seen mainly in acute pancreatitis, but also in many other disorders (Table 13-3).

The main limitation of the test is due to the fact that it may be raised in many other diseases, including diseases that cause abdominal pain (Table 13-2). In addition, it is not always elevated in acute pancreatitis.

Urine Amylase   In acute pancreatitis, tubular reabsorption of amylase may be impaired, and urine amylase may still be elevated when serum amylase has returned to normal.

Table 13-2
Diagnosis of Pancreatic Diseases

Disease	Recommended Tests	Less Specific Tests
Acute pancreatitis	Serum and urine amylase Amylase/creatinine clearance ratio Serum lipase	Serum glucose Serum calcium Serum magnesium Serum lipids
Chronic pancreatitis	Stool fat and chymotrypsin Secretin or Lundh tests	PABA test Glucose tolerance test
Carcinoma of the pancreas	Imaging and cytology techniques	Tests for pancreatic insufficiency CEA Serum immunoreactive trypsin
Cystic fibrosis	Sweat test Tests for pancreatic insufficiency	Serum immunoreactive trypsin (in newborns)

Table 13-3
Diseases in which Serum Amylase may be Elevated

Pancreatic Diseases	Diseases of Gastrointestinal Tract	Gynecologic Conditions	Diseases of the Salivary Glands	Miscellaneous
Acute pancreatitis	Esophagus perforation	Ectopic pregnancy	Mumps	Renal disease
Pseudocyst	Gastric ulcer	Ectopic pregnancy and rupture	Suppurative parotitis	Liver disease
Abscess	Duodenal ulcer	Salpingitis	Inflammation of salivary glands	Tumors of lung
Ascites	Intestinal obstruction	Papillary cystadenoma of the ovary	Calculous obstruction of salivary ducts	Diabetic coma
Carcinoma	Intestinal ischemia	Tumors of the ovary		Methanol poisoning
Calculous obstruction of pancreatic duct	Intestinal perforation			Hypoxemic and posthypoxemic conditions
	Peritonitis			Scorpion sting
	Acute cholecystitis			
	Carcinoma of colon			
	Carcinoma of biliary tract			

Normal values of urine amylase are 66–870 Somogyi units/dL. High values are found in acute pancreatitis and other diseases causing elevation of serum amylase. In macroamylasemia serum amylase will be high and urine amylase will be low.

Urine amylase values can also be given as output per time—per hour or per 24 hours (urine is collected for a period of time, at least six hours), thus eliminating concentration changes associated with high and low urine output. Normal values are 35–260 Somogyi units per hour.

Amylase/Creatinine Clearance Ratio The amylase/creatinine clearance ratio is much more specific for acute pancreatitis than either serum or urine amylase. It is presently the most reliable laboratory test for diagnosing acute pancreatitis. Blood and urine samples are taken simultaneously, and each of the samples is analyzed for both amylase and creatinine. The calculation is according to the formula:

$$\text{Amylase/creatinine clearance ratio} = \frac{\text{Urine amylase} \times \text{serum creatinine}}{\text{Serum amylase} \times \text{urine creatinine}} \times 100$$

Normal values are 1–4%. Values higher than 6% (originally higher than 5.3%) are seen in acute pancreatitis, but also occasionally in other conditions such as severe burns and diabetic ketoacidosis. High values may be found in renal disease, and low values may be found in macroamylasemia.

Isoamylases Serum and urine amylase can be raised due to diseases of the salivary glands (Table 13-3). In these conditions the high serum activity reflects the presence of the salivary isoamylase. The source of the amylase—salivary or pancreatic—can be identified either by isoenzyme electrophoresis or by specific isoamylase determination kits. In patients with high serum levels of salivary isoamylase the amylase/creatinine clearance ratio is usually within the normal range. In chronic pancreatitis the total serum amylase is usually normal, but the pancreatic isoamylase is very low. It is thus a useful screening test for chronic pancreatitis.

Macroamylasemia High serum amylase values with normal or low urine amylase values can be encountered in healthy people due to the binding of amylase (pancreatic and salivary) to serum globulins. This large molecular complex is poorly cleared by the kidneys, thus causing an elevated amylase activity in the serum. This condition can be diagnosed by a very low amylase creatinine clearance ratio (< 1%) and by isoenzyme electrophoresis.

Serum Lipase
Serum lipase was introduced as a test for acute pancreatitis, because of the uncertainties associated with the serum amylase test. Changes in serum lipase usually parallel those of serum amylase. A rise in serum lipase occurs perhaps more frequently than a rise in serum amylase. It may begin before serum amylase rises, and the abnormal levels may persist longer than those of amylase. Serum lipase rises within hours, peaks within one or two days, and disappears within three to five days from the onset of the acute pancreatitis. Normal values are 0–70 U/L using the Phadebas Kit or 0–1.5 Cherry Crandal units per liter.

Limitations Lipase values may be elevated also in perforation and diseases of the upper gastrointestinal and biliary tracts. The turbidometric method commonly used for lipase determination is fraught with technical difficulties.

Serum Glucose
Hyperglycemia may be transiently present in the early stages of acute pancreatitis in about 20% of cases.

Serum Ca^{2+}
Hypocalcemia may be present especially in the more severe cases of acute pancreatitis. It may become manifest two to five days from onset of the disease and may persist for seven to ten days. The pathogenesis is possibly multifactorial, with elevated calcitonin and glucagon, inadequate parathyroid response, and hypomagnesemia among the suggested causes. Normal Ca^{2+} levels during acute pancreatitis may suggest hyperparathyroidism as the cause of the attack, and the patients should be rechecked after the attack.

Serum Mg^{2+}
Low serum levels of Mg^{2+} have been reported in acute pancreatitis with or without hypocalcemia. In some cases this interferes with the return to normal of serum Ca^{2+}.

Serum Lipids
Hyperlipidemia may infrequently (5% to 10%) be found in acute pancreatitis, especially in alcoholic pancreatitis. In the majority, this is the result of the attack. Lipoprotein lipase activity is diminished, interfering with lipid removal. There may also be an increased production of lipids by the liver due to the alcohol. The lactescent serum usually clears over five to seven days. In a minority of patients the hyperlipoproteinemia precedes or may even cause the attack.

Immunoreactive Trypsin
Sensitive radioimmunoassays for human trypsin immunoreactivity are now available. Elevated serum trypsin levels were demonstrated in acute pancreatitis and in a relapse of chronic pancreatitis as well as in newborns suffering from cystic fibrosis. The test was suggested as a screening method for cystic fibrosis. In patients with pancreatic insufficiency serum trypsin levels may be low.

Lately, increased levels of immunoreactive trypsin in the urine were reported in pancreatic cancer. (Hoechst RiA-Gnost Trypsin Kit; normal range 140–400 mg/mL). The test was recommended for screening of pancreatic cancer.

Diagnosis of Chronic Pancreatitis

Tests for chronic pancreatitis are based on the demonstration of impaired pancreatic exocrine function. (Pancreatic endocrine function may also be impaired—see Chapter 17). Infrequently, a pancreatic tumor may obstruct the main pancreatic duct with resultant pancreatic insufficiency. The tests are, therefore, not specific.

Stool Tests

In pancreatic insufficiency stool fat will be increased because of impaired lipolysis. Stool nitrogen may be increased because of impaired proteolysis or the output of pancreatic enzymes in the stools may be diminished.

Stool Fat   Steatorrhea will be present in any significant pancreatic insufficiency. Stool fat will be in excess of 6 g/24 h (see Stool fat, below). The reduction or correction of steatorrhea by treatment with pancreatic extract proves the pancreatic origin of the steatorrhea. Pancreatic supplementation should be given in adequate or excessive doses for this therapeutic trial. The improvement, if it occurs, is almost immediate.

Chymotrypsin Output in the Stool   The enzyme chymotrypsin is secreted by the pancreas with meals and is slowly degraded during intestinal passage. It is more resistant than other enzymes, and measurable amounts appear in the stool. The analysis of chymotrypsin requires a titration system at a constant pH and is not widely performed. Normal values are more than 6000–10,000 U/24 h (or 123 U/kg of BW per 24 h). Stool collection has to be quantitated, ie, a three-day stool collection (stool kept refrigerated until analyzed). Alternatively, a nonabsorbable marker should be used to permit quantitative analysis of a single stool sample (see Stool fat, below). The simultaneous analysis of stool fat and chymotrypsin will determine whether steatorrhea exists and whether it is of pancreatic origin. Low stool chymotrypsin values are present only in marked pancreatic insufficiency, whereas normal values with minimal steatorrhea may occur in mild pancreatic insufficiency. Fecal chymotrypsin can be measured in single stool samples and expressed as activity per gram of feces. Normal values are $> 120 \mu g/g$ of stool. As a rule, tests based on the concentration of chymotrypsin are less reliable than those based on its fecal output per 24 hours. The proteolytic activity of stools can be qualitatively demonstrated by using gelatin or a piece of x-ray film.

Stool Nitrogen   Analysis of nitrogen in the stool is not easy to perform, has a limited value, and is rarely used.

Urine Tests

PABA Test   A synthetic peptide conjugated to paraaminobenzoic acid (PABA; N-benzyoyl-L-tyrosyl-PABA) is given by mouth in a dose of 15 mg/kg of BW, up to 1 g. After cleavage of the peptide by chymotrypsin, free PABA is released, absorbed, and excreted in the urine.

Normal values are more than 60% to 65% (of administered dose) in a six-hour urine collection. Lower values will appear in pancreatic insufficiency in proportion to its degree. The test obviates the need for stool collections. It is dependent, however, on kidney function (although a correction may be made), and the substrate has not yet been licensed in many countries.

Schilling Test   Recent work indicates that in about 50% of cases with chronic pancreatitis, vitamin B_{12} absorption is impaired and can be improved by therapy with pancreatic extract. Apparently the pancreatic proteolytic enzymes are important in this respect.

Tests Based on Analysis of Duodenal Contents

The direct measurement of stimulated pancreatic output into the duodenum is the most precise way to quantitate pancreatic exocrine function. These methods are invasive, require duodenal intubation, are associated with considerable discomfort to the patient, and are time consuming; thus, they are of limited use. Occasionally, there may be side effects associated with the injection of hormones.

Secretin Test After duodenal intubation under x-ray control, duodenal contents are emptied, and secretin (1 clinical unit per kg of BW) is given by bolus injection. The duodenal aspirate is collected on ice in several fractions (ie, four 20-minute fractions), and volume, bicarbonate, and amylase are analyzed. Normal values are as follows: for volume, 2–4.4 mL/kg per 80 minutes; for bicarbonate, 12.2–31.0 mEq/80 minutes; for maximal bicarbonate concentration, 90–130 mEq/L in any sample; for amylase, 6.6–35.2 U/kg/80 minutes. The test has several possible variations. (1) An augmented secretin test may be performed using 4 cu/kg. (2) The secretin may be given by a continuous infusion using 2–4 cu/kg/h. (3) Cholecystokinin-pancreozymin (CCK-PZ) may be given intravenously (1 intravenous Dog unit per kg) together with or 30 minutes after the secretin injection, and additional enzymes in the duodenal contents, trypsin, lipase, etc, may be analyzed.

The regular secretin test is the most widely used version. The test is abnormal in 96% of patients with proved chronic pancreatitis when total bicarbonate output is measured.

Lundh Test In the Lundh test the stimulus for pancreatic secretion is food, and the concentration of pancreatic enzymes in the duodenal chyme is measured. The stimulus is more physiologic and devoid of side effects, although pancreatic secretion cannot be quantitatively collected. After duodenal intubation, 300 mL of a liquid test meal is infused into the duodenum (ie, 300 mL containing 18 g of corn oil, 15 g of skim milk powder, 40 g of glucose, and 15 g of vanilla syrup). Duodenal contents are continuously aspirated for four 30-minute periods. Normal values for mean tryptic activity are around 16.8 IU/L (range 7.0–38.0 IU/L). PH, volume, and amylase activity can also be measured, but the tryptic activity is considered to have the highest diagnostic value. The test was abnormal in 90% of 168 patients with proven chronic pancreatitis.

Diagnosis of Carcinoma of the Pancreas

Carcinoma of the pancreas is diagnosed by imaging and endoscopic methods. The diagnosis may be confirmed by cytology. Laboratory tests add only indirect evidence of pancreatic insufficiency or obstruction. Serum immunoreactive trypsin may be increased. Tests of pancreatic function may be impaired. The carcinoembryonic antigen may be elevated in the serum or in pancreatic secretions.

■ Diseases of the Small Intestine

Malabsorption caused by diseases of the small bowel may be suspected on the basis of impaired serum levels of various substances but can be proven only by absorption tests.

Indicators of Malabsorption

The main indicators of malabsorption (all analyzed in the blood) are as follows: folic acid, vitamin B_{12}, iron, ferritin, carotene, vitamin A, prothrombin, calcium, and phosphorus.

Serum levels of all of these substances may be impaired in malabsorption. However, the same result may be from other causes, such as malnutrition, abnormal loss, or abnormal metabolism. Thus, impaired levels of these substances might indicate the need for performing absorption tests. They do not prove by themselves the presence of malabsorption.

Limitations

The body stores of these substances vary widely; blood levels of some will drop rapidly after the onset of malabsorption (serum levels of carotene will drop within a few weeks, and levels of vitamin A will drop within several months), whereas body stores of others are larger and may be sufficient to maintain normal serum levels for long periods of time in the presence of malabsorption. (Vitamin B_{12} level will drop only after several years.)

Tests for the Diagnosis of Malabsorption

Carbohydrate Malabsorption

D-Xylose Tolerance Test (Urine and Blood)   The D-xylose tolerance test is now the test of choice for the diagnosis of carbohydrate malabsorption. Xylose, a nonphysiological pentose, is only partially absorbed (about 50%) after a 25-g oral dose. The 5-g oral dose, often used in children, is almost completely absorbed. After absorption, it is not much metabolized in the body, and about half is excreted into the urine; thus, adequate urine levels indicate normal absorption. Alternatively, blood xylose levels may be measured one hour after ingestion. The latter method is preferable in infants in whom urine collection is difficult.

Normal values in urine are more than 4.5–5 g of xylose excreted in the urine during five hours after an oral load (in the fasting state) of 25 g of D-xylose. Lower levels indicate malabsorption. After the 5-g dose, more than 1.5–1.8 g should normally appear in the urine. Impaired renal function will result in an abnormal test (false-positive). Therefore, with low urinary values renal function must be evaluated.

Normal values in the blood are more than 20 mg of xylose per dL after one hour. Lower levels indicate malabsorption. Blood levels may be affected by gastric emptying, metabolism, and the rate of absorption and renal excretion. Whether blood or urine measurements are more advantageous in the D-xylose tolerance test is still controversial.

The monosaccharide xylose does not require digestion before absorption. Impaired absorption therefore indicates disease of the bowel wall, mostly upper small bowel. The test may also be abnormal in massive bacterial overgrowth in the proximal small bowel. It is a good screening test for diseases of the upper small bowel (celiac disease, etc).

Lactose Tolerance Test   Fifty grams of lactose is given orally in adults, and 2 g/kg of BW is given in children. A rise in blood glucose of more than 20 mg/dL is normal, and a lesser rise indicates lactose malabsorption. The sampling of capillary blood is more reliable than venous blood.

A similar test, the sucrose tolerance test, may be used when the rare sucrose malabsorption is suspected.

These tests used for the diagnosis of disaccharide malabsorption are being superseded by the hydrogen breath test, which is easier to perform and more precise.

Hydrogen Breath Test   Unabsorbed carbohydrates are fermented by colonic bacteria, and one of the products is hydrogen gas. It diffuses rapidly from the intestinal lumen into the blood and is excreted by the lungs. Its concentration can be analyzed in the expired air. Unlike the xylose tolerance test, the hydrogen breath test enables the direct examination of the malabsorption of any carbohydrate.

After an overnight fast, usually 2 g of carbohydrate per kg of BW is given in children, up to a total of 50 g in adults. A rise in breath hydrogen concentration of over 10–20 ppm above fasting levels indicates malabsorption. Upper limits of normal depend on the laboratory.

The test is neither well standardized nor widely used. Any interference with the colonic flora, such as antibiotics, enemas, laxatives, etc, may cause a false-negative test. Two to five percent of the population do not have hydrogen-producing bacteria, with resultant false-negatives. Some people digest a meal containing carbohydrate and/or protein slowly and therefore have high fasting hydrogen levels which may interfere with the test.

The hydrogen breath test is the test of choice to diagnose lactose malabsorption. It can also be used to diagnose sucrose or any carbohydrate malabsorption. The test may also be positive in massive bacterial overgrowth in the upper small bowel.

Fat Malabsorption
Stool Fat   The test of choice is the quantitative determination of fecal fat output. Normal values are less than 6 g/24 h (over a wide range of oral fat intake). Higher values indicate fat malabsorption (steatorrhea).

Stool may be quantitatively collected for three to four days, pooled, and homogenized, and a sample may be analyzed. Alternatively, a nonabsorbable marker such as cuprous isothiocyanate, chromium oxide, β Sitosterol, etc, can be used. The marker is given with meals for at least four days, and a stool sample is collected. The amount of marker recovered in the sample enables calculation of daily output without stool collection.

Stool collections are laborious and imprecise. Inadequate intake of marker will invalidate the results. A reduced fat intake during the test period will give false-negative results with both collection methods. Despite these limitations, the quantitative analysis of stool fat is still the method of choice for diagnosing steatorrhea.

The absorption of fat is a complicated process and is easily impaired. Steatorrhea is therefore likely to be present in most diseases of malabsorption (celiac disease, pancreatic disease, ileal disease, etc).

Fat absorption may be expressed as percent absorption of ingested fat (coefficient of absorption). This requires calculation or measurement of fat intake, as well as stool fat. Normal is more than 90%. The method is used mainly in a metabolic ward and for pediatric patients.

222

Microscopic Analysis of Fecal Fat The microscopic count of fat droplets after staining a stool sample on a slide is an imprecise, semi-qualitative method.

Lipid Blood Levels After a Fatty Meal Chylomicron counts, serum turbidity, or serum triglycerides may be determined after a fat-rich meal. These methods were particularly used in children. The results correlate poorly with quantitative measurements of stool fat, especially in adults.

Isotopic Tests Tests based on the absorption of labeled fat were introduced to obviate the handling of stool. ^{131}I-labeled fats gave unsatisfactory results and are seldom used. ^{14}C-labeled fats were introduced to measure fat absorption, using the analysis of $^{14}CO_2$ in the expired air (fat breath test). After absorption the labeled fatty acids are metabolized in the body, and $^{14}CO_2$ is excreted in the expired air. Normal values are more than 3.43% of the dose per hour as peak value in the ^{14}C-Triolein test. Low $^{14}CO_2$ levels indicate impaired absorption. The method is still investigational and controversial.

Protein Malabsorption
There is no good clinical test for diagnosing protein malabsorption.

Bile Acid Malabsorption
Conjugated bile acids are actively absorbed in a short segment of the terminal ileum. Unconjugated bile acids are passively absorbed through the whole length of the intestines. Only bacteria are able to deconjugate conjugated bile acids.

Bile salt malabsorption is tested by the [^{14}C]cholyl glycine breath test.

[^{14}C]cholyl Glycine Breath Test ^{14}C-labeled cholyl glycine (2.5–5 μCi; the glycine is labeled in the carboxyl group) is given orally, expired air is sampled hourly for six to eight hours, and $^{14}CO_2$ is analyzed.

Normal values are less than 3% to 4% of administered dose expired in six hours. Results may be expressed in several ways, including graphs. Abnormally high values are found after resection or disease of the terminal ileum or in bacterial overgrowth in the small intestine. False-negative results may be obtained whenever the bacterial flora is suppressed, such as after antibiotics, enemas, or laxatives or when the intestinal transit is extremely rapid (after jejunoileal bypass operation). The test is useful in evaluating the presence of ileal disease or bacterial overgrowth.

Vitamin B$_{12}$ Malabsorption
The normal absorption of vitamin B$_{12}$ is dependent upon the presence of intrinsic factor, normal ileal function, and also on normal pancreatic function. Bacterial overgrowth or the tapeworm *Diphylobotrium latum* in the small bowel may interfere with absorption.

Schilling Test See Chapter 3. Correction of vitamin B$_{12}$ malabsorption by a course of broad-spectrum antibiotics suggests the presence of bacterial overgrowth in the small bowel. The test is difficult to perform in children.

Diagnosing the Cause of Malabsorption

Absorption Tests

Absorption tests may prove the existence of malabsorption (or maldigestion). They do not tell us which disease causes it. In general, impaired absorption may be due to diseases of the bowel wall (malabsorption) or to derangements in the lumen of the bowel (maldigestion) (Table 13-4).

The tests for malabsorption may suggest the location or type of the disease; eg, an impaired xylose test suggests disease in the wall of the upper small bowel, whereas impaired absorption of bile salts and vitamin B_{12} indicates disease in the wall of the distal small bowel. However, all three tests, particularly the latter two, may be impaired in bacterial overgrowth in the small bowel.

Jejunal Biopsy

Histology   Histology is essential for the diagnosis of gluten-sensitive enteropathy. It may be helpful in diagnosing lymphoma, eosinophilic gastroenteritis, Whipple's disease, intestinal lymphangiectasia, and other conditions.

Biochemical Analysis   Analysis of enzyme activity in the biopsy material permits one to diagnose deficiency of various enzymes, particularly disaccharidases.

Aspiration of Intestinal Contents

Aspiration of intestinal contents may be helpful for counting bacteria, analyzing bile acids, and diagnosing the presence of fungi, *Giardia lamblia,* and other parasites.

Diagnosing Bacterial Overgrowth in the Small Bowel

The demonstration of more than 10^5 bacteria per mL of upper intestinal aspirate is the most direct method for diagnosing bacterial overgrowth. The demonstration of unconjugated bile acids (by extraction and thin-layer chromatography) in the aspirate supports the diagnosis.

Indirect methods include an impaired [^{14}C]cholyl glycine breath test (see above), which may show an early peak, and the D-[^{14}C]xylose breath test. In this test 5 μCi of D-[^{14}C]xylose is given orally with 1 g of unlabeled D-xylose. The appearance of more than 7% of the dose as $^{14}CO_2$ is due to bacterial overgrowth in the upper bowel causing degradation of the xylose. Results can also be expressed differently, eg, peak height. The hydrogen breath test and the Schilling test may also be impaired in bacterial overgrowth.

■ Quantitation of Gastrointestinal Losses

Occult Blood Loss

Blood loss into the gastrointestinal tract is the major cause of iron deficiency anemia in the adult. This loss may be qualitatively diagnosed or quantitatively measured.

Diagnosis of Occult Bleeding

The presently preferred method is based on guaiac-impregnated paper. It is widely available commercially (Hemoccult, Hematest, Fecatest, etc). The

Table 13-4
Diagnosing the Cause of Malabsorption

Disease	Recommended Tests	Less Specific Tests
Diseases of the Bowel Wall		
Gluten enteropathy	D-Xylose test, stool fat, small bowel biopsy, gluten withdrawal and challenge	Organ culture
Tropical sprue	D-Xylose test, stool fat, small bowel biopsy with oil red O stain, culture of duodenal aspirate.	Response to prolonged antibacterial therapy
Disaccharidase deficiency	Breath tests, small bowel biopsy with disaccharidase assay	Stool pH and reducing substances, with thin layer chromatography.
Chronic infections and infestations (eg, G. lamblia, hookworm)	Stool microscopy, duodenal aspiration and biopsy	Serologic tests
Food allergy	Response to challenge and withdrawal, specific IgE antibodies in serum, eosinophils in peripheral blood and small bowel biopsy	X-rays
Immune deficiency states	Tests of cellular and humoral immunity, plasma cells in small bowel biopsy	

Disease		
Intestinal lymphoma	X-rays, small bowel biopsy, α-heavy chain analysis in urine and plasma	
Enteropathy of dermatitis herpetiformis	Small bowel and skin biopsy, gluten withdrawal	
Intestinal lymphangiectasia	Small bowel biopsy, tests for gastrointestinal protein loss	
Whipple's disease	Small bowel biopsy with PAS stain	Electron microscopy of biopsy material
Diseases Affecting the Bowel Lumen		
Pancreatic insufficiency	Pancreatic function tests (in CF-sweat test)	Response to pancreatic supplements, glucose tolerance test.
Bacterial overgrowth	Culture of duodenal aspirate, D[14C]xylose breath test, [14C]cholyl glycine breath test	Unconjugated bile acids in duodenal aspirate, Schilling test, response to antibiotic therapy
Bile acid deficiency associated with liver disease	Decrease in postprandial serum bile acid rise (radioimmunoassay or gas-liquid chromatography)	Evaluation of liver function
Short bowel syndrome	X-rays, intestinal transit time, stool fat, [14C]cholyl glycine breath test, Schilling test.	
Post gastric surgery	X-rays, stool fat	Fecal bile acids

processing of smeared stool samples has to be done within a few days. To screen for occult bleeding, stools from three consecutive days are analyzed. The method detects blood loss in excess of 15 mL/day. False-positive results may be caused by a meat (heme)-rich diet and some peroxidase-containing foods. False-negative results may be caused by deterioration of the reagents (prolonged storage), undue delay in processing and antioxidants such as vitamin C (ascorbic acid).

Older methods using benzidine as a reagent have been abandoned because of excessive sensitivity (false-positives) and possible carcinogenic effect.

Quantitation of Occult Bleeding
Erythrocytes are labeled with ^{51}Cr and reinjected, and radioactivity in stool collections is measured. Normal values are less than 0.5–1 mL of blood per day, depending on the laboratory.

The method involves the administration of 40–100 μCi of a γ-emitting isotope. The quantitative stool collections are laborious, and the test is not widely used.

Quantitation of Protein Loss

Protein-losing gastroenteropathy may originate in any part of the gastrointestinal tract. When the loss is in the stomach or in the upper small bowel, the proteins are broken down and reabsorbed and the stool nitrogen will not be increased. Quantitation of protein loss may be performed by several methods, each with its own limitations.

^{131}I-Labeled PVP
Ten microcuries of polyvinyl pyrrolidone (PVP) is injected intravenously, stools are collected for four days, and radioactivity is measured. Normal values are not more than 1% to 1.6% of the injected PVP in the stools during four days.

PVP is a synthetic polymer similar in size to some of the smaller proteins. The iodine label may split from the polymer molecule, causing artifacts and may be absorbed by the thyroid.

^{51}C-Labeled Proteins
After injection of [^{51}Cr]albumin or [^{51}Cr]chromium chloride (in vivo labeling), stools are collected for four days and radioactivity is measured. Normal values are less than 1% of the administered dose in the four-day stools.

■ Diagnosing the Cause of Diarrhea

Diarrhea may be caused by intestinal pathogens (bacteria, viruses, parasites, etc), chronic inflammation of the bowel wall due to various causes, neoplastic diseases, drugs (sometimes taken surreptitiously), allergic and hypersensitivity conditions, hormones, and postoperative conditions. Stool analysis is essential and contributes to the diagnosis in the majority of cases.

Examination of Stools

Appearance
Bloody diarrhea indicates inflammation of the bowel wall, acute or chronic, and more rarely neoplastic conditions. *Watery diarrhea,* especially voluminous, suggests mostly small bowel disease. *Pus* usually indicates inflammation, whereas *mucus* is of large bowel origin and is nondiagnostic. *Foamy, foul-smelling stools* suggest malabsorption.

Microscopy
The presence of leukocytes is a valuable sign indicating damage to or invasion of the bowel wall. In acute diarrhea it may point toward enteroinvasive organisms. Leukocytes may also be present in neoplastic or chronic inflammatory diseases. Eosinophils are rarely seen and may indicate an allergic or parasitic origin. The presence of ova and parasites may also offer a clue to the cause of diarrhea. The presence of hematophagous trophozoites of *Enttamoeba histolytica* is diagnostic of invasive amebiasis.

Microbiology
Stool cultures are essential to diagnose the infectious cause of diarrhea. *Salmonella, Shigella, Campylobacter, Yersinia, E. histolytica,* and *Giardia lamblia* should be looked for among the enteroinvasive organisms. Enteropathogenic *Escherichia coli* are important in epidemics in pediatric patients. *Vibrio cholera* and other enterotoxigenic bacteria must be taken into account, in an appropriate clinical setting, in watery diarrheas. A cytopathic effect in cell culture, neutralized by clostridial antitoxin is diagnostic of *Clostridium difficile* toxin. This is to be looked for particularly in postantibiotic diarrheas, but also in other acute and chronic diarrheas.

Serologic Tests
Serologic tests may be of help in some conditions. Indirect hemagglutination or counterimmunoelectrophoresis tests for amebiasis may be diagnostic when stool examinations are negative. Serologic tests now exist for most bacteria and parasites.

Chemical Examination of Stools
An acid pH and reducing substances in the stool may suggest carbohydrate malabsorption.

Electrolytes and Osmolality
Sodium and potassium are the main cations in the stool. Normally, the sum of concentrations $(Na^+ + K^+) \times 2$ = osmolality of stool. This also holds true for all secretory diarrheas induced by hormones, bacterial toxins, inflammation, irritant laxatives, bile salts, etc. However, when there is an additional osmotic load in the colon, an "osmotic gap" will appear, and the stool osmolality will be more than 150–200 mOsm higher than the sum $(Na^+ + K^+) \times 2$. This occurs in malabsorption and diarrhea due to osmotic laxatives such as magnesium compounds or lactulose. The measurement of osmolality and the $Na^+ + K^+$ concentration in stool water are of diagnostic value especially in protracted diarrheas of obscure origin.

Normal values of stool osmolality are about 400 mosm. Normal concentrations for Na⁺ are 25–50 mEq/L; normal concentrations for K⁺ are 80–140 mEq/L. Diarrhea that continues after 24–48 hours of fasting is usually secretory in origin. This can be confirmed by the above analysis.

Bile Acids   The amount of bile acids in the stool can be measured (see Bile acid malabsorption, above). Bile salt-induced diarrhea is seen in ileal disease or resection and rarely in biliary-colonic fistula.

Hormonal Diarrhea   This is an exceedingly rare cause of diarrhea; it is secretory in nature and will not disappear on fasting. Some clues may exist: gastric acid hypersecretion will suggest gastrinoma, achlorhydria with hypopotasemia and hypercalcemia may suggest a vasoactive intestinal polypeptides (VIP)-secreting tumor, and increased 5-hydroxyindoleacetic acid (HIAA) in the urine may suggest carcinoid. Final diagnosis rests upon demonstration of the hormone in serum or tumor tissue. With the exception of gastrin, these hormone analyses are not widely available.

■ Selected Readings

Diseases of the Stomach

Baron JH: The clinical use of gastric secretion tests. *Scand J Gastroenterol* (Suppl) 1970;6:9–46.

Grossman MI: Gastrointestinal hormones, in Parsons JA: *Peptide Hormones.* London, Macmillan Press, 1976, p. 105.

Diseases of the Pancreas

Adrian TE: Plasma trypsin like immunoreactivity in normal subjects and in patients with pancreatic diseases. *Scand J Gastroenterol* (Suppl) 1980;15:15–20.

Arvanitakis C, Cooke AR: Diagnostic tests of exocrine pancreas: Function and disease. *Gastroenterology* 1978;74: 932–949.

Banks P: *Pancreatitis.* New York, Plenum Publishing Corp, 1979.

Gilat T, Gelman-Malachi E, Ronen O: Chymotrypsin output in the stools in pancreatic and other diseases. *Am J Gastroenterol* 1976;66:140–145.

Rolny P: Diagnosis of pancreatic disease with special reference to the secretin cholecystokinin test. *Scand J Gastroenterol* (Suppl) 1980;15:60.

Salt WB, Schenker S: Amylase—its clinical significance. A review of the literature. *Medicine* 1976;55:4, 269–289.

Warsaw AL, Fuller AF Jr: Specificity of increased renal clearance of amylase in diagnosis of acute pancreatitis. *N Engl J Med* 1975;292:325–328.

Diseases of the Small Intestine

Bliss CM: Fat absorption and malabsorption. *Arch Intern Med* 1981;141:1213–1215.

Caspary WF: Breath tests. *Clin Gastroenterol* 1978;7:351–374.

Gray GM: Carbohydrate digestion and absorption. Role of the small intestine. *N Engl J Med* 1975;292:1225–1230.

Olson WA: A pathophysiologic approach to diagnosis of malabsorption. *Am J Med* 1979;67:999–1006.

Russell RI, Lee FD: Tests of small intestinal function, digestion, absorption, secretion. *Clin Gastroenterol* 1978;7:277–315.

West PS, Levin GE, Griffin GE, et al: Comparison of simple screening tests for fat malabsorption. *Br Med J* 1981;282: 1501–1504.

Diagnosing the Cause of Diarrhea

Dobbins JW, Binder HJ: Pathophysiology of diarrhea: Alterations in fluid and electrolyte transport. *Clin Gastroenterol* 1981;10:605–625.

Evans N: Pathogenic mechanisms in bacterial diarrhea. *Clin Gastroenterol* 1979; 8:599–623.

Hamilton JR: Infectious diarrhea: Clinical implications of recent research. *Can Med Assoc J* 1980;12:29–32.

Turnberg LA: The pathophysiology of diarrhea. *Clin Gastroenterol* 1979;8: 551–568.

■ Liver Function Tests

Despite increasingly advanced technology, the experienced clinicians rely on history taking and physical examination for the basis of their diagnosis. A careful "feel" of the liver is often worth several liver function tests. Laboratory determinations alone suggest that there *is* illness. Used properly, liver function tests help considerably to confirm the clinical impression, and they may delineate the magnitude of a disorder. At present, one need not rely entirely on liver function tests, even ones with significant discriminatory value, for specific diagnosis. There are, after all, only so many biochemical responses to diverse hepatic injuries. We now have more exact diagnostic methods such as liver biopsy, peritoneoscopy, ultrasound, cholescintigraphy, computerized tomography, and several forms of cholangiography. These, however, augment but do not replace the information obtained from liver function testing.

Liver function tests confirm the clinical impression of the presence of liver disease and suggest its type; allow us to recognize subclinical or latent liver disease; in some settings allow us to determine the activity of the pathologic process, ie, determine disease severity; in some instances to allow us to infer prognosis; and finally not only to provide guidelines for therapy but also to facilitate our evaluation of response to that therapy. They are most useful when they are correlated with the clinical, laboratory, radiological, and histological findings and when they are obtained sequentially. No single liver function test meets all of the above expectations. When multiple tests are used, each should reflect a different parameter of liver function.

There may be 100 or more liver function tests for the clinician to choose from, but in practice we tend to use only the few that are rapid, inexpensive, and reproducible, cause minimal discomfort and negligible side effects, and have maximum discriminatory value. This last criterion can be expanded to include specificity, sensitivity, and selectivity.

The classical liver function tests may be divided into three major groups: those that reflect inflammatory activity, those that reflect hepatocyte synthetic function, and those that reflect hepatocyte clearance mechanisms from the circulation and the formation and flow of bile (Table 14-1). Although not usually considered among the liver function tests, tests that reflect the liver's storage function for heavy metals will also be considered.

Tests that Reflect Inflammatory Activity

SGOT (AST)
Serum glutamic-oxaloacetic transaminase (SGOT) is found

Table 14-1
Types of Liver Function Tests

Tests that Reflect Inflammatory Activity
    Serum transaminases (aminotransferases)
    Flocculation tests
    Serum globulins

Tests that Reflect Synthetic Function
    Serum albumin
    Prothrombin time
    Serum Cholesterol

Tests that Reflect Clearance Mechanisms and the Formation and Flow of Bile
    Serum bile acids
    Serum bilirubin
    Urine bilirubin and urobilinogen
    Bromsulphalein and indocyanine green
    Serum alkaline phosphatase
    Serum 5′-Nucleotidase
    Serum leucine aminopeptidase
    Serum gamma glutamyl transpeptidase

Tests that Reflect Hepatic Storage of Heavy Metals

in multiple organs. This enzyme catalyzes the reaction of L-aspartic acid and α-ketoglutaric acid to form oxaloacetic and glutamic acids. It is more properly known as aspartate aminotransferase (AST), but in North America this term has not supplanted the more firmly established SGOT.

SGOT is a test of liver cell injury and our most sensitive index of necrosis. Transaminase elevation, however, does not necessarily imply necrosis, since the activity of glutamic oxaloacetic transaminase in plasma is regulated by a releasing mechanism across the cell membranes and not by intracellular enzyme content. Injury sufficient to alter the permeability of the cell membrane may cause release into plasma without otherwise altering the cell's biochemical capabilities or its viability.

The height of the elevation does not necessarily correlate with the degree of histologic injury seen on biopsy. Enzyme elevation does not even necessarily imply that histological injury will be seen at all on liver biopsy. Transaminase elevation may be seen after several days either in patients on oral elemental diets or during total parenteral nutrition. Early in the course of such therapy liver biopsy may show no histological abnormality even though transaminases are elevated several times above baseline levels. It is uncertain whether this represents hepatotoxicity or nutrient-induced induction of enzyme synthesis.

The highest levels of SGOT are seen in acute hepatitis and in acute circulatory impairment of the liver. Values over 1000 IU are almost always a result of one of these two disorders. There are, however, reports of subclinical left ventricular failure as well as acute biliary obstruction causing similar elevations. In the latter circumstance, there is a rapid return toward the more characteristic range even when obstruction continues. Alcohol may rarely cause very high levels of SGOT; however, the higher the elevation of this enzyme, the more likely one of the first two causes.

The test is highly sensitive—several days of alcohol intake will result in mild elevations of SGOT in normal persons at a time when liver biopsy will show minimal or no histologic changes. In viral hepatitis SGOT elevation is one of the earliest abnormalities noted.

Below levels of 300 IU, the SGOT allows for little selectivity among various liver diseases or specificity between diseases of other organs such as heart or skeletal muscles. Specificity is also impaired by factors that may interfere with its determination. With some colormetric methods, an artifactual increase in SGOT may be seen in patients taking drugs such as erythromycin or para-aminosalicylic acid, and an artifactual decrease may be seen in azotemic patients.

SGPT (ALT)

Serum glutamic pyruvate transaminase (SGPT) or alanine aminotransferase (ALT) is responsible for the reaction of alanine with ketoglutarate to form pyruvic and glutamic acids. SGPT is also found in kidney and skeletal muscle, but its highest concentration is in the liver. It therefore offers greater specificity than SGOT. In acute hepatitis or circulatory injury, its value equals or exceeds that of SGOT. In myocardial infarction, it is considerably lower. In two special situations the greater specificity of SGPT for liver injury seems not to hold. In alcohol-induced liver disease the SGPT is almost always less than the SGOT. It has been found that the SGOT/SGPT ratio is over 1.5 in over 90% of patients with alcohol-induced liver injury. It is less than 1 in under 2%. The reasons are not fully understood. A reduction in pyridoxal phosphate, a co-factor upon which both transaminase activities are dependent, results in values of SGOT in alcohol-induced disease which are low relative to the degree of necrosis. SGPT levels are even more affected, and the result is the characteristic reversal of the usual ratio of these enzymes. The other setting for the frequent reversal of the SGOT/SGPT ratio is in hepatoma, especially when accompanied by tumor necrosis. There appears to be preferential leakage of SGOT across the cell membranes.

In the setting of alcohol-induced injury, the determination of both enzymes may be justified. In most other circumstances one enzyme seems to serve just as well. The older clinicians seem to prefer SGOT because their clinical experience with it is longer. Other physicians opt for SGPT because of its greater specificity.

Flocculation Tests

Since we can now quantify albumin and globulin and perform protein electrophoresis on a routine basis, the flocculation tests have begun to disappear from general use.

Serum Globulins

Elevation of globulins can occur in many diseases unrelated to the liver and must therefore be regarded as not specific. Globulin determinations are also not particularly sensitive. Elevations are seen in all forms of parenchymal liver disease; therefore, globulin elevation has little discriminatory value.

In chronic active hepatitis, elevated levels may sometimes serve as a marker of continuing inflammatory activity. Globulin elevations may also indicate the progression of acute viral hepatitis to a chronic form.

In cirrhotic liver disease globulin elevation, rather than signifying ongoing inflammation, may reflect significant extrahepatic and intrahepatic portal venous shunting. Antigens from the gut normally removed by hepatic Kuppfer cells are instead taken up by antibody-producing tissues such as the spleen where a continuous anamnestic stimulation to immunoglobulin production may occur.

Separation of globulin into its separate classes, in general, provides little additional information. The α globulins may be elevated, normal, or decreased in liver disease. The $\alpha 1$ fraction is diminished or absent in $\alpha 1$ antitrypsin deficiency. The $\alpha 2$ fraction is occasionally elevated in secondary carcinoma of the liver; β globulins are increased in all types of liver disease, but may reach extremely high levels in protracted obstructive jaundice. The hyperglobulinemia of cirrhosis is from elevation of the gamma globulins. The hypergammaglobulinemia of liver disease produces a wide electrophoretic band rather than the high narrow band typical of the paraproteinemias. Elevations of gamma globulin can also be seen in any active inflammatory disease and are not specific for liver disease.

Some selectivity can be found in the pattern of immunoglobulins. While immunoglobulin A (IgA) is elevated most frequently in alcoholic liver disease and is raised in approximately 75% of patients with biliary tract disease, it is also seen in almost every other cause for liver disease and cannot be relied upon to be of value in an individual patient. High IgG levels are seen most often in chronic hepatitis, but are better used as markers for activity rather than for etiology. Spectacular elevations may be seen in visceral leishmaniasis. Marked elevations of IgM are seen in 80% of patients with primary biliary cirrhosis, but 20% of patients with persistent extrahepatic obstruction also have elevated IgM. Antimitochondrial antibody has for the most part supplanted IgM as a specific marker for primary biliary cirrhosis; however, the combination of increased IgM and the presence of antimitochondrial antibody makes a strong case for primary biliary cirrhosis.

Tests that Reflect Synthetic Function

Serum Albumin

Serum albumin is low in patients with liver disease for any of several reasons. Impaired formation may result from damaged liver cells or inadequate amounts of dietary protein. Distribution may be abnormal due to edema or ascites. Increased loss of albumin may occur from hemorrhage, paracentesis, or exudation of protein into the intestinal tract. The most important of these mechanisms is failure of the damaged liver cells to synthesize adequate amounts of albumin. The finding of low albumin does not necessarily implicate liver disease. It may be low entirely on the basis of a poor protein intake, a general catabolic state, or increased degradation and loss. When these are ruled out, a fall in serum albumin correlates roughly with the degree and duration of liver disease. Alterations are infrequent in acute disease unless severe. The half-life of albumin is 17–20 days. Complete cessation of albumin production for a week is therefore required to reduce the serum albumin concentration by 25%. In evaluating the albumin level, the clinician should remember that a recent hemorrhage or paracentesis can produce a fall of 1 g/dL in the albumin level.

Remember that the usual salting out technique used by laboratories for albumin determination tends to overestimate serum albumin concentration. The albumin filtrate contains most of the α globulin and a portion of the β globulin as well. The albumin values obtained from more accurate electrophoretic methods are often as much as 1 g/dL less than the fractionation technique.

Despite these pitfalls, one can estimate prognosis from the serum albumin. Patients with a persistent serum albumin less than 2 g/dL have a poor prognosis. Patients capable of raising the serum albumin in successive months of observation have a good prognosis. Patients with serum albumin levels below 3 g/dL are at increased risk for surgery and general anesthesia.

Prothrombin Time
The liver synthesizes factors I, II, V, VII, IX, and X. Of these factors II, VII, IX, and X are vitamin K dependent. The standard prothrombin time (one stage prothrombin time of Quick) will be prolonged if any of the contributing factors, singly or in combination, is significantly deficient because of decreased synthesis as a result of either hepatic damage or unavailability of vitamin K.

A prolonged prothrombin time may also be seen in various congenital deficiencies of coagulation factors, in clotting factor consumptive disorders, and after the injection of certain drugs. Vitamin K, which is fat soluble, may be deficient in prolonged obstructive jaundice, steatorrhea, or, rarely, on a dietary basis. When these are excluded hepatic parenchymal disease can be inferred. One ought, nonetheless, to administer vitamin K to exclude hypovitaminosis, in which case the prothrombin time will return to normal or increase by at least 30% within 24 hours after a dose of 5–10 mg parenterally. Administration of large doses of vitamin K in an attempt to correct the hypoprothrombinemia of severe liver disease may result in a paradoxical further depression of prothrombin concentration. The mechanism is unknown.

The prothrombin time is not a sensitive test, since it may be normal with advanced cirrhosis or with significant infiltrative disease. When prothrombin time is abnormal and nonhepatic causes are excluded, however, it invariably means significant parenchymal disease. Unlike serum albumin, which also reflects synthetic function, the prothrombin time may become abnormal quickly and reflect acute injury. Some laboratories report actual prothrombin time and a control value; others report patient values as a percentage of control.

Prothrombin time may have prognostic significance. Values below 40% of control after parenteral administration of vitamin K have been found to be the best single indicator of progression of acute hepatitis to the fulminant disease. Values below 10% suggest that recovery is unlikely. In alcoholic hepatitis prothrombin time also has prognostic value. In a group of patients in which prothrombin time remained prolonged by four seconds or more after parenteral administration of vitamin K, the mortality was near 50%. When the prothrombin time corrected to less than four seconds beyond control value, mortality was less than 10%.

Another application of the prothrombin time is its use in helping to determine whether liver biopsy can be safely performed. In the absence of other contraindications to biopsy, a prothrombin time above 70% usually indicates that biopsy can be performed with safety. With a prothrombin time between 50% and 70%, biopsy can often still be performed with safety by an experienced operator, but increased caution is in order. Below a value of 50%, the risk-benefit ratio should be carefully examined, and both patient and physician must be prepared for an increased likelihood of bleeding.

Serum Cholesterol

The majority of the body's cholesterol is synthesized by the liver from the metabolic pool, but other sources of serum cholesterol exist. Besides synthesizing cholesterol, the liver degrades it, principally by conversion into bile salts and acids. The liver may be responsible for changes in cholesterol concentration by either altered synthesis, altered biliary excretion, or altered liver metabolism. Yet changes in serum cholesterol values have little specificity for liver disease. The interplay of genetic factors, dietary factors, and this complex metabolism makes determination of serum cholesterol of limited value in the diagnosis of liver conditions. Elevations in serum cholesterol are seen, however, with cholestasis from either extrahepatic or intrahepatic obstruction, with values increasing as the process becomes chronic. In cirrhotic patients, perhaps reflecting malnutrition, cholesterol values tend to be low. Low values can also reflect severe liver cell disease, and a falling cholesterol in biliary cirrhosis, either primary or secondary, may herald the onset of hepatocellular failure. A high cholesterol level in the cirrhotic patient (who does not have cholestatic alcohol hepatitis) ought to make one consider hepatoma, which has increased cholesterol as one of its metabolic manifestations. The ratio of free to esterified cholesterol is no longer used.

Tests that Reflect Clearance Function and Bile Formation

Serum Bile Acids

The clinical use of bile acid tests has been severely limited by the methods available for measuring them, but commercial radioimmunoassay kits are now increasingly available. Bile acids do not have an established clinical track record, but look promising.

Four bile acids form over 99% of the bile acid pool: cholic acid, chenodeoxycholic acid, deoxycholic acid, and lithocholic acid. All are derivatives of cholesterol and differ from one another only by the number and sites of hydroxylation. Cholic acid and chenodeoxycholic acid are termed primary bile acids because they are formed from cholesterol by the liver. They are metabolized by intestinal bacteria to form the secondary bile acids, deoxycholic acid and lithocholic acid. The relative concentration of these acids (cholic: chenodeoxycholic: deoxycholic: lithocholic) is 10:10:5:1.

Bile acids are synthesized by hepatocytes and form part of an enterohepatic circulation. Because their total amount is significantly greater than the daily bilirubin pool, they may form the basis of a more sensitive measure of hepatic and biliary tract function. They have the further advantage of being highly specific for liver disease. The concentration of total serum bile acids indicates the fraction reabsorbed from the intestine that has escaped extraction on first passage through the liver. The fraction reabsorbed is essentially constant over a large range of blood levels. Bile acid concentration may be measured in the fasting state, two hours postprandially, or by determining the disappearance rate of intravenously injected bile acid. The latter procedure remains for the moment strictly an investigative tool. Many studies suggest that the two hour postprandial determination is a more sensitive indicator of hepatic dysfunction than the fasting level. This enhanced sensitivity results from the greater load on hepatic excretory function that occurs in the postprandial period from enterohepatic recycling. During the course of the digestion of a meal, the bile acid pool is absorbed and resecreted at least once. Serum bile acids may rise two- to sixfold. The two hour postprandial serum bile acid level, which is more or less an endogenous tolerance test, may be elevated in patients with minimal liver disease and normal fasting bile acid levels.

An elevation of total serum bile acid is thought by some to be the most sensitive indicator of the presence of hepatic disease. Although this may be true in comparison with other standard liver function tests taken individually, it does not appear to be true when compared to the collective use of standard liver function tests—all of which are better standarized than the measurement of serum bile acids. There is no need, however, to use bile acids in isolation. They may be used to supplement other liver function tests.

Information can be gained from total serum bile acids or the ratio of primary bile acids. Total serum bile acids are elevated in anicteric acute or chronic liver diseases and can be a sensitive clue to their presence. They also have selectivity in distinguishing types of liver disease. Some authors have suggested the absence of an elevation in serum bile acids as a necessary condition for the diagnosis of Gilbert's syndrome. Total bile acids may also be used to follow the course of a disease or for identifying recurrence in chronic hepatitis. The Mayo Clinic group found a rise in total bile acids to be more sensitive than bilirubin, proteins, alkaline phosphatase, prothrombin time, and bromsulphthalein (BSP)—and slightly more sensitive than the transaminase activity—in predicting disease activity in patients who relapsed. This change preceded histologic change.

Determination of the primary bile salt ratio may be useful in some circumstances. It has been claimed that the cholic/chenodeoxycholic acid ratio is less than 1.5 in portal cirrhosis and greater than 1.5 in large duct obstruction jaundice. If one uses a ratio of 0.5 for cirrhosis and 3.5 for obstruction, a complete separation of the disorders is possible. This separation is probably based on impairment of cholic acid synthesis in cirrhosis, owing to damage to the 12_α-hydroxylating mechanism, and a relative increase in cholic acid production in large duct obstruction. There is no evidence, however, that measurement of bile acids or determination of their ratios is sufficiently selective to allow separation of patients with intrahepatic cholestasis from those with extrahepatic cholestasis.

Still another role for the primary bile salt ratio is in the staging of disease. Patients with primary biliary cirrhosis have falling values as the disease progresses; as illness become terminal, the cholic/deoxycholic acid ratio falls to less than 1. In alcoholic liver disease the ratio progresses from low to high as cirrhosis changes from active to inactive. Patients with chronic active hepatitis sometimes have an increase in the ratio from abnormally low values as the disease enters remission.

Bile acid determinations promise to provide noninvasive liver function tests that may offer sensitivity, specificity, and some selectivity, but further experience is necessary.

Serum Bilirubin

Serum bilirubin is the oldest of the determinants of the liver's clearance and bile formation functions. Each day bilirubin, formed from the breakdown of senescent red blood cells and a smaller percentage from myoglobin and directly from the bone marrow from ineffective erythropoesis, enters the plasma. In plasma it binds to albumin and is delivered by the circulation to the hepatic sinusoids, where it is taken up, conjugated, excreted, and drained along with other constituents of bile down the biliary passages into the intestines, where some of it, by an enterohepatic circulation, reenters the system. Elevation of bilirubin in serum can occur at any one of these steps: production, delivery, uptake, conjugation, excretion, and drainage. At the production, delivery, uptake, and conjugation stages, bilirubin is unconjugated. In the excretion and drainage steps it is conjugated. While unconjugated it is not water soluble, is albumin bound, and does not appear in the urine. After conjugation it is water soluble and when present in excess gives rise to bilirubinuria.

The classic differentiation between these two forms of bilirubin has been the Van den Bergh reaction. In this reaction a diazo reagent reacts promptly with the water-soluble conjugated moiety and can be measured by its spectral absorptive characteristics. The unconjugated moiety is lipophilic and must be solubilized with alcohol before it reacts with the diazo reagent. The terms direct and indirect reacting bilirubin are therefore used synonymously with conjugated and unconjugated. The direct bilirubin measured by this technique is thought to be most accurate when the value is read at exactly one minute. Thus, one-minute bilirubin is also used as a synonym for conjugated bilirubin.

Knowing whether elevated bilirubin is predominantly direct or indirect, helps to determine etiology. Indirect (unconjugated) hyperbilirubinemia occurs with increased breakdown of red blood cells as in hemolysis or an increase in the bone marrow component as in ineffective erythropoiesis (increased production). If for some reason bilirubin does not reach the liver efficiently as in circulatory failure or with extensive shunting of blood away from the liver, in portal hypertension from cirrhosis and other causes, unconjugated bilirubin will also be elevated (impaired delivery).

Once bilirubin reaches the hepatic sinusoids, uptake by hepatocytes begins. Elevations in bilirubin can occur when other organic anions or drugs (such as BSP, biliary contrast media, flavaspidic acid, rifampicin) compete with the carrier system (impaired uptake).

Once inside the cell a relatively small fraction of the bilirubin diffuses back out again. This amount is about 25%. In the hereditary disorders Crigler-Najjar syndrome (type I) and Arias syndrome (type II), UDP glucuronyl transferase is either absent or markedly diminished. Hyperbilirubinemia may occur in neonates because the UDP glucuronyl transferase system has not yet matured or because inhibitors of bilirubin conjugation are transferred from the mother to the neonate as in the Lucey-Driscoll syndrome and "breast-milk jaundice." In Gilbert's syndrome there is also a deficiency of UDP glucuronyl transferase.

Disorders at any of these steps (production, delivery, uptake, conjugation) can cause unconjugated hyperbilirubinemia. Disorders of the next two steps (excretion and drainage) cause conjugated hyperbilirubinemia. The number of causes for defects at these steps is large.

Excretion is an active carrier-mediated secretory process. The most common cause of jaundice at this step is hepatocellular disease such as alcoholic or viral hepatitis and cirrhosis. Some drugs and toxins may also cause hepatocellular disease. There are, however, also hereditary abnormalities of excretion of bilirubin such as the Dubin-Johnson and Rotor syndromes. A final cause of conjugated hyperbilirubinemia at the excretion step is injury from drugs, such as methyl-testosterone, and other 17-alpha-alkyl-steroids which alter the canalicular membrane.

The second major cause of conjugated hyperbilirubinemia is a defect at the drainage step leading to cholestasis. Elevated plasma levels of bile salts, and often cholesterol and alkaline phosphatase as well as conjugated bilirubin, distinguish cholestasis from the hepatocellular form of jaundice. The cholestatic disorders may be either intrahepatic or extrahepatic and are further classifiable by etiology. Causes of intrahepatic cholestasis include various hepatic storage syndromes and congenital diseases, drug-induced injury (such as estrogenic steroid hormones, phenothiazines, diazepoxides, sulfonylureas, antithyroid preparations, and many other drugs capable of causing hypersensitivity reactions), and sometimes certain cholestatic forms of viral and alcoholic hepatitis, granulomatous diseases, intrahepatic space occupying lesions, and bile duct destructive processes such as primary biliary cirrhosis. Extrahepatic obstruction includes stones, strictures, tumors, and poorly understood phenomena such as sclerosing cholangitis.

We can thus see that direct bilirubin is a specific test of liver function though neither very sensitive nor selective. In some automated techniques, the partition of bilirubin into direct and indirect is not always entirely accurate at concentrations below 5 mg/dL and this possibility should be considered before yielding to the confusion which an unexpected partition may engender. The presence or absence of urine bilirubin is sometimes a simple way of sidestepping the confusion.

Indirect bilirubin is not sensitive, specific, or selective, but nonetheless can be used constructively to arrive at an understanding of its etiology if the steps at which disorders in bilirubin metabolism can occur are kept in mind (Table 14-2).

Urine Bilirubin and Urine Urobilinogen
Several commercial products allow rapid determination of bilirubinuria on the ward. Although these tests are usually sensitive for bilirubinuria, bilirubinuria itself is not a sensitive test for hepatic disorders. Bilirubinuria may be absent in moderately advanced liver disease. Like bilirubin, it is quite specific, but not selective. Many hepatic disorders cause it.

The last step in the metabolism of bilirubin is its breakdown in the intestine and absorption of its derivatives. Theoretically, urinary urobilinogen is reduced in the presence of excretory or drainage disorders, absent with

Table 14-2
Causes of Elevations in Serum Bilirubin

Step in Bilirubin Metabolism	Fraction Elevated	Causes
Production	Indirect	Hemolysis Ineffective erythropoiesis
Delivery	Indirect	Portal systemic shunting (surgical, cirrhosis) Congestive heart failure
Uptake	Indirect	Competition by drugs or diagnostic agents
Conjugation	Indirect	UDP glucuronyl transferase immaturity (neonatal jaundice) UDP glucuronyl transferase diminished or absent (Gilbert's syndrome, Arias's syndrome, Crigler-Najjar syndrome) Inhibition of UDP glucuronyl transferase (Lucey-Driscoll syndrome, breast milk jaundice)
Excretion	Direct	Hepatocellular disease Hereditary abnormalities (Dubin-Johnson syndrome, Rotor syndrome) Drug injury (17-alpha alkyl steroids)
Drainage	Direct	Intrahepatic cholestasis (hepatic storage syndromes, congenital diseases, drug induced injury, infiltrative and granulomatous diseases, hepatocellular disease, cholangiolytic processes) Extrahepatic cholestasis (obstruction from stones, strictures, tumors, bile duct destructive processes)

complete biliary obstruction, and increased in hemolytic states or whenever there is increased bilirubin production, as well as in any hepatic dysfunctional state where a decrease in hepatic excretion of urobilinogen leads to an increase in blood levels and increased excretion into the urine. The test, however, is beset with pitfalls that have the accumulative effect of making urinary urobilinogen determination a less than satisfactory routine procedure. It is most likely to be helpful when urinary urobilinogen is persistently completely absent, which usually suggests cancerous obstruction of the biliary tree. Cholangiolytic hepatitis and biliary tract stones, however, may on occasion cause a similar absence of urobilinogen. Today the enlightened practice of medicine is entirely possible without ever once ordering a urine urobilinogen test.

BSP and Indocyanine Green
BSP is taken up, conjugated, and excreted by the liver in much the same way as bilirubin. Long a favorite test of the liver's metabolic function, BSP has fallen into disfavor among certain groups. This disfavor is the result of several factors. In spite of its sensitivity and its relative specificity, requiring only integrity of the circulation, it is not very discriminating.

More important, a number of fatal anaphylactic reactions have occurred. For this reason it is the view of many that its advantages are still inadequate to make an acceptable risk/benefit ratio. Nonfatal reactions are also reported, and extravasation can cause severe necrosis.

The standard test is performed by injecting BSP intravenously (5 mg/kg) and drawing a venous sample at 45 minutes from the contralateral arm. At 45 minutes the concentration remaining in the blood is determined, and the result is usually expressed in terms of percent retention based on the assumed initial concentration.

Since BSP is widely regarded as the most sensitive test of liver function (but even with BSP more than half the liver may need to be diseased to cause abnormal results), an almost mystic reverence is given by some for the results of the BSP, a reverence altogether undeserved. In a very thin person, plasma volume is probably more than 5% of total body weight, and these patients may get too small a dose of BSP; on the other hand, patients who are markedly over 70 kg may receive far too large a dose, since plasma volume will be less than the 5% estimate.

Most hepatologists have found clinical uses for the standard 45-minute BSP test, although more sophisticated BSP clearance studies remain a highly useful research technique. Even for research purposes, BSP has in some instances been replaced by indocyanine green. Indocyanine green is handled much the same way as BSP (except that it does not require conjugation in order to be excreted), but lacks its toxicity. Most clinicians give 0.5 mg/kg of body weight intravenously; a sample is taken after 20 minutes. While it is safer than BSP, it is not often that reliance on the test can give information that thoughtful analysis of the history, physical, and more specific tests cannot also provide.

Serum Alkaline Phosphatase
The alkaline phosphatases are a ubiquitous group of enzymes, generally found on the absorptive or secretory surfaces of cells. The alkaline phosphatases found in normal serum come predominently from the liver, bone, intestine, and placenta.

Serum alkaline phosphatase is most sensitive as a liver function test as an indicator of disruption in bile flow, either intrahepatic or extrahepatic obstruction, infiltration, or cholestasis from other causes (such as drugs). It has some differential function in that hepatocellular diseases usually result in less than a twofold increase in alkaline phosphatase. Cholestatic mechanisms of all causes, on the other hand, usually result in more than a twofold increase. Some caution is needed, however, in that as many as 20% of cases of clearly established obstructive jaundice may have alkaline phosphatase values in the "hepatocellular" range, whereas some 5% of hepatocellular jaundice may be associated with alkaline phosphatase elevations greater than 5 times the upper limit of normal.

The cause for alkaline phosphatase elevation in the serum of patients with liver disease appears to be enhanced de novo synthesis, since in experimental animals alkaline phosphatase response to liver and bile duct injury can be blocked by drugs that inhibit protein or RNA synthesis.

Although alkaline phosphatase may be relatively sensitive and somewhat discriminatory, it is not always specific. In bone disease with osteoblastic activity, alkaline phosphatase may also be increased, and there are also reports of increased alkaline phosphatase activity after pulmonary infarction and with congestive heart failure, thyrotoxicosis, intraabdominal infections, diabetes, and in stage I or II of Hodgkins' disease without evidence of liver or bone involvement. In normal pregnancy it is expected to be increased. A falling alkaline phosphatase in the third trimester, in fact, may be viewed as a sign of fetal distress. Some manufacturers of serum albumin use human placenta, and such albumin infusions can be expected to raise alkaline phosphatase (placental isoenzyme).

The cause of an increase in alkaline phosphatase—whether bone, liver, or placenta (intestinal alkaline phosphatase may constitute a sizable portion of circulating alkaline phosphatase in some patients, especially after a fatty meal, but is seldom a cause for major elevation of alkaline phosphatase)—can be determined by several techniques: heat stability, electrophoretic mobility, and various inhibition studies. In practice, however, one does not always get a clear-cut answer. Other confirmatory enzymes may be needed if the hepatic source of alkaline phosphatase is not certain. One advantage of these new fractionation studies has been our recognition of an additional cause of increased serum alkaline phosphatase. In some patients with cancer, particularly of the lung, an elevated alkaline phosphatase corresponding to the placental isoenzyme has been identified and is referred to as the Regan isoenzyme. This enzyme can be found in the tumor itself and is thought to represent the derepression of a gene. More recently, additional tumor alkaline phosphatases have been identified that do not correspond to placental alkaline phosphatase; these may be phylogenetically immature forms.

One must also remember that some patients may have a mild elevation of alkaline phosphatase that has no pathologic significance—even though one may establish that it is the liver isoenzyme that is elevated. It should also be borne in mind that the upper limit for normal alkaline phosphatase increases with age, and by the sixth decade of life, values of one and one-half times greater than the usual upper limit of normal may be seen in apparently healthy persons. Therefore, be wary of diagnosing liver disease on the basis of enzymology alone.

5'N

The 5' nucleotidase (5'N) in human serum comes principally from liver canalicular and sinusoidal membranes. This group of enzymes is, however, ubiquitous and is found in heart and blood vessels, skeletal muscle, pancreas, intestine, testes, the central nervous system, lung, posterior pituitary, and in human leukocytes and lymphocytes.

These enzymes are related to the alkaline phosphatases and may be artifactually elevated if the technique for measuring it does not inhibit alkaline phosphatase activity. Even so, it is often elevated in the same conditions as one finds elevations in the isoenzyme of alkaline phosphatase; however, 5'N elevation seems to be related to simple regurgitation, whereas alkaline phosphatase elevation is the result of de novo synthesis. The elevation of 5'N is not prevented by drugs that inhibit protein or RNA synthesis. Some authors suggest that 5'N reflects either bile duct proliferation or intensity of bile ductule destruction or bile ductule inflammation (5'N activity is high in cholangitis), whereas alkaline phosphatase mirrors the degree of biliary stasis. Whereas 5'N may parallel alkaline phosphatase in extrahepatic obstruction, it may fall more rapidly when the obstruction is relieved.

Why so ubiquitous an enzyme should be elevated primarily in serum in hepatobiliary disease and not in a wide range of other disorders is not known. One theory is that the enzyme, found in so many plasma membranes, is soluble only on treatment with detergents or bile salts, and the combination of a large surface area of plasma membrane and a high local concentration of bile salts exists uniquely in the liver and biliary tree.

When methods that inhibit alkaline phosphatase are utilized, 5'N is seldom elevated in osteoblastic bone disease. 5'N is normal in infants and children and probably normal in pregnancy, although this is not unequivocally established. Elevation of 5'N is most likely to be useful, therefore, in diagnosing liver disease in children in whom alkaline phosphatase values are already high and to confirm that an elevated alkaline phosphatase is hepatobiliary in origin when bone disease is being considered. Unless one is sure of the specificity of this test in his or her own laboratory (whether the method completely inhibits alkaline phosphatase activity) its use in pregnant women should be discouraged. A normal 5'N does not exclude hepatobiliary disease or hepatobiliary origin of elevated alkaline phosphatase and the test should not be used in such a manner.

In most circumstances 5'N is less sensitive than alkaline phosphatase. Certainly 5'N is less frequently elevated than alkaline phosphatase when the bilirubin is also elevated. In some cases, however, 5'N is more sensitive than alkaline phosphatase in the early detection of hepatic metastases when bilirubin is not elevated. Some workers also suggest it is superior to alkaline phosphatase in monitoring antitumor therapy.

Because 5'N is so universally distributed it would be surprising if it were entirely specific. Elevations of 5'N have been reported, but usually of small degree, in rheumatoid arthritis, central nervous system disorders, congestive heart failure, myocardial infarction, and acute pancreatitis, in some patients with carcinoma but no clinical evidence of liver involvement, and in patients with damage to the blood vessels such as polyarteritis nodosa and temporal arteritis.

The selectivity of the enzyme has been alluded to, in that it is more likely to be elevated in cholestasis or bile duct inflammatory disorders than in hepatocellular disease, but mild elevations are frequent in the latter. Some authors have presented evidence that very high values of 5'N are more likely to be found in surgical than in medical jaundice, and it has been reported that 5'N discriminates between biliary atresia and neonatal hepatitis. Since these two disorders may coexist, 5'N should not be called upon to bear the burden of such an important differential diagnosis. It is unnecessary and probably unwise to rely upon enzymology for any such critical decision.

Although 5'N is a specialized liver function test, it can be useful when alkaline phosphatase cannot be depended upon, such as with children and pregnant women (if the laboratory techniques adequately inhibit alkaline phosphatase) and when the hepatic origin of alkaline phosphatase needs confirmation. This latter condition usually occurs only when alkaline phosphatase is the only abnormality of liver function. An elevation of direct (but not necessarily of indirect) bilirubin should contravene the need for confirmation of the hepatic origin of alkaline phosphatase in most circumstances.

Serum Leucine Aminopeptidase

Leucine aminopeptidase is a proteolytic enzyme which has been found in all human tissues assayed, with its highest activity in the biliary epithelium. Elevation of leucine aminopeptidase activity has the same diagnostic significance in liver disease as that of alkaline phosphatase and 5'N. In most studies it has been at least as sensitive as alkaline phosphatase, but may be more specific than alkaline phosphatase because it is not present in bone. The normal range is the same in children and adults, but it is, like alkaline phosphatase, increased in pregnancy. Its principal use, therefore, is the confirmation of the hepatic origin of alkaline phosphatase. Elevated levels of leucine aminopeptidase have been reported in acute pancreatitis, malignancy, certain skin diseases, and the nephrotic syndrome. It is therefore one more nonspecific enzyme which has little to offer in any but specialized circumstances.

Serum Gamma Glutamyl Transpeptidase

Gamma glutamyl transpeptidase is found in renal and hepatobiliary tissue and in the endothelial cells of many other tissues. Most of the enzyme circulating in normal serum is of hepatobiliary origin.

It is the most sensitive indicator of cholestasis, in which it may increase 40-fold. It may be elevated in biliary disease without jaundice up to 5–10 times the normal level even when alkaline phosphatase is normal or only slightly elevated. It is not specific for cholestasis and may be elevated in hepatocellular disease of all kinds, but never to the levels seen in cholestasis. In hepatocellular disease it is frequently the last enzyme to return to normal. Its specificity for liver disease is enhanced by its absence in bone and placenta, and values are therefore normal in children and pregnant women. This advantage is offset, however, by its being elevated in pancreatic disease, certain neurological diseases, and after myocardial infarction and by its tendency to be induced, even without organ damage, by the intake of both alcohol and certain drugs. It is therefore a highly sensitive test, but lacks specificity unless levels are truly spectacularly elevated. In general it offers little new information, and there is little reason to recommend its general routine use.

Table 14-3 is a comparison of some of the features of the various tests of bile flow.

Tests that Reflect Hepatic Storage of Heavy Metals

The liver stores many constituents of the body including minerals, copper and iron. When these are present in excess, liver disease may result. These tests are not general screening tests as are the preceding ones; they are obtained when the clinical situation suggests their appropriateness. Unexplained liver disease in a young adult is often sufficient to consider a disorder of copper storage.

Tests for Disorders of Hepatic Copper Storage

Copper, found in the human body in relatively small amounts, is essential for health. Its major function is its association with enzymes involved in oxidation. In excess it inhibits the activity of the enzyme ATPase and has other toxic consequences.

Table 14-3
Comparative Features of Tests of Bile Flow

Test	Sensitivity	Specificity	Selectivity	Same Range of Normal Values in Children	Same Range of Normal Values in Pregnant Women
Bile acids	High	High	Mild	Yes	Yes
Conjugated bilirubin	No	High	Mild	Yes	Usually
Urine urobilinogen	No	No	Mild	Yes	Yes
BSP	High	Moderate	No	Yes	No
Indocyanine green	High	Moderate	No	Yes	?
Alkaline phosphatase	Moderate	No	Mild	No	No
5'-Nucleotidase	Moderate	Moderate	Mild	Yes	Technique dependent
Leucine aminopeptidase	Moderate	Moderate	Mild	Yes	No
Gamma glutamyl transpeptidase	High	Mild	Moderate	Yes	Yes

The efficiency of the absorption–transport–clearing system for copper is such that within hours almost 90% of the absorbed copper is deposited in the liver, where it is taken up by various proteins or by lysosomes.

Copper is mobilized from the liver by two principal routes; (1) synthesis of the glycoprotein ceruloplasmin, which is then released into the blood where it plays a role as an oxidase enzyme; and (2) excretion into the bile bound to a carrier which prevents its reabsorption. Hepatic copper will therefore increase either if there is a defect in synthesis or incorporation of copper into ceruloplasmin, as in Wilson's disease, or if there is diminished bile flow, as in primary biliary cirrhosis and various forms of prolonged cholestasis.

It is generally known that liver copper concentration is increased to high levels in Wilson's disease (in untreated patients usually 250–3000μg [4–47 μmol] of copper per gram [dry weight] of liver), but even higher levels may sometimes be found in primary biliary cirrhosis, extrahepatic biliary atresia, Indian childhood cirrhosis, and the various cholestatic syndromes, as well as in vineyard sprayers who inhale copper salts.

A normal hepatic copper concentration (lower than 100 μg/g or 1.6 μmol/g) excludes the diagnosis of untreated Wilson's disease; it does not excude early primary biliary cirrhosis. An elevated hepatic copper concentration does not establish any diagnosis since it is consistent with several. In all liver diseases except Wilson's disease, however, the concentration of serum ceruloplasmin (see below) is almost always either normal or elevated. Liver copper may be increased in Wilson's disease even when hepatic histology is normal. Rubeanic acid stains for copper may be negative even when total hepatic copper is increased, and a negative stain does not necessarily mean normal copper stores.

Although liver biopsy is often a necessary diagnostic technique for disorders of copper storage, it is not always a sufficient technique. Not only are other tests of copper metabolism often necessary to assist in interpreting the liver biopsy, but, along with the clinical history, they help determine the need for biopsy. These tests include serum ceruloplasmin, total serum copper, and urinary copper excretion.

Serum levels of ceruloplasmin reflect hepatic synthesis and copper incorporation. The concentration of ceruloplasmin in normal healthy adults is 20–40 mg/dL. It may be increased as a result of endocrine influences on body proteins as in pregnancy, during stress, and in patients taking estrogens, or it may reflect an increase in α globulin as part of a response to inflammation as in rheumatoid arthritis and in patients with infections, malignancy, leukemia, and hepatocellular necrosis.

Serum ceruloplasmin is decreased or absent classically in patients with Wilson's disease in whom the value falls below 20 mg/dL in 95% of patients (and between 20 and 30 mg/dL in the rest). Heterozygous carriers of Wilson's disease may have low values without having manifestation of the disease. Ceruloplasmin is also decreased in neonates since hepatic copper seems to be localized to lysosomes for the first few months of life. Transient mild decreases in serum ceruloplasmin may be associated with nephrosis, sprue, kwashiorkor, and other deficiency states and in liver disease with impaired synthetic function, but seldom do the values fall below 25 mg/dL in these conditions.

Serum copper concentrations reflect both ceruloplasmin-bound copper and "free" copper that is loosely bound to albumin or amino acids. Serum copper may be elevated when serum proteins increase, as in pregnancy or in other circumstances in which ceruloplasmin itself is elevated. Serum copper levels also rise in pellagra.

Decreases in serum copper are associated with hypoproteinemia (such as kwashiorkor, protein malabsorption, and nephrosis) and in Menke's X-linked copper deficiency (kinky hair syndrome or trichopoliodystrophy). It is characteristic of early Wilson's disease. In more advanced Wilson's disease, however, total serum copper may be only slightly less than normal since the decrease in ceruloplasmin copper may be balanced by an increase in nonceruloplasmin copper as a result of diffusion from liver to blood.

Urinary copper excretion in patients with symptoms of Wilson's disease is almost always increased to levels of 100 μg/24 h (1.6 μmol/24 h) or greater. Urinary copper excretion may also be increased in heterozygote carriers, in pellagra, and in other types of liver disease. One must be sure that elevated urinary copper levels do not represent contamination with copper.

Tests for Disorders of Hepatic Iron Storage

The metabolism of serum iron is discussed in the hematology section. The major concern about serum iron in patients with liver disease is whether total body iron stores are increased. Deposition of excess iron in the liver may result in tissue damage.

An increase in total body iron is termed hemochromatosis. Tissue damage need not be present at the time of diagnosis. Hemosiderosis is the increase of iron in a tissue without an increase in total body iron. Hemochromatosis may be idiopathic and familial, or it may be acquired. Essential to all of these diagnoses, however, is the demonstration of an increase in total body iron stores.

The suspicion of hemochromatosis is usually on the basis of clinical manifestations. The definitive diagnosis is based on liver biopsy, but we rely on screening tests to help decide when liver biopsy may be appropriate. The laboratory studies that are most often used for screening are the serum iron concentration and the serum transferrin saturation. If one uses a serum iron level greater than 170 μg/100 mL (> 30 μmol/L), one may correctly assess iron stores in most patients, but one will diagnose iron storage excess in 10% in whom it is not present (false-positive) and fail to diagnose it in 24% in whom it is present (false-negative). Elevations in serum iron are particularly seen in patients with alcoholic liver disease without iron overload. If one uses a serum transferrin saturation of greater than 90% as a criterion for increased total body iron stores, one will have 33% false-positives but no false-negatives. These two studies are therefore useful screening tests, but they have limited specificity.

Recently, much attention has focused on serum ferritin, an iron storage protein present in tissues and in serum. Serum ferritin levels are proportional to body iron stores and, in males, rise progressively with age. The false-positive rate for the diagnosis is of elevated total body iron stores is 2%, and the false-negative rate is 3%. Elevation of ferritin out of proportion to body stores may be seen in patients with infection, malignancy, leukemia, and hepatocellular necrosis.

One can therefore conclude that serum ferritin should be obtained in any patient suspected of having hemochromatosis who has an elevation of either serum iron concentration or percentage transferrin saturation. If neither is elevated one is unlikely to find an elevation of serum ferritin, but it is worth obtaining if clinical suspicion for hemochromatosis is high. If all three tests are normal, do not consider liver biopsy.

For the detection of total body iron increase in the asymptomatic relatives of a patient with idiopathic hemochromatosis, serum iron concentration and percentage transferrin saturation are not satisfactory screening tests. One needs to obtain serum ferritin even if the other tests are normal. Serum ferritin will be raised in all but 2% of such asymptomatic relatives who have increased iron stores. When looking for evidence of total body iron excess in such individuals, liver biopsy should be considered if either serum iron concentration, transferrin saturation, or serum ferritin concentration is elevated.

If serum ferritin levels are unavailable one can estimate iron stores by an iron chelation test with desferrioxamine. When 0.5 g of desferrioxamine is injected intramuscularly, a 24-hour urine iron excretion in excess of 2.0 mg (36 μmol) indicates excess total iron stores.

If either the serum ferritin or the urinary excretion test is abnormal, liver biopsy should be performed. The definitive test for the diagnosis of hemochromatosis is the demonstration of hepatic iron concentration in excess of 1 g/100 g (180 μmol/g) dry weight. A semiquantiative determination can be made by examining tissue prepared with Perl's Prussian blue stain (for hemosiderin). When the majority of parenchymal cells contain abundant stainable iron, an increase in total body iron may be presumed.

In some circumstances an estimation of total body iron stores can be made retrospectively after a trial of phlebotomy. With each 500 mL of blood removed, approximately 250 mg of iron is also removed. If more than 2 g of iron is removed without inducing iron deficiency, one can presume total iron stores were in excess.

The distinction between secondary and idiopathic hemochromatosis can usually be suggested by the clinical history. It is sometimes particularly difficult, however, to distinguish idiopathic hemochromatosis aggravated by alcoholism and alcoholic cirrhosis with secondary iron overload. There is frequently overlap between the two groups in clinical manifestations and in the values for estimates of total body iron stores. The values tend, however, to be higher in idiopathic hemochromatosis. When there is active hepatocellular necrosis in alcoholism, serum iron concentration, percentage saturation of transferrin, and serum ferritin concentration are particularly unreliable. However, when serum transaminase levels are elevated, a serum ferritin level of less than 1000 μg/L, which fluctuates widely, strongly suggests alcoholic liver disease rather than idiopathic hemochromatosis. The finding of evidence for elevation in total body iron stores in family members is strongly suggestive of idiopathic hemochromatosis. More than 25% of first-degree relatives of patients with idiopathic hemochromatosis have iron store increases. In some circumstances HLA typing may be necessary for diagnosis. There is an increased incidence of HLA A3 in hemochromatosis. In France there is a further association with HLA B14. In the United States,

United Kingdom, and Australia there is an association with HLA B7. The finding of HLA markers alone is not, however, clinical evidence of hemochromatosis; the frequency of HLA A3 is 20% in the white general population. When seeking to identify family members with hemochromatosis, one should note that affected members often have HLA haplotypes identical to the identified patient, regardless of whether HLA A3 is present. HLA typing is too costly for routine use.

The Selection of Liver Function Tests

The use of tests that reflect hepatic storage of heavy metals is usually dictated by specific clinical situations. The choice of other liver function tests depends on the use to which they will be put. Indiscriminate laboratory tests should not replace careful thought. In some circumstances, a single, carefully chosen liver function test may be all that is required, as in previously diagnosed anicteric hepatitis with a normal course—for which a single transaminase level test at intervals would be sufficient to document improvement. In a patient with known hepatic cancer, either the alkaline phosphatase or 5′N may be followed to document response to therapy. Even in these circumstances, however, more than one liver function test would have been needed for initial diagnosis and occasionally during follow-up. Under most circumstances, a combination of tests is necessary, since no single test provides information about all aspects of liver structural and metabolic integrity. When using multiple tests, therefore, one should ensure that the tests reflect different aspects of liver function. In general one can obtain adequate information using only the following tests: SGOT (or SGPT), serum bilirubin (total and direct), alkaline phosphatase, albumin, globulin, and the prothrombin time. Usually, additional studies provide only one more nonspecific test. Occasionally, an additional study can add auxiliary information, such as the addition of SGPT to SGOT when alcohol-induced disease is suspected or the use of 5′N in an adolescent with elevated alkaline phosphatase. On the other hand, in a patient with elevated direct bilirubin and an elevation of alkaline phosphatase, there is nothing to be gained by ordering leucine aminopeptidase, gamma glutamyl transpeptidase, or even 5′N. In most circumstances BSP and indocyanine green make no useful contribution, but where a general screening test is needed, eg, for hepatotoxicity in an industrial plant, the sensitivity of these compounds at the expense of specificity becomes an asset.

■ Serology of Viral Hepatitis

The diagnosis of viral hepatitis was once simple. One recognized a clinical syndrome, noted consistent elevation of liver function tests, and, depending on clear-cut epidemiological features, labeled it either "infectious" or "serum" hepatitis. It was straight-forward and unlikely to be proved wrong.

Now we have in abecedarian classification hepatitis A and hepatitis B, and, less felicitously, hepatitis non-A, non-B. Almost surely C, D, and so on will appear.

Diagnosis of Hepatitis A

Hepatitis A is an infection of relatively short (two- to six-week) incubation period, transmitted predominantly by a fecal-oral route, not associated with prolonged viremia, and not associated with a carrier state. It is caused by a 27-nm virus for which a simple antigen-antibody system has thus far been described. The World Health Organization has recommended, however, that the term hepatitis A antigen and antibody to hepatitis A antigen be supplanted by hepatitis A virus (HAV) and antibody to hepatitis A virus (anti-HAV).

A competitive inhibition radioimmunoassay test kit for anti-HAV is available commercially. An enzyme-linked immunoabsorbent assay for anti-HAV is also being developed for commercial distribution. These techniques make the serological diagnosis of hepatitis A available to most practicing physicians.

The appearance of antibody to HAV usually coincides with acute liver necrosis—just before or at the same time as elevation in transaminases. It is seldom present during the incubation period. Titers continue to rise after the acute illness, reach a peak in two to three months, and gradually fall over several more months, but may remain detectable indefinitely.

The anti-HAV which is present during acute illness is predominantly of the IgM class and is transient, becoming progressively less after two to three months, but may remain detectable for a year or more. There is gradual development of IgG antibody until high levels are reached three to six months after the onset of illness. This IgG antibody to HAV is detectable for many years and perhaps for a lifetime. Its presence prevents reinfection with HAV.

The diagnosis of acute viral hepatitis A can be confirmed by either seroconversion of recently negative serum or by a fourfold rise in titer of total anti-HAV (no distinction between IgM and IgG) between acute and convalescent serum. An interval of one to two months is recommended.

When convalescent serum is not available or when confirmation is desired without waiting for a convalescent sample, one need only demonstrate high levels of anti-HAV of the IgM class. Methods to discriminate between IgM and IgG anti-HAV are available. Anti-HAV IgM is the technique of choice for the determination of recent HAV infection. Since it may be detected for up to a year, however, some caution is in order in interpreting its presence. Maximum titers are found shortly after the onset of clinical symptoms and then decline; therefore, one can be less certain that a patient's symptoms are related to HAV infection when anti-HAV IgM is present at less than 1:4000 dilutions.

With assay systems which do not discriminate between IgM and IgG anti-HAV, one can only document that there has been exposure to HAV, which may not necessarily be recent. A rising titer would then be essential to document recent acute illness.

Diagnosis of Hepatitis B

Hepatitis B is an infection of longer incubation period (one to five months) associated with prolonged viremia, and in which there is a carrier state in 5% to 10% of those infected.

The hepatitis B virus (HBV) is identical to the spherical Dane particle. It contains an inner core which, when the Dane particle is solubilized, can be identified with hepatitis B core antigen. HBV is associated with at least three major antigen systems: hepatitis B surface antigen and antibody (HB$_s$Ag and anti-HB$_s$), hepatitis B core antigen and antibody (HB$_c$ and anti-HB$_c$), and hepatitis B "e" antigen and antibody (HB$_e$Ag and anti-HB$_e$).

HB$_s$Ag circulates in serum not only as the surface component to the virion (whole infective virus) but also as incomplete particles composed entirely of capsid which has been produced in excess. HB$_c$Ag is derived from the inner core of the virion. It does not circulate freely in serum, but is located in the nuclei of the hepatocytes of patients infected with hepatitis B. HB$_e$Ag is either a subcomponent or a breakdown product of HB$_c$Ag. It may be found in serum. Antibodies to all three antigens can be detected in serum.

One's understanding of the diagnostic usefulness of these antigens and the antibodies to them depends upon an understanding of the time course over which they are detected when susceptible persons are exposed to HBV infection (Figure 14-1).

In most adults who develop symptomatic hepatitis B, HB$_s$Ag appears in the serum several weeks after exposure and precedes by several weeks the appearance of clinical symptoms and subsequent clearance of surface antigen, usually within six weeks. HB$_e$Ag appears at about the same time as HB$_s$Ag. Its disappearance usually precedes that of HB$_s$Ag. HB$_e$ usually develops at the height of clinical illness and biochemical evidence of hepatitis. Titers decline over several months, but may persist at low levels for several years. Most patients with HB$_s$Ag develop anti-HB$_c$ (HB$_c$Ag, however, is usually not detected in serum). Anti-HB$_c$ rises to a peak and begins to decline with clearance of HB$_s$Ag and clinical recovery, but may persist at low titers for years. For a period between the time of HB$_s$Ag disappearance and the appearance of anti-HB$_s$, the serum may be positive for anti-HB$_c$ only. The appearance of anti-HB$_s$ usually coincides with the onset of clinical recovery. Its appearance sometimes may be late—several months to a year after the disappearance of HB$_s$Ag. Anti-HB$_s$ rises to high titers and diminishes slowly over many years.

HB$_s$Ag persisting for more than six months in a person with clinical hepatitis indicates that the illness has become chronic. Anti-HB$_c$ persists, but

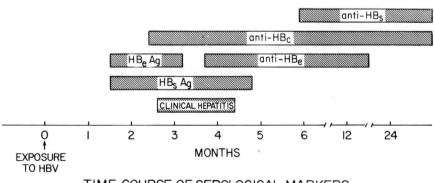

TIME COURSE OF SEROLOGICAL MARKERS
IN ACUTE HBV INFECTION

Figure 14-1 The appearance and disappearance of HBV antigens and antibodies in a representative patient exposed to HBV is depicted.

252

anti-HB$_s$ does not develop. HB$_e$Ag is likely to be positive. If it seroconverts to anti-HB$_e$ this may presage resolution of the illness, clearance of HB$_s$Ag, and clinical recovery.

In some patients the response to HBV exposure is characterized by either the absence of HB$_s$Ag or its presence in low titers for only a brief period, followed by the appearance of anti-HB$_s$ alone several weeks after exposure. The titers of this antibody are both high and sustained. This phenomenom is referred to as "seroconversion" or "primary antibody response" (Figure 14-2). Anti-HB$_c$ and anti-HB$_e$ also develop in low titer for short periods of time. Patients with this type of response generally do not develop clinical symptoms, but occasionally there are mild and transient elevations of transaminase.

Rarely, after exposure to HBV, a carrier state develops in which HB$_s$Ag persists in the serum of an asymptomatic person (Figure 14-3). Chronic carriers characteristically develop high titers of anti-HB$_c$, but anti-HB$_s$ is not detected. HB$_e$Ag rises to quite high titers. Although HB$_e$Ag positivity may persist for years, its longevity is not as great as that of HB$_s$Ag. This same pattern is seen in persons whose acute hepatitis becomes chronic.

From the preceding information and from clinical studies I suggest the following interpretation of the various serological markers.

Interpretation of HB$_s$AG

The confirmed presence of HB$_s$Ag in the serum indicates hepatitis B infection and potential infectivity to others. One does not know, however, where in the course of hepatitis B infection the patient may be or the relative degree of infectivity. For this information one must seek clues from HB$_e$Ag, anti-HB$_e$, and anti-HB$_c$.

If all three are negative one may assume that the patient is in the incubation period or early course of hepatitis B infection. The coexistence of appropriate symptoms in the patient is reassuring. The blood from such patients is probably highly infective.

When HB$_s$Ag is present one cannot be sure from a single determination whether the infection is acute or chronic. If HB$_s$AG persists beyond 12 weeks, it is likely that the infection will become chronic. If HB$_s$Ag persists beyond six months, long-term infection is established, and the patient either has chronic liver disease or has become an asymptomatic carrier. Although

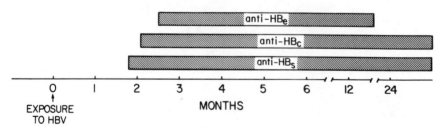

TIME COURSE OF SEROLOGICAL MARKERS IN SEROCONVERSION

Figure 14-2 The appearance and disappearance of antigens and antibodies is depicted for a patient with "seroconversion" or a "primary antibody response" to HBV exposure. Such patients are usually asymptomatic.

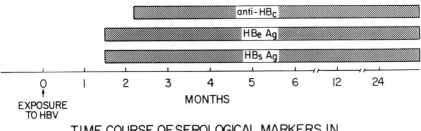

TIME COURSE OF SEROLOGICAL MARKERS IN
CHRONIC CARRIERS AND CHRONIC HEPATITIS

Figure 14-3 Antigen and antibody pattern for a representative patient who is an asymptomatic chronic carrier of HBV. This same pattern may be seen in patients with symptomatic chronic hepatitis.

all such patients are presumed to be infective, one can gain a clearer idea of relative infectivity by determining the status of HB_eAg and anti-HB_eAg.

Interpretation of HB$_e$AG

In acute hepatitis, HB_eAg is almost universally present when a sensitive assay is used (such as radioimmunoassay or enzyme-linked immunosorbent assay). It normally disappears within six weeks. High titers of > 1:1000 by radioimmunoassay or enzyme-linked immunosorbent assay indicate the possibility of development of chronic disease, or at least the chronic carrier state, a possibility that is greater if the HB_eAg titers, even when not high, persist for more than 10 weeks after the acute phase of illness. Furthermore, the presence of HB_eAg in serum indicates persisting active viral replication, and blood from such patients, especially with medium to high titers, must be considered highly infectious.

The presence of HB_eAg in patients who are chronically positive for HB_sAg, at least when measured by less sensitive techniques, is associated with increased likelihood of ongoing liver damage. It is not known whether this correlation will hold up when large numbers of patients are examined by the more sensitive radioimmunoassay and enzyme-linked immunosorbent assay. In any event, liver biopsy is the only method for determining the degree of histological damage in the individual patient.

Interpretation of Anti-HB$_e$

Most acute cases of hepatitis B seroconvert from HB_eAg to anti-HB_e during the clinical illness. The disappearance of HB_eAg and development of anti-HB_e is generally a good prognostic indicator, but does not guarantee complete clearance of HBV. In most patients who seroconvert, anti-HB_e develops within two weeks of clearance of HB_eAg, and these patients, in general, seem to have an uncomplicated course. The clinical characteristics of those patients with delayed appearance of anti-HB_eAg remain unestablished.

Since most acute cases of hepatitis B seroconvert from HB_eAg to anti-HB_e during the acute illness, seroconversion of e antigen suggests that seroconversion from HB_sAg to anti-HB_s will also occur.

Studies on infectivity titers of sera containing anti-HB_e have indicated that the likelihood of transmission of HBV, although still possible, is far less likely than when HB_eAg is present. Nonetheless, transmission of hepatitis B from HB_sAg-positive, anti-HB_e-positive plasma has been documented.

In persons chronically positive for HB_sAg, the presence of anti-HB_e is more likely to be associated with negligible liver disease than when HB_eAg is present. In patients with HB_sAg-associated chronic hepatitis, there is some evidence that seroconversion from HB_eAg to anti-HB_e, which may be preceded by a rise in transaminase values, may herald the elimination of HB_sAG and clinical recovery.

Interpretation of Anti-HB_c

Anti-HB_c in high titers may be detected in the sera of patients with acute hepatitis B and in chronic carriers. In lower titers it is a marker of previous HBV infection that persists indefinitely.

In acute hepatitis its appearance in serum generally follows that of HB_sAg, but when patients have clinical hepatitis the two are generally coexistent. Their presence together indicates active viral replication and either acute or chronic disease. Antibody to core antigen generally appears about three to five weeks after the appearance of HB_sAg and remains detectable for long periods, perhaps for life.

The presence of anti-HB_c alone may be the only marker of active infection in patients in whom serological studies are obtained during the "window period" between the clearance of HB_sAg and the appearance of anti-HB_s. In these circumstances anti-HB_c is generally present in high titers. Anti-HB_e may also be present. Some cases of the chronic carrier state have also been described in which there is continuous high-titer anti-HB_c but in which HB_sAg is detectable only intermittently even by sensitive methods.

Low-titer anti-HB_c with no other serological markers may sometimes indicate remote HBV infection. More commonly it coexists with anti-HB_s.

Interpretation of Anti-HB_s

The presence of anti-HB_s indicates past infection and, in adequate titers, immunity to subsequent infection. These patients are not infective for HBV. Anti-HB_s may also be present as a result of passive (eg, gamma globulin) or active (eg, vaccine) immunization. If anti-HB_s is the consequence of infection having occurred, anti-HB_c will usually also be present, but in some patients a remote HBV infection, especially if subclinical, may result in anti-HB_s without anti-HB_c; therefore, this distinction is not absolute.

Table 14-4 illustrates the usual interpretation of several combinations of serological markers. It is not necessary to order every serological marker in every patient in whom the diagnosis of hepatitis B is sought.

The practicing physician will want to know whether an acute hepatitis is or is not hepatitis B, and for this he or she may need only a hepatitis B surface antigen. If it is positive, the physician will have the answer.

If the HB_sAg is negative, one can usually presume the illness is unrelated to hepatitis B. Should the epidemiological features suggest hepatitis B strongly, however, one would need also to establish that anti-HB_c was not present to be certain one was not dealing with hepatitis B. Some investigators believe that the screening of transfused blood for anti-HB_c would cause a further decrement in the incidence of posttransfusion hepatitis B beyond that resulting from the measurement of HB_sAg alone.

Table 14-4
Representative Serological Patterns in Viral Hepatitis

Serological Markers*					Interpretation
HBsAg	HBeAg	Anti-HBc	Anti-HBe	Anti-HBs	
+	−	−	−	−	Incubation period or early hepatitis B, infective
+	+	+	−	−	Acute hepatitis B or chronic carrier, infective
+	−	+	+	−	Resolving acute hepatitis or chronic carrier, low infectivity
−	+	+	−	−	Acute hepatitis in "window period" or low grade chronic carrier, infective
−	−	+	+	−	Convalescence from acute hepatitis, low infectivity
−	−	+	+	+	Recent recovery from acute hepatitis, not infective, immune
−	−	+	−	+	Post recovery from hepatitis, not infective, immune
−	−	−	−	+	Past subclinical infection or active/passive immunization, not infective, immune

+, Present; −, Absent.

One might want to know about anti-HB$_s$ in the setting of a patient exposed to HBV infection, by needle stick or through a sexual partner, in whom hepatitis B immune-globulin prophylaxis is contemplated. If antiHB$_s$ is present, the patient can be presumed to be immune, and prophylaxis is unnecessary.

There is rarely any need to determine HB$_e$Ag in usual clinical practice. In chronic hepatitis, however, it may be useful in patients under therapy since seroconversion might herald clearance of HB$_s$Ag. Although anti-HB$_e$ correlates statistically with diminished infectivity, it is probably insufficiently reliable to use for making clinical decisions in an individual patient. Similarly, even though HB$_e$Ag correlates in large groups of chronic HB$_s$Ag carriers with likelihood of significant liver disease and anti-HB$_e$ correlates with lack of significant liver disease, serologic determinations should never supplant liver biopsy in the individual patient.

Diagnosis of Hepatitis Non-A, Non-B

Hepatitis non-A, non-B, an infection with a usual incubation period of 6 to 10 weeks (but with a range between 2 and 26 weeks). It is not possible to distinguish hepatitis non-A, non-B from hepatitis A or B on purely clinical grounds in the individual patient. From series of cases, however, one notes certain special characteristics. There is a high incidence (65% to 75%) of anicteric cases; enzymes are usually only mildly elevated, but tend to fluctuate markedly over brief periods of time; and the incidence of progression to chronic hepatitis may approach 50%.

Several candidates have come forth as a virus specific antigen-antibody system for hepatitis non-A, non-B, but none has yet proved reliable. The present diagnosis of hepatitis non-A, non-B, therefore, retains the older virtues once shared by all forms of hepatitis. One recognizes a clinical syndrome, notes consistent abnormalities of liver function tests, clinically excludes nonviral causes of hepatocellular injury, and serologically excludes known hepatitis viruses. The exclusion of hepatitis A and B requires the absence of IgM antibody to HAV and absence of both circulating HB$_s$Ag and anti-HB$_c$. One also needs to exclude mononucleosis. Theoretically one should also exclude cytomegalovirus, herpes simplex virus, coxsackievirus B, adenovirus, and Rubeola; however, except in special situations where the clinical setting may suggest these viruses, the diagnosis of hepatitis non-A, non-B can be comfortably entertained by the exclusion only of HAV, HBV, and mononucleosis.

■ Laboratory Diagnosis of the Porphyrias

The porphyrias are a group of disorders characterized by partial deficiencies of the various enzymes involved in the production of heme. These defects result in the accumulation of porphyrins, porphyrin precursors, or both (Figure 14-4).

Heme may be produced in all types of cells, but is produced mainly in the red cell and the liver; the disorders of heme synthesis are therefore classified as erythropoietic, hepatic, or erythrohepatic, depending on whether the major defect in synthesis is expressed in the red blood cell, the liver, or both (Table 14-5).

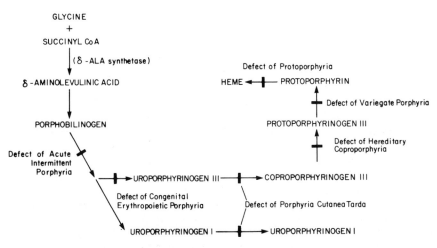

Figure 14-4 The biosynthetic pathway of heme is illustrated, and the sites of the enzymatic defects in the various porphyrias are indicated. The actual substrates are porphyrinogens. These are easily converted to the respective porphyrins by weak oxidizing agents such as light in the presence of air.

Table 14-5
Classification of the Porphyrias

Erythropoietic Defect
    Congenital erythropoietic porphyria
Hepatic Defect
    Acute intermittent porphyria
    Porphyria cutanea tarda
    Coproporphyria
    Variegate porphyria
Erythrohepatic Defect
    Protoporphyria

    The intermediate compounds in heme synthesis, depending on their relative water solubility, are found in urine, feces (by way of bile), or both in a pattern unique to each defect of porphyrin metabolism. The porphyrin precursors δ-aminolevulinic acid (ALA) and porphobilinogen (PBG) are found only in urine; uroporphyrin is usually found only in urine; coproporphyrin is found predominantly in feces but also in urine and protoporphyrin is found only in feces. In erythropoietic porphyria and erythrohepatic protoporphyria, increased metabolites are also found in red blood cells.

    All of the enzymatic defects are partial since it is assumed that complete block of metabolism at any of the steps would be lethal. Defects at some sites, however, seem to be more crucial than others because they result in a reduction in the production of heme. These are the "heme-deficient" porphyrias. The others do not reduce heme production substantially and are known as "heme-compensated" porphyrias. The heme-deficient porphyrias are acute intermittent porphyria, variegate porphyria, and coproporphyria. In these disorders the resultant decrease in heme production, presumably by a feedback mechanism, is associated with increased activity of ALA synthetase, the rate-limiting step in heme production (Figure 14-4). The intermediates ALA and PBG are therefore increased—further contributing to ALA and PBG production in acute intermittent porphyria and accumulating in addition to the metabolite preceding the enzymatic defect in variegate porphyria and coproporphyria.

The major categories of manifestation of the porphyrias are either neuropsychiatric abnormalities (which may include abdominal pain) or skin lesions or both. Table 14-6 lists the clinical and laboratory manifestations according to which disorders of prophyrin metabolism are present.

Familiarity with the site of the specific enzyme defect associated with each porphyria (Figure 14-4), helps to predict what metabolic intermediates will be found in stool and urine (Table 14-6).

Acute intermittent porphyria is a defect in the enzyme (uroporphyrinogen I synthetase) that catalyzes the formation of uroporphyrinogen from ALA and PBG. Therefore, these precursors, both of which are found in the urine, are elevated in the disorder. This is always true during acute attacks and usually true between attacks.

Porphyria cutanea tarda is a deficiency of the enzyme (uroporphyrinogen decarboxylase) that catalyzes the formation of coproporphyrinogen from uroporphyrinogen; therefore, one finds an increase in uroporphyrin in the urine.

Coproporphyria is a deficiency in the enzyme (coproporphyrinogen oxidative decarboxylase) that catalyzes the formation of protoporphyrinogen from coproporphyrinogen. One sees the expected increase in coproporphyrin in feces and urine. One also finds an increase in urinary ALA and PBG, since coproporphyria is one of the heme-deficient porphyrias. Between attacks porphyrins may be present only in the stool.

Variegate porphyria is a defect in the enzyme (protoporphyrinogen oxidase) that catalyzes the formation of protoporphyrin from protoporphyrinogen. One finds protoporphyrin in feces, but also one finds its precursor, coproporphyrin, in feces and urine. Since this is a heme-deficient porphyria, ALA and PBG are also increased. Between acute attacks protoporphyrin and coproporphyrin in the stool may be the only findings.

Protoporphyria is a defect in the synthesis of heme from protoporphyrin because of deficient heme sythetase (also known as ferrochetolase). The result is an elevation of heme's precursor, protoporhyrin, which is found in feces—its only mode of excretion—in increased amounts. Protoporphyrin is also increased in red blood cells since this is an erythrohepatic porphyria.

Congenital erthropoietic porphyria is a deficiency of the enzyme uroporphyrinogen III cosynthetase and results in defective conversion of PBG to uroporphyrinogen III. The conversion of PBG to uroporphyrinogen I and coproporphyrinogen I (which are not biologically active) is not affected, however, and these accumulate in excess. Uroporphyrin I and coproporphyrin I therefore accumulate in red cells and urine, and coproporphyrin I accumulates in feces.

The analysis of body fluids for porphyrins is difficult; therefore, one utilizes qualitative screening tests before requesting quantitative analysis. Quantitation of ALA in urine is usually not necessary. The usual screening test for PBG is the Watson-Schwartz test. PBG condenses with Ehrlich's

Table 14-6
Manifestations of the Porphyrias

Disorders	Clinical Manifestations		Laboratory Manifestations			Watson-Schwartz (or Hoesch) Test Positive
	Neuropsychiatric Symptoms	Skin Lesions	Biochemical Elevations			
			RBC	Urine	Feces	
Acute intermittent porphyria*	+	0	0	ALA PBG	0	Yes
Congenital erythropoietic porphyria	0	+	Uroporphyrin Coproporphyrin	Uroporphyrin Coproporphyrin	Coproporphyrin	No
Porphyria cutanea tarda	0	+	0	Uroporphyrin	0	No
Coproporphyria*	+	+	0	ALA PBG Coproporphyrin	Coproporphyrin	Yes, in acute attacks
Variegate porphyria*	+	+	0	ALA PBG Coproporphyrin	Protoporphyrin Coproporphyrin	Yes, in acute attacks
Protoporphyria	0	+	Protoporphyrin	0	Protoporphyrin	No

*Heme-deficient porphyrias.
Adapted from tables in Bloomer JR: *Gastroenterology* 1976;71:689–701 and Riely CA, Brenner DA: *Diagnosis* July 1982:51–61.

260

reagent to form a magenta complex which cannot be extracted with butanol and chloroform (as can urobilinogen, which also reacts with Ehrlich's reagent). More recently, the Hoesch test has also been used to screen for PBG. This test is an inverse Watson-Schwartz test in which a small urine volume added to a large Ehrlich's reagent volume (instead of vice versa) results in a cherry-red color. The screening test for porphyrins themselves is fluorescence upon exposure to ultraviolet light.

One should note that the Watson-Schwartz and Hoesch tests are not positive in porphyrias in which PBG does not accumulate. Even in those in which it does accumulate, it may be negative if the level of PBG is less than 3 times normal.

It should be noted that porphyrinogins are reduced forms of porphyrins. They are easily converted to porphyrins by weak oxidizing agents such as light in the presence of air; it is the oxidation to fluorescent and colored porphyrins that results in the dramatic pink-red appearance of the urine when they are present in high levels and in ultraviolet fluorescence even at lower levels. In AIP the compounds in the urine, ALA and PBG, are not porphyrins, and they are therefore colorless. With acidification or prolonged standing in light, however, polymerization to uroporphyrinogen and porphobilin may occur resulting in dark urine. The urine in protoporphyria contains no porphyrins (protoporphyrin is found in feces only) so no color will be imparted to the urine.

During acute attacks all the porphyrias with neuropsychiatric involvement (acute intermittent porphyria, variegate porphyria, coproporphyria) will be characterized by an increase in PBG, and the Watson-Schwartz and Hoesch screening tests for PBG in the urine will be positive. Screening tests for stool prophyrin are always positive in variegate porphyria and coproporphyria, and specific analysis will allow distinction between the two.

Porphyrias associated with skin lesions will not have a positive Watson-Schwartz or Hoesch test, since PBG is not elevated in these diseases, except during acute attacks of variegate porphyria and coproporphyria.

■ Selected Readings

Angelico M, Attili AF, Capocaccia L: Fasting and postprandial serum bile acids as a screening test for hepatocellular disease. *Am J Digest Dis* 1977;11:941–946.

Bloomer JR: The Hepatic Porphyrias—Pathogenesis, Manifestations, and Management. *Gastroenterology* 1976;71:689–701.

Bouchier IAD, Pennington CR: Serum bile acids in hepatobiliary disease. *Gut* 1978;19:492–496.

Burrell CJ: Serological markers of hepatitis B infection. *Clin Gastroenterol* 1980;9:47–163.

Clermont RJ, Chalmers TC: The transaminase tests in liver disease. *Medicine* 1967;46:197–207.

Dienstag JL: Viral hepatitis type A: Virology and course. *Clin Gastroenterol* 1980;9:135–154.

Hill PG, Simmons HG: An assessment of 5'nucleotidase as a liver function test. *Quart J Med* 1967;36:457–468.

Hoofnagle JH: Serological markers of hepatitis B virus infection. *Annu Rev Med* 1981;32:1–11.

Javitt NB: Diagnostic value of serum bile acids. *Clin Gastorenterol* 1977;6:219–226.

Kaplan MM: Alkaline phosphatase. *Gastroenterology* 1972;62:452–468.

Killenberg PG, Stevens RD, Wilderman RF, et al: The laboratory method as a variable in the interpretation of serum bilirubin fractionation. *Gastroenterology* 1980;78:1011–1015.

Mathiesen LR: The hepatitis A virus infection. *Liver* 1981;1:81–109.

Ostrow JD: Bilirubin and jaundice, in Becker F (ed): *The Liver: Normal and Abnormal Functions.* New York, Marcel Dekker, Inc, 1974.

Overby, LR: Serology of liver diseases, in Gitnick GL (ed): *Current Hepatology,* vol 2. New York, John Wiley & Sons, Inc, 1982.

Powell LW, Bassett ML, Halliday JW: Hemochromatosis: 1980 update. *Gastroenterology* 1980;78:374–381.

Skrede S, Blomhoff JP, Elgjo K, et al: Biochemical tests in the evaluation of liver function. *Scand J Gastroenterol* (Suppl 19) 1973;8:3745.

Whitfield JB, Pounder RE, Neale G, et al: Serum γ-glutamyl transpeptidase activity in liver disease. *Gut* 1972;13:702–708.

Zimmerman HJ, West M: Serum enzyme levels in the diagnosis of hepatic disease. *Am J Gastroenterol* 1963;40:387.

CSF

The subarachnoid space is the brain's sewer. The choroid plexus generates the fluid and the pressure to flush the system. Just as archeologists learn much about a civilization from its garbage, scientists and physicians learn much about the brain's function and its diseases from cerebrospinal fluid (CSF). In 1891, Quincke introduced the technique of percutaneous puncture of the lumbar subarachnoid space by a needle with a stylet, measured CSF pressure with a manometer, and pioneered the basic analyses of CSF for blood cells, protein, and glucose.

Proper handling of the specimens is essential. Because CSF should be examined for cells within one hour of lumbar puncture, the physician himself or herself must do the analysis, or the physician or a trusted delegate (rarely the hospital's dispatch system) should take the specimen straight away to the laboratory. Save an extra specimen until the basic analyses have been completed so that a laboratory accident or the unexpected need for additional tests does not necessitate a second lumbar puncture. The physician should record the opening pressure, the clarity and color of the fluid, and what tests were ordered. Clean slides and filtered strains will prevent artifacts.

Clarity and Color

Clarity and color should be determined with at least 1 mL of CSF in a glass tube by daylight if possible. Any cloudiness or tint is abnormal. Opalescence requires at least 200 to 400 white blood cells (WBC) per mm^3 of CSF. The presence of fewer cells may be detected by the scatter of direct sunlight which produces a snowy appearance. A pink-tinged fluid contains 500 to 6000 red blood cells (RBC) per mm^3. Grossly bloody CSF contains more than 6000 RBC/mm^3. A pink-tinged fluid may be due to a "traumatic tap," in which case the supernatant of a certrifuged specimen will be clear and colorless.

Xanthochromia is pivotal evidence in the diagnosis of a suspected subarachnoid hemorrhage. The presence of a yellow tint to the clear supernatant indicates the presence of red cells in the subarachnoid space for at least six hours before the procedure. Slight differences in color are best detected with a specimen of 5 mL in a glass tube. A physician who believes that he or she has probably caused a traumatic puncture, in a patient strongly suspected of having had a subarachnoid hemorrhage in the preceding 12 hours, should immediately do another puncture one interspace higher. Usually the second fluid is colorless if the bloody fluid of the first procedure was due to a traumatic procedure. Xanthochromia may also be due to hypercarotenemia, jaundice with plasma bilirubin concentrations in excess of 15 mg/dL, and CSF protein concentrations greater than 250 mg/dL.

15

The Laboratory in Neurological and Muscular Diseases

James Donaldson

Cell Count and Differential

All CSF cell counts should be done within one hour after the procedure because thereafter at room temperature red and white cells begin to lyse. No cells will be viable after 24 hours. If a traumatic tap has occurred, usually 1 WBC/mm³ can be subtracted from the total WBC count for every 700 RBC/mm³; this correction for anemic patients can be determined by the ratio of peripheral blood white and red cell counts. More than 5 mononucleated WBC/mm³ is abnormal. Any granulocytes are abnormal. Cell type cannot be determined in a counting chamber. The sediment of a centrifuged specimen must be stained. Crenated red cells have no diagnostic significance.

Cytology

Tumor cytomorphological studies are dependent upon the quantity of CSF submitted, the method of harvesting cells, and upon the freshness of the cells. Do not hesitate to send 5 to 10 mL of CSF. Cytocentrifugation destroys many cells. Membrane microfilters are preferred for cytological studies.

Glucose

The glucose level of lumbar CSF is normally 60% of the blood glucose. CSF glucose concentrations below 45 mg/dL are abnormal. Hyperglycemia may mask hypoglycorrhachia. Whenever the CSF glucose concentration is of great importance (eg, the diagnosis and follow-up of chronic meningitides), the patient should fast for at least four hours, preferably overnight. Random simultaneous blood and CSF glucose levels are misleading; CSF glucose peaks lag approximately two hours behind blood glucose peaks.

A low CSF glucose concentration in the absence of hypoglycemia indicates a widespread disorder of the meninges which inhibits active transport of glucose into the CSF. In addition, anaerobic glycolysis by bacteria, mycobacteria, fungi, tumor cells, and parasites consumes glucose and produces lactic acid. Viral diseases do not cause hypoglycorrhacia with the exception of a few cases of mumps meningoencephalitis and rare cases of herpetic encephalitis.

Lactic Acid

The CSF lactate concentration, which is independent of the blood lactate level, increases in purulent meningitides and usually remains at normal levels in viral meningitis. There is enough overlap among conditions that it is not a reliable differential point. There is no clinical advantage in following CSF lactate in addition to, or in place of, CSF glucose during the recovery from meningitis.

Protein

The total protein concentration of CSF varies with the source of the sample: ventricular fluid from 5 to 15 mg/dL, cisternal fluid from 15 to 25 mg/dL, lumbar fluid from 20 to 45 mg/dL. Low lumbar CSF protein levels occur in young children and in patients with pseudotumor cerebri. CSF protein concentrations between 50 and 400 mg/dL occur in a long list of conditions. CSF protein concentrations greater than 400 mg/dL are caused by meningitis, acoustic neuromas and other tumors, bleeding, severe Guillain-Barré syndrome, and blockage of CSF circulation by tumor or inflammation. CSF with a protein concentration greater than 1 g/dL can clot (Froin's syndrome). All cell counts and bacterial stains should be done before clotting occurs lest the clot sweep cells with it.

Gamma Globulin

CSF concentrations of immunoglobulins, particularly immumoglobulin G (IgG), are important in the diagnosis of inflamatory conditions of the central nervous system, especially neurosyphilis and multiple sclerosis. A monoclonal gammopathy of serum may be reflected in the CSF.

The Lange colloidal gold test was the first method to detect increased gamma globulins. The paretic, first-zone curve, which was reported as 5555444321, indicated an increase in CSF gamma globulin with relatively normal total protein and albumin levels. Pandy's test also indicated excess gamma globulin in specimens in which total CSF protein was less than 100 mg/dL. Both tests have been supplanted by electrophoretic and radioimmunologic assays for albumin, IgG, and other immunoglobins.

IgG-Albumin Index

The CSF IgG-albumin index is the ratio of CSF and serum proteins which has proven to be a valuable aid in determining whether an increased CSF IgG concentration is due to greater amounts crossing the meninges or due to synthesis of IgG within the central nervous system.

$$\text{IgG-albumin index} = \frac{\text{IgG (CSF)} \times \text{albumin (serum)}}{\text{IgG (serum} \times \text{albumin (CSF)}}$$

An IgG index greater than 0.7 (in most laboratories) indicates IgG synthesis within the central nervous system as occurs in neurosyphilis, multiple sclerosis, subacute sclerosing panencephalitis, and meningeal sarcoidosis.

Oligoclonal Bands

Electrophoresis of concentrated CSF with agarose gel or other gels may produce a spectrum of bands in the gamma globulin zone. The presence of these oligoclonal bands in CSF in the absence of similar bands in serum usually indicates an inflammatory condition within the central nervous system, although this finding may be seen infrequently in other conditions. Approximately 80% of patients with definite multiple sclerosis have an increased CSF IgG-albumin index and oligoclonal banding in their CSF.

Myelin Basic Protein

Myelin basic protein may be present in the CSF in increased amounts after damage to the central nervous system by stroke or trauma or during demyelination of axons by active multiple sclerosis and acute disseminated encephalomyelitis. Its value in the diagnosis of multiple sclerosis is limited because increased levels may be detected for only a few days after the clinical symptoms of a regressing multiple sclerosis. A normal level is not evidence against the diagnosis of multiple sclerosis.

"Serological" Tests for Syphilis

Immunological assays for the nonspecific reagin-globulin complex and specific treponemal antibodies can use CSF or serum. The tests developed by Wassermann, Kolmer, and the Venereal Disease Research Laboratory are reagin tests. A patient whose CSF has a positive reagin test should be assumed to have neurosyphilis. A leak or serum reagin into CSF due to meningitis or a bloody puncture will cause a false-positive CSF test.

The fluorescent treponemal antibody absorption test is usually not performed with CSF because a positive result does not indicate neurosyphilis, only that enough serum antitreponemal IgG has crossed a normal blood-brain barrier to be detected. A false-positive CSF fluorescent treponemal antibody absorption test can be caused by only 0.8 μL of blood.

Microbial Tests

Gram stains and aerobic and anaerobic bacterial cultures of CSF are standard procedures. Blood should also be cultured in patients suspected of having bacterial meningitis. Remember that patients with early pneumococcal meningitis, especially patients with granulocytopenia, may have a clear, colorless CSF filled with bacteria.

CIE

Countercurrent immunoelectrophoresis (CIE) can detect antigens of the major bacterial antigens. This test in conjunction with repeated lumbar punctures is helpful in distinguishing partially treated meningitis from early viral meningitis. CIE can be applied to the diagnosis of fungal and parasitic diseases.

A value of CIE is the rapidity with which it can be performed. The combination of CIE and routine Gram staining made a specific bacterial diagnosis within one hour in 85% of 170 patients with meningitis. Specific antibiotic treatment should not be based on CIE of CSF alone due to the limits of antigen detection and cross-antigenity among bacterial antigens.

Mycobacteria

Acid-fast stains of CSF are unlikely to be positive except in severe cases of tuberculous meningitis. The yield can be slightly increased by putting many drops of CSF on the slide, drying the slide after each drop. Because cultures for mycobacteria may not show growth for six weeks, patients with meningitis characterized by a CSF containing a mononuclear pleocytosis, hypoglycorrhacia, no tumor cells, and no cryptococcal antigen should be treated for tuberculous meningitis at least until culture results are known. Before starting treatment at least two lumbar punctures should be done, with large amounts of CSF sent for mycobacterial and fungal cultures and cytological examination for tumor cells. The response to therapy is monitored by serial CSF examinations. Low CSF chloride levels are not specific for tuberculous meningitis.

Fungi

Cryptococcus neoformans is the fungus that most commonly infects the central nervous system and is the only capsulated fungus to do so. CSF filled with yeast may be viscous. Yeast cells surrounded by halos in well-filtered India ink preparations establish the diagnosis, but false-negative results are common, especialy with indolent infections and localized granulomas. The detection of cryptococcal antigen in CSF is a more reliable diagnostic method and can be used to monitor response to therapy. A CSF cryptococcal antigen titer of eight or more dilutions is an indication for antifungal treatment. Fungal cultures in Sabouraud's agar may take 10 days to show growth.

Muscle Disease

CPK
Breakdown and inflamation of muscle increases the serum concentration of sarcoplasmic enzymes: creatine phosphokinase (CPK), aldolase, serum glutamic-oxaloacetic and glutamic-pyruvic transaminases, and lactic acid dehydrogenase. CPK is the most reliable enzyme in the diagnosis of polymyositis, rhabdomyolysis, Duchenne's muscular dystrophy, and McArdle's myophosphorylase deficiency. Repeated CPK determinations are useful for following the course of polymyositis. Serum CPK elevations sometimes two or three times normal levels occur after paralytic strokes due to skeletal muscle breakdown and not due to the addition of brain CPK to serum. Polymyositis due to trichinosis is accompanied by eosinophilia and high titers of anti-trichinella antibodies.

Myoglobinuria
Severe rhabdomyolysis can produce myoglobinuria and a dark urine, but acute tubular necrosis may be caused by minimal myoglobinuria undetected by the eye. Myoglobinuria must be distinguished from hemoglobinuria. In both instances the benzidine test is positive. In hemoglobinuria the serum may be pink because of hemolysis and the serum haptoglobin is low. In myoglobinuria, the serum is of normal color, has a normal haptoglobin level, and has elevated levels of muscle enzymes. Early in the course of renal failure after rhabdomyolysis, the serum creatinine will be disproportionately higher than the serum blood urea nitrogen because of the release of muscle creatine. Myoglobin can be measured in small amounts by immunodiffusion (> 9 mg/L) and by CIE (> 3 mg/L).

Myasthenia
Most patients with myasthenia gravis have antibodies against the nicotinic acetylcholine receptors of skeletal muscle. Patients with purely ocular myasthenia have low titers; patients with generalized myasthenia gravis have a wide range of titers with little relation to severity of disease. The anti-AChR antibody titer of patients who improve after thymectomy usually decreases by 50% within one year. Patients treated with penicillamine for rheumatoid arthritis or Wilson's disease may develop anti-AChR antibody.

Antibody against the striations of skeletal muscle occurs in myasthenia gravis, and titers of 60 or more dilutions are associated with thymoma.

■ Selected Readings

Cohen SR, Brooks BR, Herndron RM, et al: A diagnostic index of active demyelination: Myelin basic protein in cerebrospinal fluid. *Ann Neurol* 1980;8: 25–31.

Colding H, Lind I: Counterimmuno-electrophoresis in the diagnosis of bacterial meningitis. *J Clin Microbiol* 1977;5: 405–409.

Dubo H, Park DC, Pennington RJT: Serum creatine-kinase in cases of stroke, head injury, and meningitis. *Lancet* 1967; 2:743–748.

Fishman RA: *Cerebrospinal Fluid in Diseases of the Nervous System.* Philadelphia, The W.B. Saunders Co, 1980.

Glass JP, Melamed M, Chernick NL, et al: Malignant cells in cerebrospinal fluid (CSF): The meaning of a positive CSF cytology. *Neurology* 1979;29:1369–1375.

Jaffee HW: The laboratory diagnosis of syphilis: new concepts. *Ann Intern Med* 1975;83:846–850.

Johnson KP, Nelson BJ: Multiple sclerosis: Diagnostic usefulness of cerebrospinal fluid. *Ann Neurol* 1977;2:425–431.

■ Diabetes Mellitus

Diagnosis

The laboratory diagnosis of diabetes mellitus (DM) is relatively straightforward. Despite the fact that insulin deficiency alters many aspects of fuel metabolism, the sine qua non of DM is an abnormally elevated blood glucose level. Testing for urine glucose is a useful screening procedure, but the detection of glycosuria must be followed by measurements of blood glucose.

Laboratory Methods

Most clinical laboratories use serum or plasma for glucose determinations, having replaced the older whole blood glucose assays. The significance of this change is that the "classical" diagnostic criteria for DM must be adjusted upward by about 15%; this difference is accounted for by the lower glucose concentration in red blood cells compared with that in extracellular fluid. Serum or plasma should be separated from cells promptly since glucose levels may fall up to 25 mg/dL per hour due to red blood cell and leukocyte glycolysis. Alternatively, tubes containing fluoride may be used to inhibit glycolysis, but fluoride may interfere with some assays based on the glucose oxidase technique.

There are many different methods for measuring serum or plasma glucose levels, each with its own normal range. The most widely employed chemical technique, which has been adapted to automated equipment, is the Hoffman ferricyanide procedure. Not specific for glucose, this measures total reducing substances. "True" glucose can be measured by specific enzymatic methods (eg, glucose oxidase or hexokinase). The practicing physician should be aware of the method used and the normal range for plasma glucose in the local laboratory.

FPG and OGTT

There are standardized criteria for the diagnosis of "overt DM" based upon either the fasting plasma glucose (FPG) or the response to an oral glucose tolerance test (OGTT) (Table 16-1). The latter test is completely unnecessary, however, in the presence of an elevated FPG. Blood for a FPG determination should be drawn after an overnight (10 to 14-hour) fast; no other preparation is necessary. Transient elevations of FPG may occur in severely stressed patients.

The diagnosis of "impaired glucose tolerance" is based on the results of an OGTT (Table 16-1), but the use of this test should be selective. First, many factors can alter glucose tolerance (Table 16-2), so that the results are often not reproducible and may be difficult to interpret. Second, less than half of

Kenneth L. Cohen
Richard D. Kayne

269

270

Table 16-1
Diagnostic Criteria (Plasma or Serum Glucose) of Overt DM and Impaired Glucose Tolerance in Patients with Normal Fasting Glucose Levels*

Time After Glucose (min)	Fajans and Conn	NIH International Workshop†	
		Overt DM	Impaired Glucose Tolerance
30			
60	> 195 mg/dL	One value over 200	One value over 200
90	> 165		
120	> 140	Over 200	> 140 < 200

*There is no need to do an OGTT in patients with elevated FPG levels. In patients over age 50, add 10 mg/dL for each decade above the fifth.
†Data from the National Diabetes Data Group. *Diabetes* 1979;28:1039–1057.

Table 16-2
Factors Which Impair Glucose Tolerance

Physiologic—Increased Age, Pregnancy

Diet—Severe Carbohydrate Restriction (less than 100 g/day)

Inactivity

Intercurrent Illness or Stress

Drugs—Glucocorticoids, Oral Contraceptives, Diuretics, Phenytoin, Alcohol

the patients found to have impaired glucose tolerance will go on to develop overt DM (1% to 5% per year). Third, labeling someone as having impaired glucose tolerance may adversely affect his or her social or psychological well being. The situations in which an OGTT can be useful are (1) screening women at risk for DM during pregnancy (see below), (2) the occurrence of "diabetic" complications, such as peripheral neuropathy or mononeuropathy, in the presence of a normal FPG, and (3) possibly in the obese patient for whom the documentation of impaired glucose tolerance may be an impetus to weight reduction.

Preparation for an OGTT should include (1) at least three days *without* severe carbohydrate restriction, ie, consumption of at least 100 g of carbohydrate per day (equivalent to about six slices of bread), (2) an overnight fast, and (3) abstention from exercise and smoking during the test. The adult patient is given either 75 or 100 g of glucose (1.75 g/kg of ideal body weight for children) to be consumed over a five-minute period. Blood samples are obtained at 30, 60, 90, and 120 minutes. If reactive hypoglycemia is suspected, additional samples should be obtained at three, four, and five hours.

Primary (Idiopathic) Versus Secondary DM
Labeling DM as "primary" or "idiopathic" indicates our ignorance concerning the genetic and environmental factors which have led to the impairment of insulin secretion and/or action. In a few patients, however, the cause of

the DM can be defined and, if treated, may lead to cure. Most of these conditions will be apparent from the patient's history and physical examination, but are included here to indicate the importance of considering these diagnoses and ordering the appropriate laboratory tests. The secondary causes of DM can be divided into several categories: (1) excess antiinsulin hormones, (2) impairment of insulin release, and (3) pancreoprivic diabetes (Table 16-3).

DM in Pregnancy
Overt DM and impaired glucose tolerance during pregnancy are both risk factors for fetal morbidity and mortality. Periodic screening for glycosuria should be a routine part of all obstetrical practices. Detection of glucose in the urine should be followed by measurements of fasting and postprandial plasma glucose levels since false-positive urine tests can occur due to a

Table 16-3
Etiology of DM

I. Primary—Idiopathic
II. Secondary

Mechanism	Associated Findings	Laboratory Evaluation
A. Excess antiinsulin hormones		
1. Catecholamines	Hypertension	24-hour urine catecholamines (see pheochromocytoma, Chapter 17.)
2. Growth Hormone (GH)	Acral enlargement	Basal serum GH level (see acromegaly, Chapter 17.)
3. Glucocorticoids	Hypertension Obesity Striae	24-hour urine cortisol dexamethasone suppression test (see Adrenal section, Chapter 17.)
4. Glucagon	Skin rash	Basal glucagon level (see MEN 1, Chapter 17.)
B. Impaired insulin release		
1. Hypokalemia		
a. Aldosterone excess	Hypertension	Plasma renin, urine aldosterone (see adrenal section, Chapter 17.)
b. Diuretics		
2. Drug induced a. Beta blockers b. Phenytoin		
C. Pancreoprivic		
1. Pancreatitis	Malabsorption	
2. Hemochromatosis	Hyperpigmentation Cirrhosis	Serum iron/IBC (see Hematology, Chapter 3.)

lowered renal threshold for glucose or the presence of lactose (see Monitoring, below). Some obstetricians also recommend routine screening for impaired glucose tolerance by using an OGTT at about the 26th week of gestation. Others are more selective and will screen women with a positive family history for DM, previous delivery of a large infant, or obesity. (See also Chapter 19.)

Monitoring of DM

Once a diagnosis of DM is made, the patient is committed to lifelong dietary therapy, with or without insulin or oral hypoglycemic agents. Chronic monitoring of urine and/or blood glucose is also necessary, but should be as convenient as possible to insure compliance and to avoid major disruptions of the patient's life.

Urine Glucose

Before beginning regular urine glucose testing, it is necessary to determine the correlation between blood and urine glucose levels in each patient, ie, the renal threshold. This is most easily done by obtaining several fasting and random plasma glucose levels with simultaneous "double-voided" urine specimens—having the patient void just before the blood sampling and then testing the urine passed one-half hour later. Some patients will have a high threshold (over 250 or 300 mg/dL), so that urine testing will only serve to document very elevated plasma glucose levels. The corollary to this statement is that negative urine tests do not necessarily imply good glucose control. In addition, patients with large residual urine volumes due to diabetic autonomic neuropathy may be unable to utilize urine monitoring due to a complete lack of correlation between blood and urine glucose levels.

"Close" monitoring of urine fractional samples involves testing preprandial and nighttime "double-voided" urine specimens. Single-voided specimens may be more convenient to obtain during the workday and can give a general guide to glucose control since the preceding test. The frequency of testing can be adjusted according to the ease of glucose control in the individual patient. For example, a mild, diet-controlled diabetic patient may test only once a day. However, even in that setting, tests should be done at various times, rather than only in the morning, to provide information concerning the degree of glucose control throughout the entire day. Occasionally, quantitative glucose measurements in either 24-hour or 8-hour specimens can be useful in assessing glucose control. For example, quantitation of glucose in an 8-hour overnight specimen can help distinguish the patient with poor control (with many grams of glucose in the specimen) from the one with nocturnal hypoglycemia followed by rebound morning hyperglycemia (with relatively little glucose in the overnight collection).

The two methods commonly available for urine glucose testing utilize either copper sulfate reduction (Clinitest tablets) or the glucose oxidase reaction (Testape, Clinistix, etc). Each technique has its own advantages and disadvantages which make it acceptable to different groups of patients. Since the color reactions occur at different urine glucose concentrations (Table 16-4), it is advisable for patients to report urine tests as "percent glucose" rather than "number of pluses" in order to avoid confusion.

The copper sulfate method is not specific for glucose, but measures total reducing substances in the urine; this may lead to false-positive and false-negative tests (Table 16-5). In addition, some consider the test to be cumbersome and time consuming. The advantages of the test are that the color distinction between various glucose concentrations is clear cut and is relatively stable after the chemical reaction is complete. The glucose oxidase test is a glucose-specific reaction, but certain chemicals can interfere with the enzyme, giving false-negative values (Table 16-5). The main advantage of these test strips is their simplicity and convenience. However, the color separation between different glucose levels is less clear cut, and the timing of the reaction is critical; since the enzymatic process does not stop, the strips tend to get progressively darker after the recommended 30- or 60-second test period.

Urine Ketones
Testing the urine for ketones is important in monitoring type I (insulin-dependent, ketosis-prone) diabetics. All current methods are based on the nitroprusside reaction, which measures acetoacetic acid and acetone, but not beta-hydroxybutyric acid. In the presence of large amount of reducing

Table 16-4
Interpretation of Clinitest (Total Reducing Substances)
and Testape (Glucose Oxidase) Urine Tests

Clinitest (5-drop method)			Testape	
Color Reaction	*Pluses*	Glucose (%)	*Pluses*	*Color Reaction*
Blue	−	0	−	Yellow
		1/10 (0.10)	+	Light green
Green	Trace	1/4 (0.25)	+ +	Green
Light green	+	1/2 (0.50)	+ + +	Dark green
Olive green	+ +	3/4 (0.75)		
Brown	+ + +	1 (1.0)		
Orange	+ + + +	≥ 2 (2.0)	+ + + +	Black

Table 16-5
False-Positive and False-Negative Urine Tests

	Urine Test Method	
Compound	*Reducing Substances*	*Glucose Oxidase*
Lactose	+	
Ascorbic Acid	+	−
Salicylates	+	−
Cephalothin	+	
Nalidixic Acid	+	
L-Dopa	+	−
Homogentisic acid (alcaptonuria)	+	

substances, as in lactic acidosis, most of the ketones may be in the reduced form (beta-hydroxybutyric acid), leading to a falsely low urine (and serum) ketone level as determined by the nitroprusside reaction. A far more common reason for false-negative tests, however, is that nitroprusside dipsticks have a very short shelf life once the bottle is opened. Therefore, unless ketone testing is being done on a daily basis, the more stable nitroprusside tablets should be used.

Blood Glucose
The measurement of FPG was discussed above. In long-term monitoring of patients, random specimens taken at various times during the day are useful in addition to fasting tests to get a better picture of the 24-hour glucose control. With recent advances in insulin delivery systems and attempts to normalize glucose control in type I diabetics, there has been renewed interest in home capillary blood glucose monitoring using glucose oxidase strips (Dextrostix, Chemstrips) with or without reflectance meters. The skill required and the inconvenience imposed by these systems require a highly motivated patient and a readily available physician to make the program successful.

Glycosylated Hemoglobin
It has been known for some time that glucose can become covalently attached to hemoglobin in circulating red blood cells via a chemical reaction dependent mainly upon the plasma glucose concentration. The reaction is relatively irreversible, so the level of the glycosylated hemoglobin rises gradually during the life span of the erythrocyte. Therefore, the level of glycosylated hemoglobin will reflect the average or integrated plasma glucose over the preceding four to six week period. Such a measurement can be useful in documenting the overall success or failure of a given regimen in achieving near-normal blood glucose levels. The test will not reflect the hour-to-hour or day-to-day variability in glucose levels.

Complication of DM

DKA
When diabetic ketoacidosis (DKA) is suspected, the diagnosis can rapidly be confirmed with appropriate laboratory tests. The combination of glucose oxidase dipsticks and nitroprusside tablets can reduce the time required to a few minutes, and treatment can be started before the results of arterial pH and "routine" plasma glucose measurements are available. (Table 16-6).

The differential diagnosis of DKA initially includes all forms of metabolic acidosis. Once a large concentration of ketones is documented in blood and urine, the major diagnosis to be ruled out is alcoholic ketoacidosis (AKA). The laboratory distinction between AKA and DKA generally rests upon the plasma glucose determination. The glucose level in DKA is elevated, usually well above 200 mg/dL, whereas it is generally less than 200 mg/dL in AKA. In about 30% of cases of AKA, hypoglycemia is present.

The sequential measurement of glucose, potassium, and bicarbonate is critical during the treatment of DKA. Repeated measurement of serum and urine ketones is less helpful since the gradual conversion of beta-hydroxybutyrate (not measured in the nitroprusside reaction) to acetoacetic

Table 16-6
Laboratory Diagnosis of DKA

	Method	Results
Rapid Tests		
Urine glucose	Glucose oxidase	> 2% (4+)
Urine ketones	Nitroprusside tablet	Large
Blood glucose	Glucose oxidase stick	> > 200 mg/dL
Serum ketones	Nitroprusside tablet	Large undiluted
Confirmatory and Additional Tests		
Arterial blood gases		pH ≤ 7.30
		pCO_2 ≤ 40 mmHg
Serum glucose, sodium, bicarbonate chloride, potassium, phosphate, etc.		

acid and acetone may create the false impression of a lack of response to therapy. Urine ketones often remain positive for days after therapy of DKA. Serum phosphate levels fall precipitously with insulin administration, often to levels less than 1 mg/dL. However, there are still no definitive data to suggest that this requires specific therapy. Serum amylase levels are frequently elevated in DKA, but some or all of this enzyme may be of salivary gland origin and may not reflect pancreatitis.

During the recovery from DKA, the anion gap acidosis caused by the ketoacids may be replaced by a hyperchloremic acidosis. The apparent explanation for this phenomenon involves the loss of bicarbonate equivalents during DKA due to the ketonuria and the subsequent therapy with saline solutions.

HNKC
The clinical diagnosis of hyperglycemic non-ketotic coma (HNKC) is often initially overlooked since patients may have no previous history of DM and may present with focal or generalized seizures. The laboratory report of marked hyperglycemia (over 600 mg/dL), azotemia (average blood urea nitrogen of 80 mg/dL), and serum hyperosmolarity (over 320 mOsm/L), will lead to the proper diagnosis. Although ketosis is classically absent, mild elevations of serum ketones in association with marked hyperglycemia may still be appropriately labeled HNKC. Lactic acid levels are frequently elevated due to tissue hypoperfusion, but measurements of lactate are clinically unnecessary. Assays for serum amylase are important, however, since acute pancreatitis can be found in up to one-fourth of patients with HNKC.

■ Hypoglycemia

Hypoglycemia is categorized as fasting, reactive, or spurious. Fasting hypoglycemia is defined as a serum glucose obtained after a 12-hour overnight fast which is below 60 mg/dL in both men and women and a serum glucose obtained after a 72-hour fast which is below 50 mg/dL in men and below 40 mg/dL in women. Normally, fasting leads to suppression of insulin secretion and low serum insulin levels, although there are some persons whose fasting serum glucose values fall below those stated above but who have normal suppression of insulin secretion. This is particularly so in healthy young women in whom serum glucose values after a 72-hour fast occasionally fall to 25–30 mg/dL in the absence of symptoms.

Fasting hypoglycemia accompanies states of decreased glucose production, increased glucose utilization, and insulin excess. The first two conditions are associated with very low serum insulin levels which lead to ketosis and ketonuria. *States of hypoglycemia caused by insulin excess will not be associated with ketonuria.* Insulinoma is the disease of major concern in this category. Thus, the finding of ketonuria in a hypoglycemic patient prompts laboratory investigation for primary or secondary adrenal insufficiency, growth hormone deficiency, liver failure, alcoholic hypoglycemia (elevated serum alcohol level in a patient with ketonuric hypoglycemia which is nonrecurrent during alcohol deprivation), early pregnancy (serum or urine HCG levels), or bulky mesenchymal tumors (nonspecific laboratory abnormalities of complete blood cell count or liver function tests may be present). The causes of hypoglycemia reviewed above are generally suggested by history and physical examination and distinguished by the presence of ketonuria.

If ketonuria is absent on initial evaluation, a period of fasting with measurement of serum glucose and insulin levels is required to eliminate insulinoma. The five-hour OGTT is not a substitute for fasting, nor does it offer any useful information in the evaluation of *fasting* hypoglycemia. Both serum glucose and insulin values obtained during the OGTT are highly variable in patients with insulinomas, and insulin/glucose ratios obtained in this setting are meaningless. Most patients with insulinoma will have an overnight fasting serum glucose below 50 mg/dL with a plasma insulin level above 20 μU/mL, values diagnostic of insulinoma. Additional patients will be identified by extending the overnight fast for 18 hours. Ten percent of patients require a 72-hour fast. Prolonged fasting (beyond 12 hours) should be performed under close observation, as patients with insulinomas may develop seizures or coma. Serum samples for glucose and simultaneous insulin levels are obtained every four to six hours or until hypoglycemic symptoms appear; glucose-free fluid intake is unrestricted, and all urine voided is assayed for ketones. Samples for insulin determination are not processed unless the serum glucose is less than 50 mg/dL or hypoglycemic symptoms are present. *The development of ketonuria excludes the diagnosis of insulinoma, warrants discontinuation of the test, and eliminates the need to process the samples for serum insulin levels.* Should neither ketonuria nor a fall in serum glucose to below 50 mg/dL occur, the last two or three sets of sera for glucose and insulin should be processed. The diagnosis of insulinoma is suggested when the ratio of serum insulin to serum glucose exceeds 0.3. The finding of rising insulin and falling glucose level also suggests an insulinoma. An amended insulin/glucose ratio [(plasma insulin level × 100)/(fasting plasma glucose − 30)] can be used for obese patients in whom basal hyperinsulinemia may lead to a false-positive diagnosis of insulinoma if the standard ratio is applied. A normal value for the amended ratio is less than 50 in an obese patient with a fasting serum glucose below 60 mg/dL. The prolonged fast may be extended for an additional two hours with the patient exercising; in normal persons, serum glucose rises with exercise, whereas glucose declines further with exercise in patients with insulinomas. Almost all patients with insulinomas will be identified by these maneuvers. The tests discussed below are needed when the diagnosis is still unclear.

Patients with insulinoma will have parallel elevations of serum insulin and serum C-peptide, a segment of the proinsulin molecule that is secreted on an equimolar basis with insulin. When plasma insulin is fractionated into insulin and proinsulin, proinsulin constitutes more than 20% of total serum insulin in the majority of patients with insulinoma. Rarely, insulin suppression or stimulation tests are required. The infusion of fish insulin, not measured by the human plasma insulin assay, normally results in suppression of serum insulin levels, whereas suppression is absent in patients with insulinoma. Similarly, the infusion of commercial insulin normally suppresses C-peptide levels (reflecting suppression of pancreatic insulin secretion), whereas suppression does not occur in patients with insulinoma. Stimulation tests involving the injection of tolbutamide, leucine, glucagon, or calcium to provoke diagnostically elevated serum insulin levels can also cause severe and prolonged hypoglycemia, and false-negative results occur in a significant number of patients with insulinoma.

Insulin excess may be induced by (self-) administration of insulin or oral hypoglycemic agents. This form of hyperinsulinemic hypoglycemia must be distinguished from hypoglycemia due to an insulinoma. Patients with factitious hypoglycemia tend to have intermittent hypoglycemia associated with elevations of serum insulin levels higher than those seen in patients with insulinoma, ie, often in the range of 200–1000 μU/mL. The presence of antiinsulin antibodies in the serum of a patient with hypoglycemia suggests self-administration of commercial beef or pork insulin. However, these antibodies may not develop until insulin has been injected for several months. (Conversely, in the rare patient with the autoimmune insulin hypoglycemia syndrome, antiinsulin antibodies may be present without insulin administration.) Serum C-peptide levels are suppressed by insulin administration to a normal patient; thus, C-peptide levels are low in patients with factitious hypoglycemia, but are high in patients with insulinoma. Insulin-requiring diabetic patients who have factitious hypoglycemia may have antibodies to the proinsulin contaminants contained in their commercial insulin preparations; such antibodies may cross-react in the measurement of C-peptide and give falsely high values suggestive of an insulinoma. Urinary C-peptide determinations or special assay systems for C-peptide circumvent this problem. The abuse of oral hypoglycemic agents which may cause hyperinsulinemic hypoglycemia by stimulating pancreatic insulin secretion can be detected by serum sulfonylurea drug levels or, if tolbutamide is being used, by acidification of the urine which forms carboxytolbutamide, a white precipitate.

A small subset of patients with symptomatic fasting hypoglycemia will have hypoglycemia in the absence of ketonuria due to the production of an insulin-like growth factor (IGF1 or 2) or related peptides which comprise "nonsuppressible insulin-like activity" (NSILA-s); these factors are insulin-like substances and produce hypoglycemia while inhibiting ketosis.

278

Laboratory evaluaton of these patients, who often have bulky mesenchymal tumors, reveals hypoinsulinemia and, in the majority of patients, increased levels of IGF1 or 2 or NSILA-s.

Reactive hypoglycemia describes a situation in which serum glucose falls after the ingestion of large amounts of glucose-rich food; serum glucose is normal during a fast in such patients. Only 5% of normal patients will experience a decrease in serum glucose below 50 mg/dL in response to a 75- to 100-g oral glucose load. The diagnosis of reactive hypoglycemia requires the development of postprandial hypoglycemia (serum glucose below 50 mg/dL), simultaneous symptoms of hypoglycemia, and prompt resolution of these symptoms by the ingestion of glucose and normalization of the serum glucose. The finding of an isolated low serum glucose value in the absence of the other two criteria is not diagnostic of reactive hypoglycemia. Serum glucose levels are obtained every 30 to 60 minutes for five hours after the oral glucose load. Serum insulin levels should not be measured during this test, as the results are not interpretable. There are three prominent patterns of hypoglycemia provoked by ingesting glucose. (1) Patients with alimentary hypoglycemia usually have had prior gastric surgery and experience hyperglycemia 30–60 minutes after glucose loading, followed by symptomatic hypoglycemia at 90–120 minutes. (2) Some patients with early diabetes have fasting normoglycemia, hyperglycemia during the first two hours of the test, and hypoglycemia at four to five hours. (3) Patients with idiopathic or functional hypoglycemia do not manifest hyperglycemia during the test and have hypoglycemia at three to four hours which will persist throughout the remainder of the test in some patients. These three patterns are summarized in Figure 16-1. The OGTT is of no value in the diagnosis of an insulinoma, as any pattern of glucose values may be seen.

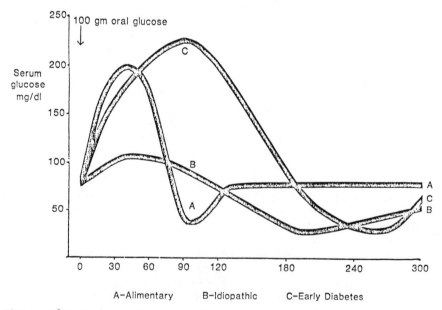

Figure 16-1 Patterns of oral glucose tolerance test in patients with reactive hypoglycemia.

Spurious hypoglycemia occurs in vitro when serum collected from patients with chronic myelogenous leukemia and marked leukocytosis is allowed to remain in contact with the white blood cells long enough for significant metabolism of glucose by the leukocytes to occur. Prompt separation of serum from whole blood eliminates this confusion. Prolonged exposure of serum glucose to erythrocytes can lead to spurious hypoglycemia due to erythrocytic glycolysis. This effect is less than that which occurs in vitro in some leukemic patients and is prevented by prompt processing or by collecting the sample in a tube which contains sodium fluoride.

■ Selected Readings

Diabetes Mellitus

Koenig RJ, Peterson CM, Jones RL, et al: Correlation of glucose regulation and hemoglobin A_1c in diabetes mellitus. *N Engl J Med* 1976;295:417–420.

National Diabetes Data Group: Classification and diagnosis of diabetes mellitus and other catagories of glucose intolerance. *Diabetes* 1979;28:1039–1057.

Sayegh HA, Jarrett RJ: Oral glucose tolerance tests and the diagnosis of diabetes: Results of a prospective study based on the Whitehall survey. *Lancet* 1979;2: 431–433.

Hypoglycemia

Cahill GF, Soeldner JS: A non-editorial on non-hypoglycemia. *N Engl J Med* 1974;291:905.

Faber OK, Kehlet H: Strategy in the diagnosis of insulinoma. *Scand J Gastroenterol* Suppl 53 1979;14:45–48.

Fajans S, Floyd JC: Fasting hypoglycemia in adults. *N Engl J Med* 1976;294: 766.

Farriss BL: Prevalence of post-glucose-load glycosuria and hypoglycemia in a group of healthy young men. *Diabetes* 1974;23:189.

Hoekstra JBL, van Rijn HJM, Erkelens DW, et al: C-peptide. *Diabetes Care* 1982;5:438–446.

Permutt MA: Postprandial hypoglycemia. *Diabetes* 1976;25:719.

Scarlett JA, Mako ME, et al: Diagnosis of factitious hypoglycemia. *N Engl J Med* 1977;297:1029.

Seltzer HS: Drug-induced hypoglycemia. A review based on 473 cases. *Diabetes* 1972;21:955.

Service FJ, Dale AJD, Elveback LR, et al: Insulinoma. Clinical and diagnostic features of 60 consecutive cases. *Mayo Clin Proc* 1976;51:417.

Pituitary Disease

Many physicians are reluctant to evaluate patients with possible pituitary disease because the workup is "too complicated." Such statements are unwarranted. Simple screening tests can reliably rule out pituitary disease or indicate the need for more detailed testing. If additional provocative or suppression tests are necessary, straightforward protocols are available which allow accurate and safe collection of specimens.

Pituitary disease can present in one of three ways: (1) hormone deficiency—single or multiple, (2) hormone excess, or (3) mass effect. The possibility of pituitary dysfunction is raised whenever a patient has signs and symptoms of thyroid hormone or sex hormone deficiency. Although these conditions are most often due to end organ dysfunction, it is important to do screening tests which confirm the diagnosis of primary thyroid or gonadal failure or suggest the presence of pituitary disease. If evidence of pituitary disease is found, additional testing is necessary to search for multiple hormone deficiencies and to screen for pituitary mass effect. The signs and symptoms of acromegaly, amenorrhea-galactorrhea syndrome, and Cushing's disease are due to the hypersecretion of growth hormone, prolactin, and adrenocorticotropic hormone (ACTH), respectively. Deficiencies of other pituitary hormones may coexist and must be screened for in these patients. Pituitary disease may also present with headache, visual field disturbance, or simply the accidental discovery of an abnormal sella on skull x-ray—all suggesting a mass effect. The key objectives of the pituitary workup are similar for all three modes of presentation of pituitary disease (Table 17-1).

■ Specific Laboratory Tests in the Evaluation of Pituitary Function and Pituitary Disease

Pituitary-Adrenal Axis

Basal Tests
Plasma or Serum Cortisol Levels Cortisol, the major glucocorticoid in humans, is the key compound in the feedback regulation of ACTH secretion. Obviously, the measurement of circulating cortisol is of major importance in the evaluation of the pituitary adrenal axis. However, cortisol levels are affected by the diurnal cycle of ACTH secretion and by the disturbance of this cycle caused by stress. Therefore, *random determinations of serum cortisol are not useful.*

Pulsatile secretion of cortisol, in response to ACTH spikes, peaks in the morning (10–25 μg/dL at 8 AM) and then tapers off during the rest of the day. Serum cortisol may be undetectable around midnight in normal subjects. An AM cortisol level within

Kenneth L. Cohen
Richard D. Kayne

the normal range does not, however, guarantee a normal pituitary adrenal axis since (1) there may be a deficiency of ACTH reserve such that the pituitary may not respond normally to stress, and (2) serum cortisol should be elevated in stressed patients (eg, hypotensive, nauseated, etc) and values within the "normal range" are inappropriate. Clearly, provocative testing of ACTH is required in most patients being screened for hypopituitarism. The exception may be in patients with random cortisol values over 20 µg/dL, since that is the minimum normal response to provocative stimuli.

Twenty-Four-Hour Urine Steroid Levels Measurements of either glucocorticoid metabolites (as 17-hydroxysteroids) or free cortisol in 24-hour urine collections serves as an index of the integrated daily secretion rate of cortisol. Unfortunately, both assays discriminate poorly between low and low-normal values; they are much more useful in the evaluation of cortisol hypersecretion-Cushing's syndrome (see Adrenal Gland, below). In addition, cortisol metabolism is altered in patients with hypothyroidism or malnutrition and those receiving phenytoin (Dilantin) therapy, leading to falsely low urine 17-hydroxysteroid levels. These tests are therefore of limited value in the workup of possible ACTH deficiency.

ACTH Level The radioimmunoassay of ACTH is relatively difficult and therefore less available and more expensive than measurements of other peptide hormones. In addition, since ACTH is unstable in plasma and adheres to glass, blood must be drawn into chilled heparinized plastic syringes, promptly centrifuged in the cold, and frozen in plastic tubes. The assay may not distinguish low from low-normal values and thus is of limited use in evaluating ACTH deficiency. There is no advantage in measuring ACTH during provocative tests over the simpler cortisol assay. A single ACTH determination can be useful in (1) documenting primary adrenal disease (with markedly elevated ACTH levels) versus secondary adrenal dysfunction and (2) helping to evaluate the etiology of Cushing's syndrome (see Adrenal Gland, below).

Stimulation Tests Due to technical difficulties with ACTH assays, provocative tests of ACTH reserve rely on cortisol or 11-deoxycortisol determinations as indirect measures of ACTH secretion; for the test results to be valid, the adrenal gland must be capable of responding to ACTH. The distinction between primary versus secondary (pituitary) causes of adrenal insufficiency should therefore be made before testing. Hyperpigmentation, hyperkalemia, and severe volume contraction, indicating glucocorticoid *and* mineralocorticoid deficiency, would lead to adrenal testing; more nonspecific complaints of anorexia and nausea caused by low glucocorticoid levels, usually in association with evidence of deficiency of other pituitary hormones or of pituitary mass effect, will lead to tests of ACTH reserve.

Cosyntropin (Synthetic ACTH) Injection Test Although originally designed as a test for primary adrenal disease, the ACTH injection can also serve as a rapid, simple test of pituitary function. ACTH does more than acutely stimulate cortisol secretion; it is a trophic hormone which can stimulate the growth and metabolism of adrenal cortical cells. Thus, the

Table 17-1
Key Objectives in the Evaluation of Pituitary Function

1. Distinguish pituitary diseases from end organ failure in patients with hypothyroidism, hypogonadism, or hypoadrenalism
2. Confirm or rule out pituitary hypersecretion in patients with amenorrhea/galactorrhea, acral enlargement, or Cushing's syndrome
3. Determine the status of ACTH and TSH secretion since deficiencies of these hormones may be life threatening
4. Screen for mass effect
5. Retest after definitive therapy to determine the need for chronic hormone replacement

maximal cortisol response to a pharmacologic challenge with ACTH is actually set by the endogenous ACTH level. With endogenous ACTH excess, as in Cushing's disease, there is a hyperresponsiveness of the adrenal gland to exogenous ACTH; with ACTH deficiency, the adrenal response is impaired. It has been demonstrated that the serum cortisol value obtained 30 minutes after a cosyntropin injection is closely correlated with the peak cortisol response after insulin hypoglycemia. Thus, this simple screening test, which has essentially no contraindications or side effects, can often provide the same information as the more involved provocative tests. However, some patients with only partial ACTH deficiency and mild impairment of adrenal reserve may have a cortisol response to cosyntropin that approaches or exceeds the minimum normal level; borderline normal values in these subjects require further study with the tests described below.

The cosyntropin test can be done any time of the day without special patient preparation. The test is performed by (1) obtaining a basal serum or plasma cortisol level, (2) injecting 250 μg of synthetic ACTH intravenously in a 1-minute bolus, and (3) obtaining a 30-minute cortisol determination. The cortisol level at 30 minutes should exceed 20 μg/dL. If it does not, additional confirmatory tests of decreased ACTH reserve should be pursued.

Insulin Hypoglycemia—Insulin Tolerance Test (ITT) Insulin hypoglycemia is the production of a hypoglycemic stress by the injection of insulin. This stress, impinging upon the hypothalamic pituitary axis, stimulates the release of ACTH and the consequent secretion of cortisol. The test is done in the fasting patient after the insertion of an intravenous line containing saline. Baseline specimens for glucose and cortisol determination are obtained, and a bolus of 0.1 U of regular insulin per kilogram of body weight is injected. This dose may be increased to 0.2 U/k for insulin-resistant patients (obese, acromegalic) or decreased to 0.05 U/kg for insulin-sensitive patients (known cortisol or growth hormone deficiency). Repeat blood specimens are obtained at least every 30 minutes until one hour after the occurrence of hypoglycemic symptoms. A peak serum cortisol level over 20 μg/dL, usually occurring about 30 minutes after hypoglycemic symptoms, is a normal response.

Criteria for an adequate hypoglycemic stress include (1) at least a 50% decline in plasma glucose levels, (2) a nadir less than 50 mg/dL, and

(3) symptoms of hypoglycemia. Inadequate hypoglycemia may result in a subnormal cortisol response, whereas excessive hypoglycemia may provoke seizures or coma. A physician must be present during the test, prepared to reverse excessive symptoms with intravenous glucose; this usually does not affect the subsequent cortisol response.

The ITT is also useful as a provocative test of growth hormone and prolactin reserve (see below). However, the peak growth hormone response will be blunted if hypoglycemic symptoms are treated with intravenous glucose. In addition, reliable prolactin stimulation requires more severe degrees of hypoglycemic stress than those required to stimulate ACTH secretion.

Metyrapone Test Metyrapone inhibits adrenal 11 beta-hydroxylase, which is the last step in cortisol synthesis. The resulting decrease in serum cortisol provokes ACTH secretion and a subsequent rise in adrenal steroid production, particularly 11-deoxycortisol (compound S), which accumulates behind the 11-hydroxylase block. The original three-day protocol is cumbersome and may precipitate or aggravate symptoms of cortisol deficiency in patients with borderline pituitary function. A simpler overnight test is available, although the larger single dose of metyrapone required may cause nausea and vomiting and invalidate the test. In addition, phenytoin (Dilantin) accelerates the metabolism of metyrapone, leading to an incomplete 11-hydroxylase block and a false-positive test result.

The protocol for the three-day metyrapone test is as follows: (1) Collect a 24-hour urine specimen for baseline 17-hydroxysteroids (17-OHS) and creatinine determination; (2) Administer 750 mg of metyrapone (300 mg/m^a in children) by mouth every four hours for six doses; (3) Collect urine on the day of and the day after metyrapone ingestion for 17-OHS and/or 11-deoxycortisol determination; (4) Measure plasma cortisol four hours after the last metyrapone dose. A normal response is a 2.5- to 3-fold increase in 17-OHS or a peak 11-deoxycortisol value of greater than 8 mg/24 h. In addition, the plasma cortisol level should be less than 8 μg/dL, thus ensuring adequate 11-beta-hydroxylase blockade.

The overnight metyrapone test is done by (1) giving 3 g (30 mg/kg) of metyrapone by mouth at midnight, and (2) drawing plasma samples for cortisol and 11-deoxycortisol determination at 8 AM. A normal response is indicated by an 8 AM plasma cortisol level of less than 10 μg/dL and a simultaneous 11-deoxycortisol level above 7 μg/dL.

Vasopressin (ADH) Injection Antidiuretic hormone (ADH) can directly stimulate the release of ACTH from the pituitary gland, with subsequent rise in plasma cortisol levels. It is not, however, as reliable a test as those discussed above. In addition, problems with abdominal pain, nausea, high blood pressure, and precipitation of angina limit its usefulness. The test is performed injecting 10 U of aqueous vasopressin subcutaneously and obtaining specimens for plasma cortisol determination at 0, 30, and 60 minutes. The peak plasma cortisol response should exceed 20 μg/dL.

Suppression Test
Dexamethasone suppression testing for the evaluation of Cushing's syndrome is discussed below (see Adrenal Gland).

Pituitary-Thyroid Axis

Basal Tests

Resin Uptake/Free T₄ Index These screening tests of thyroid function are discussed in detail in Thyroid, below. Free thyroxine index measurements in the midnormal to upper-normal range reliably rule out pituitary-thyroid dysfunction. Low values require a basal thyroid-stimulating hormone (TSH) determination. The patient with signs or symptoms of hypothyroidism and a low-normal free thyroxine index should also have a TSH measurement performed.

Serum TSH The radioimmunoassay for TSH is discussed elsewhere. The important point to reiterate is that a serum TSH measurement should be obtained in any patient with newly diagnosed hypothyroidism in order to screen for the smaller but definite possibility of a secondary (pituitary) cause of the disease.

Stimulation Test

TRH Injection The indications and protocol for the thyrotropin-releasing hormone (TRH) test are outlined below (see Thyroid Disease). The TRH injection was initially promoted to distinguish secondary (pituitary) from tertiary (hypothalamic) hypothyroidism. The "classical response" in patients with pituitary disease is an absent or blunted TSH release after TRH injection; patients with organic or functional hypothalamic disease demonstrate a delayed but quantitatively normal TSH response to TRH. Since there is significant overlap in these patterns of response between the two groups of patients, the TSH response to TRH may give a little additional information beyond that provided by the basal TSH level in the individual patient evaluated for pituitary disease. TRH injections, however, have diagnostic value in the workup of hyperprolactinemia or growth hormone excess (see below).

Suppression Test

Triiodothyronine The triiodothyronine suppression test, designed to evaluate the patient with hyperthyroidism, has been replaced by the TRH injection test.

Pituitary-Gonadal Axis

Basal Tests

Testosterone, Estradiol The testis and ovary produce a variety of steroid compounds, but the key hormones measured in screening for hypogonadism are testosterone in men and estradiol in women. This may be done on random plasma specimens; these assays are described below (see Gonadal Disease). Two points need to be emphasized here. (1) Testosterone is fairly tightly bound to sex hormone binding globulin in plasma so that changes in the level of total testosterone are not necessarily accompanied by abnormalities of free (active) testosterone—assays which provide an estimate of free as well as total testosterone are necessary in the evaluation of possible male hypogonadism. (2) Estradiol levels in women change dramatically at various stages of sexual development as well as during the normal menstrual cycle so the appropriate normal range needs to be applied in the interpretation of laboratory reports.

LH and FSH Levels   Although most patients with hypogonadism have end organ (testicular or ovarian) failure, it should be routine practice to obtain gonadotropin measurements which will either conform the diagnosis or suggest the possibility of pituitary disease. Despite the periodic secretion of gonadotropins, a random determination is usually diagnostically high (in primary hypogonadism) or low (in pituitary disease). Borderline results can usually be clarified by obtaining three separate specimens 20 minutes apart and either assaying them individually or pooling them for a single gonadotropin determination. Of the two gonadotropins, luteinizing hormone (LH) tends to be more elevated in men with hypogonadism, and follicle-stimulating hormone (FSH) tends to be more elevated in women with hypogonadism; however, both LH and FSH measurements are usually obtained in screening hypogonadal patients. Details of the radioimmunoassay for gonadotropin are described elsewhere.

The gonadotropin levels must be interpreted in light of the plasma testosterone level in men or the estradiol level in women. For example, a normal LH level in an infertile man is not interpretable by itself. If that patient's testosterone level is low then the "normal" LH level is inappropriate signifying pituitary or hypothalamic disease.

Stimulation Tests
GnRH Injection   Although gonadotropin-releasing hormone (GnRH) is used as a research tool, it is currently not widely available in clinical practice. The GNRH injection was initially conceived to distinguish pituitary from hypothalamic hypogonadism; unfortunately, it usually cannot make this distinction.

Growth Hormone (GH)

Basal Tests
Serum GH Level   GH in serum is measured by radioimmunoassay; the older bioassay (rat tibial epiphysis growth) and the newer radioreceptor assays are limited to research laboratories. Small peaks of GH may be seen during the day, although most GH secretion occurs during deep sleep. In men, basal levels of GH (after an overnight fast) are less than 5 ng/mL, whereas in women they are less than 8 ng/mL. With currently available radioimmunoassays, many normal persons will actually have nondetectable basal GH levels; documentation of GH deficiency generally requires provocative testing. In testing for possible GH hypersecretion, basal GH levels of less than 5 ng/mL reliably rule out that diagnosis, whereas levels over 50 ng/mL are vitually diagnostic of acromegaly. Mild elevations of GH (10–50 ng/mL) can be seen with stress, starvation, anorexia nervosa, chronic renal failure, cirrhosis, poorly controlled diabetes mellitus, and with exercise (in children); suppression tests would be required in the elevation of such patients.

Somatomedin Levels   The somatomedins are a family of proinsulin-like polypeptides which are synthesized in the liver after GH stimulation. They in turn stimulate cell growth and division in many different tissues. Since the serum level of somatomedin is relatively steady throughout the day (due to binding to a carrier protein), it was hoped that a single measurement would be a more reliable guide to GH excess or deficiency than the measurement of fluctuating GH levels. In fact, the radioimmunoassay or radioreceptor assay for one of these somatomedins, somatomedin C, correlates relatively well with GH status. However, several factors have limited the usefulness of this test including (1) the continued need to document GH excess and nonsuppressibility in the workup of acromegaly and (2) the high cost of the test.

Stimulation Tests
Provocative tests of GH secretion have had two major applications: (1) the documentation of GH deficiency in children with short stature and (2) a confirmatory test of pituitary disease in adults with evidence for deficiency of other pituitary hormones or of mass effect. The results in children have routinely been used to select appropriate subjects for GH therapy. In adults, impaired GH reserve is the most frequently observed hormone deficiency in patients with pituitary tumors. However, the value of provocative tests of GH secretion in this setting is lessened by several factors: (1) no test is uniformly effective in provoking GH release in normal subjects; (2) some of the tests are uncomfortable or inconvenient; (3) obesity, thyroid disease, and glucocorticoid therapy all blunt GH responsiveness; and (4) the basal serum prolactin level has emerged as the best marker for pituitary tumors.

Although the provocative stimuli for a GH are quite varied, peak serum GH of at least 8 ng/mL would generally be considered a normal response in the tests described below. TRH-induced GH secretion, a pathological response, is very useful in the evaluation of patients with acromegaly.

Insulin Hypoglycemia—ITT   This ITT uses the same protocol described above for ACTH. GH levels are measured at 30-minute intervals until one hour after hypoglycemic symptoms. Hypoglycemia is the single best stimulus of GH release. The peak GH response may be blunted if glucose is given to reverse excessive symptoms.

L-Dopa Ingestion   Enhanced dopaminergic activity leads to increased GH secretion. L-Dopa is administered by mouth (500 mg in adults, 250 mg if 30–70 lb, [ca 13.6–31.8 kg], 125 mg if less than 30 lb [13.6 kg]) to a fasting subject, and blood samples for GH are obtained at 0, 60, 90, 120, 150, and 180 minutes. Peak GH levels are usually achieved 90–150 minutes after L-Dopa ingestion. The major side effect of the test is nausea and vomiting, which may occur in up to one-fourth of all subjects. Tricyclic antiemetics can blunt the GH response during the test.

Arginine Infusion Test   Hyperaminoacidemia after meals can stimulate GH secretion. This stimulus can be provided by an intravenous infusion of L-arginine hydrochloride (30 or 0.5 g/kg in 30 minutes) with measurement of GH levels at 0, 30, 60, 90, and 120 minutes. This response is greater in women than in men, and pretreatment with estrogens may be necessary to demonstrate growth hormone secretion in some normal men.

Glucagon-Propranolol Test   The changes in blood glucose after glucagon injection provide a weak stimulus for GH secretion which may be enhanced by beta blockade in the central nervous system. One milligram of glucagon is given intramuscularly or subcutaneously in the fasting patient two hours after administration of 40 mg of propranolol (not done in children). GH is measured hourly for four hours, and peak levels are usually obtained at two to three hours after glucagon.

Exercise   In children, vigorous exercise is a fairly reliable stimulus of GH secretion. A single GH measurement after exercise may be a useful screening procedure in children with short stature.

TRH Test   TRH does not stimulate GH release in normal subjects. However, most patients with acromegaly have a significant increase in GH levels 15 to 30 minutes after TRH injection (for protocol, see Thyroid Disease, below). This response can be very useful in (1) confirming a diagnosis of acromegaly and (2) screening for tumor recurrence in patients with normal basal GH levels after surgery and/or radiation therapy. Patients with malnutrition, renal failure, anorexia nervosa, and cirrhosis may demonstrate a GH rise after TRH injection, although the responses are often delayed with peak GH levels at 45 to 60 minutes after TRH.

Suppression Test
OGTT   When the basal serum GH level is elevated but not diagnostic of acromegaly (in the 10–50 ng/mL range), the next step in confirming the diagnosis is to demonstrate lack of suppressibility of GH secretion. Hyperglycemia normally suppresses GH levels to less than 2 ng/mL within two hours; a 75- or 100-g oral glucose tolerance test (OGTT) with measurement of serum glucose and GH levels at 0, 0.5, 1, 2, and 3 hours provides a standard protocol. Patients with acromegaly may demonstrate incomplete suppression, a complete lack of suppression, or even a paradoxical rise in serum GH levels. Similar responses may be seen in starvation, anorexia nervosa, renal failure, cirrhosis, and depression, but these should not pose a clinical problem in the workup of acromegaly.

Prolactin

Basal Tests
Serum Prolactin Level   The development of specific and senstive radioimmunoassays for prolactin led to the observation that up to 80% of pituitary adenomas previously labeled "nonfunctional" actually hypersecreted prolactin.For this reason, *the basal prolactin level has become the single most useful screening test for pituitary dysfunction,* particularly in women with amenorrhea and/or galactorrhea and in patients with evidence of a pituitary mass lesion but without apparent hormonal abnormalities. Basal prolactin levels over 200 ng/mL (normal less than 20 ng/mL) are generally diagnostic of pituitary tumors. Prolactin levels in the range of 100–200 ng/mL correlate well with the presence of pituitary adenomas, provided several other possibilities are excluded: (1) phenothiazine or tricyclic antidepressant drug use, (2) primary hypothyroidism, (3) renal

failure, and (4) normal postpartum lactation. Prolactin levels in the range of 20–100 ng/mL are more difficult to interpret since many factors can cause mild prolactin elevations including (1) "stress", (2) chest wall trauma, (3) sleep, (4) certain drugs (methyldopa, reserpine, cimetidine, opiates, and estrogen), and (5) cirrhosis. In addition, women with amenorrhea and moderately elevated prolactin levels but without radiographically demonstrable pituitary lesions are said to have "functional hypoprolactinemia." Some of these patients eventually develop evidence of pituitary adenomas, whereas others may have an abnormality in hypothalamic control of prolactin secretion.

A basal prolactin measurement should be obtained in patients when a pituitary lesion is suspected. In addition to providing further evidence for the presence of a tumor, an elevated prolactin level can serve as an invaluable marker in the follow-up of these patients. Successful surgery or radiation therapy should normalize the prolactin level; persistent or recurrent prolatin elevation indicates the presence of residual tumor.

Stimulation Tests

Although several provocative tests of prolactin secretion are available, they provide little additional information. Application of these tests is described below.

TRH Injection TRH directly stimulates prolactin secretion from the pituitary gland. The protocol is the same as described below (see Thyroid Disease) with prolactin levels measured at 0, 20, and 60 minutes after intravenous injection of 500 μg of TRH. The prolactin level should rise at least threefold over the basal level and should exceed 20 ng/mL at 20 minutes; the rise is greater in women than in men. It has been stated that patients with hyperprolactinemia due to pituitary adenomas have a blunted or absent rise in prolactin after TRH, whereas patients with "functional hypoprolactinemia" demonstrates a normal response. Unfortunately, there are many exceptions to this observation. One situation in which the TRH test may be useful is in the evaluation of patients who cannot be withdrawn from psychotropic medication (phenothiazines, tricyclic antidepressants) for pituitary testing. In the absence of pituitary disease, these patients have mild to moderate basal hyperprolactinemia and have an exaggerated prolactin rise in response to TRH.

Chlorpromazine Ingestion Phenothiazines, as dopaminergic antagonists, cause a rise in prolactin levels. Chlorpromazine in a dose of 25 mg is given orally, and prolactin is measured at 0, 60, and 90 minutes. Prolactin rises two- to threefold in men and two- to fivefold in women. This test provides little useful information, however, and the drug may cause hypotension and dizziness.

Insulin Hypoglycemia—ITT The same test used to measure ACTH and GH reserve can be used to stimulate prolactin secretion, providing a relatively severe degree of hypoglycemia is achieved. It is not a discriminatory test since prolactin levels do not rise in many normal persons during the ITT.

Suppression Test
Dopaminergenic Agonist The only reproducible way of suppressing prolactin secretion is via the dopaminergic agonist L-Dopa (see protocol under GH testing, above) or bromocriptine (2.5 mg by mouth). These tests do not discriminate between tumor and "functional" elevation. The test with bromocriptine may, however, be useful in predicting the subsequent response to long-term therapy with this drug.

ADH

ADH is synthesized in hypothalamic nuclei, transported down nerve axons, and stored in the posterior pituitary. Since nerve terminals high on the pituitary stalk are capable of releasing ADH, it is uncommon for pituitary lesions to affect ADH unless (1) they have significant suprasellar extension or (2) they arise principally in a suprasellar location, eg, craniopharyngioma. There is one other important way in which ADH secretion is affected by anterior pituitary disease. Cortisol appears to have an inhibitory effect on ADH release; patients with ACTH deficiency and therefore cortisol deficiency may have excessive ADH secretion. Clinically and biochemically, the picture is that of the syndrome of inappropriate antidiuretic hormone secretion (SIADH) with hyponatremia, low serum osmolarity, high urine osmolarity, and inability to excrete a free water load. Unlike other causes of SIADH, however, the abnormality in this setting is reversible with cortisol replacement therapy.

Basal Tests
Serum and Urine Osmolarity Serum osmolarity is normally maintained within narrow limits. In a patient with a pituitary tumor, polyuria and a high normal or elevated serum osmolarity strongly suggests a diagnosis of diabetes insipidus; a low or low normal serum osmolarity might be due to SIADH. Serum osmolarity can either be measured directly via a freezing point depression or can be calculated according to the following formula:

$$\text{Serum osmolarity} = 2 \times \text{Na} + \frac{\text{plasma glucose}}{18} + \frac{\text{blood urea nitrogen}}{2.8}$$

Urine osmolarity varies tremendously depending upon the state of hydration and can range between 50 and 1500/kg, measured by freezing point depression. The osmolarity of the first voided morning specimen generally exceeds 600. Values less than this in a patient being evaluated for possible pituitary disease should lead to more detailed testing for possible diabetes insipidus.

Serum ADH Levels Until recently, ADH was measured by a cumbersome bioassay; sensitive and specific radioimmunoassays are now performed in a few research laboratories. Several reports have suggested that the routine indirect test of ADH secretion (see below) may lead to incorrect diagnoses in borderline cases. Greater availability may make these radioimmunoassays for ADH more useful clinically.

Stimulation Test

Dehydration Test (Miller-Moses Test)   Total fluid and food deprivation is begun at 6 AM in patients with polyuria or at 8 PM the preceding night in asymptomatic patients. The subject is weighted, the baseline specimens are obtained for serum and urine osmolarity measurements. Beginning at 6 AM, urine osmolarities are determined at hourly intervals. A plateau of urine osmolarity is reached when two consecutive samples do not differ by more than 30 mOsm. If the patient loses more than 3% of his initial body weight before a plateau is reached, the collection period should be terminated to avoid excessive dehydration. The next step involves the injection of 5 U of exogenous ADH subcutaneously or intramuscularly (10 U if cortisol secretion is also being tested—see above) or the intranasal application of 0.1 mL of DDAVP. One hour later, a final urine and serum osmolarity is determined.

Criteria for a normal response are (1) a plateau of urine osmolarity greater than 500 mOsm/kg, (2) serum osmolarity consistently below 300 mOsm/kg, and (3) an increase in urine osmolarity of less than 5% after ADH injection. The last requirement is critically dependent upon having achieved a plateau in urine osmolarity. In the normal person, endogenous ADH will then be maximal, and little or no change in urine concentration will occur with exogenous ADH. Urine osmolarity in patients with diabetes insipidus will plateau at a subnormal level. The response to exogenous ADH will then separate these subjects into two groups: (1) central diabetes insipidus (ADH deficiency), with a significant increase in urine osmolarity after ADH, and (2) nephrogenic diabetes insipidus, in which the kidney will not respond to the ADH injection.

Suppression Test

Water Loading Test   The water loading test is occasionally useful in documenting the existence of SIADH and distinguishing it from other causes of hyponatremia. The test is performed by having the subject consume 20 mL of tap water per kg of body weight over a 30-minute period. A normal person will excrete over 80% of the water load over the subsequent four to five hours. In a patient with pituitary disease, hyponatremia suggests either hypocortisolism or hypothyroidism. It is usually safer to approach these possibilities directly than to perform a water load test which could precipitate symptomatic or even fatal hyponatremia.

■ Practical Use of Laboratory Tests in the Diagnosis of Pituitary Disease

A practical approach to ordering pituitary function tests is to separate the clinically useful and available protocols described above into (1) screening and (2) confirmatory tests (Table 17-2). Screening tests can be used individually or together under various clinical circumstances: (1) screening all newly diagnosed hypothyroid patients with low thyroxine levels for possible pituitary disease (serum TSH), (2) screening all newly diagnosed hypogonadal patients (low testosterone or estradiol) for possible pituitary disease (serum LH and FSH), (3) testing all aspects of pituitary function in a patient with multiple suggestive complaints or with an abnormal sella on

Table 17-2
Endocrine Testing for Pituitary
Hormone Deficiency or Excess

	Screening Tests	Confirmatory Tests
Hormone Deficiency		
ACTH	Cosyntropin stimulation test	ITT Metyrapone
TSH	TT_4 T_3RU } FT_4I TSH	(TRH test)*
FSH/LH	Testosterone (men) Estradiol (women) LH/FSH	(GnRH test)*
Growth hormone	Exercise-induced rise (children)	ITT L-Dopa L-Arginine
ADH	AM urine osm	Dehydration
Hormone Excess		
Prolactin	Basal PRL	(TRH)*
Growth hormone	Fasting GH	OGTT TRH (Somatomedin level)*
ACTH	24-hour UFC Overnight DST	DST ACTH levels (ITT)* (Metyrapone)*

*Only occasionally useful.

x-ray, or (4) reevaluating pituitary function regularly in patients with known pituitary disease. These endocrine screening tests should be supplemented with an evaluation for pituitary mass effect (visual field examination and coned-down x-ray view of the sella).

Any abnormality found on a screening test should be pursued with the more detailed confirmatory tests. Some of these require hospitalization for accurate and safe collection of specimens. Additional radiologic procedures such as sella tomography or, preferably, computed axial tomography of the sella may be appropriate in this setting.

Thyroid Disease

In the last decade there has been a rapid proliferation of laboratory tests designed to help evaluate thyroid function. The wide variety of commercially available methods has led to confusion. Much effort has been directed toward obtaining a simple and accurate measurement of serum free thyroxine. Before discussing the individual tests, it is necessary to review the concept of "free thyroxine" and its application to clinical practice.

Most of the thyroxine (T_4) and triiodothyronine (T_3) circulating in serum is bound to large proteins and, therefore, does not have direct access to the intracellular space. These hormones are in equilibrium with tiny amounts of free (unbound) T_4 (FT_4) and T_3 (FT_3) that can enter cells, bind to nuclear receptor sites, and set in motion multiple biochemical reactions. The homeostatic feedback loops in the hypothalamus and pituitary gland are concerned with the maintenance of a normal level of FT_4 and FT_3. In theory, therefore, assessment of a patient's thyroid status would be most accurately determined by measurement of free hormone levels. In practice, however, such determinations are difficult, and there may be poor correlation between values obtained with different methods. Clinicians must, therefore, rely upon measurement of total (bound plus free) thyroid hormones plus some indirect assessment of the binding capacity of the serum thyroid binding proteins.

If the concentration and affinity of the thyroid binding proteins in serum were constant, the total T_4 (TT_4) and total T_3 (TT_3) levels would be directly proportional to the free hormone concentrations. However, there are many factors which can alter either the absolute level of these proteins or their affinity for thyroid hormone (Table 17-3). These factors will alter the free hormone concentration unless there is a compensatory change in the levels of TT_4 and TT_3. For example, if the level of T_4 binding globulin were to double without a change in the TT_4, then proportionately more T_4 would become bound, lowering the FT_4 to one-half its original concentration. To compensate for this change, additional T_4 must be produced to fill some of the new binding sites and to raise the FT_4 back to its original level; this adjustment is brought about via a transient change in thyroid stimulating hormone (TSH) secretion by the pituitary gland. The end result of these changes is an elevated level of bound T_4 (biologically inactive), but a normal level of FT_4 (biologically active), ie, the patient is euthyroid. Measurement of only the TT_4 in this setting, however, will lead to the incorrect diagnosis of thyroid disease.

The procedure most commonly used to assess the thyroid hormone binding affinity and capacity is the T_3 resin uptake test (T_3RU). This is *not* a measure of serum TT_3; the reason that the word "T_3" is part of the name of the test is that radioactive T_3 is used as the tracer hormone (for technical

Table 17-3
Factors Affecting Serum Thyroid Hormone Binding Capacity and T_3 RU Test Results

Increased Binding Capacity (Decreased T_3RU Test Results)	Decreased Binding Capacity (Increased T_3RU Test Results)
Estrogen	Nonthyroidal illness or stress
Pregnancy	Chronic liver disease
Acute hepatitis	Androgen
Perphenazine	Hypoproteinemia
Acute intermittent porphyria	Glucocorticoid excess
Genetic TBG excess	Heparin
	Acromegaly
	Genetic TBG deficiency

reasons, it is preferable to radioactive T_4). The procedure measures the relative distribution of the radioactive hormone between the patient's binding proteins and the added binding resin. The greater the affinity and capacity of the patient's binding protein, the less uptake by the resin; the lower the binding affinity and capacity, the greater the uptake by the resin.

When the TT_4 or TT_3 level is multiplied by the T_3RU, a number is obtained which is proportional to the free hormone concentration; this is the FT_4 index (FT_4I) or the FT_3 index (FT_3I), respectively. Table 17-4 illustrates the way in which the T_3RU test can permit the proper interpretation of TT_4 levels even in the presence of alterations in binding proteins. This correction factor is not fail-safe, however. The greater the alteration in binding proteins, the less likely the FT_4I will fall within the normal range. However, a rough rule of thumb is that when abnormalities in the TT_4 and the T_3RU are concordant (both up or both down), thyroid disease is likely; if they are discordant (one high, one low), the abnormality is probably due to an alteration in binding proteins. When only one test (TT_4 *or* T_3RU is abnormal, one may be dealing with (1) mild thyroid disease, (2) a combination of thyroid disease plus a binding protein abnormality (Table 17-4), or (3) stress-induced changes in thyroid function tests (see below).

■ Specific Laboratory Tests in the Evaluation of Thyroid Function and Thyroid Disease

TT_4

The methodology for measuring TT_4 has evolved over many years to the point where it is now a highly specific, routine test done in most clinical laboratories. Protein-bound iodine and butanol-extractable iodine assays were plagued by interference by inorganic and organic iodides. T_4 measure-

Table 17-4
TT_4, T_3RU, and Calculation of FT_4I in Normal and Pathological States*

	TT_4	×	T_3RU	=	FT_4I
A. Subjects with normal binding proteins who are:					
1. Euthyroid	N	×	N	=	N
2. Hyperthyroid	↑	×	↑	=	↑
3. Hypothyroid	↓	×	↓	=	↓
B. Subjects with increased binding proteins who are:					
1. Euthyroid	↑	×	↓	=	N
2. Hyperthyroid	↑↑	×	N	=	↑
3. Hypothyroid	N	×	↓↓	=	↓
C. Subjects with decreased binding protein who are:					
1. Euthyroid	↓	×	↑	=	N
2. Hyperthyroid	N	×	↑↑	=	↑
3. Hypothyroid	↓↓	×	N	=	↓

*N, Normal; ↑, increased; ↓, decreased.

ments by column chromatography removed the problem of inorganic iodide, but were still affected by organified iodine. The competitive protein binding (CPB) assay (Murphy-Patee) eliminated almost all of the problems associated with the measurement of TT_4. It, of course, is still subjected to the actual change in TT_4 caused by changes in thyroid binding proteins (Table 17-3). However, technical factors make the method less than ideal in terms of the serum volumes required and the expense. Therefore, with the current availability of antibodies with high affinity and specificity for T_4, most laboratories are using some variation of a radioimmunoassay (RIA) as the preferred method for TT_4 determination. In both the CPB and the RIA methods, the patient's TT_4 is chemically stripped from the binding proteins. Thus, all of the T_4 is free in solution and can compete with the radioactive tracer T_4 for binding to exogenous thyroxine binding protein (CPB assay) or to the antibody (RIA).

The normal range for TT_4 varies significantly with age (Table 17-5). This is of particular importance in the interpretation of thyroid function tests in infants and children. The normal range of TT_4 levels in the elderly is the same as in younger adults, although the serum T_3 level may decline due to decreased peripheral conversion of T_4 to T_3.

Thyroid Hormone Binding Proteins
(T_3RU Test and TBG Assay)

Thyroid binding proteins can be assessed by measurement of their affinity and capacity (T_3RU) or by direct quantitation of their serum level (thyroxine binding globulin [TBG] RIA). The details of the T_3RU test were discussed above. Two points should be reemphasized. First, this test has nothing to do with measurement of serum T_3 levels. Second, this test or some variant of it is critical for the proper interpretation of the TT_4 level since alterations in T_4 binding proteins are common (Table 17-3).

Recently, a RIA for TBG has become available commercially. This assay measures the absolute level of TBG in serum, but does not reflect the binding affinity. There is no method for calculating a FT_4 index from this number. In addition, other proteins, namely, T_4 binding prealbumin and albumin, contribute to the total thyroid hormone binding capacity. The TBG RIA is occasionally useful in the evaluation of a persistent, unexplained abnormality of the T_3RU or for confirming a diagnosis of congenital absence or excess of TBG.

Table 17-5
Changes in T_4 Levels With Age

	Normal Range (μg/dL)
Cord Blood	7–15
1–3 Days	10–21
1–3 Weeks	10–17
1–3 Months	7–15
1–6 Years	6–13
Adult	5–11

FT₄I and FT₄ Measurements

The level of free T_4 in serum can either be estimated from the TT_4 and T_3RU measurements (ie, the FT_4I) or can be measured more directly by equilibrium dialysis or RIA. The theory behind the FTI was discussed above. The actual calculation of the FT_4I can be done in two different ways:

$$\text{``}T_{12}\text{''} = TT_4 \times T_3RU$$

$$\text{``}T_7\text{''} = TT_4 \times \frac{T_3RU}{\text{Mean laboratory } T_3RU}$$

The major difference is that the normal range for the "T_7" will approximate that of the TT_4, whereas the "T_{12}" will have its own normal range. Both calculations allow the proper interpretation of thyroid functions tests in the face of changes in T_4 binding proteins.

The FT_4 level can be measured by placing serum and radioactive T_4 in a dialysis sac and determining the ratio of radioactivity in the dialysate versus the serum at equilibrium. This "free fraction of T_4" is then multiplied by the TT_4 to give the "FT_4 by dialysis." Recently, the RIA for TT_4 has been modified in an attempt to directly measure the FT_4 level. Instead of stripping the T_4 off of TBG, as in the TT_4 assay, untreated serum is used so that only the free fraction of T_4 can bind to the antibody. After separation of antibody and serum, the antibody-bound T_4 can be quantitated by using radioactive T_4 tracer.

All three methods—FT_4I, FT_4 by dialysis, and the FT_4 by RIA—give reliable data in normal persons and in hyperthyroid and hypothyroid patients; the widest experience is with the FT_4I. In the setting of acute or chronic illness, however, there may be changes in thyroid hormone binding proteins with concomitant alterations in the FT_4 level. Unfortunately, there has been poor correlation in the FT_4 values obtained when sera from such patients has been assayed by all three techniques. The differences are due, no doubt, to technical factors, but the "true FT_4" during stress is unclear. The interpretation of these stress-related changes in thyroid function tests is discussed below.

T₃ RIA

T_3 is the most potent of the thyroid hormones, but its low concentration in serum (90–180 ng/mL) made measurement difficult until specific RIAs were developed. Most laboratories simply report the TT_3 level. However, T_3 is highly protein bound (99.7%) and is in equilibrium with a tiny amount of free hormone (FT_3), which is the active fraction. It is important to note that the TT_3 and the FT_3 can be affected in the same way as the TT_4 and FT_4 by alterations in thyroid binding proteins (Table 17-3). For example, a rise in binding protein concentration due to estrogen therapy will cause a proportionate rise in both TT_4 and TT_3, although the free hormone concentrations will not be affected; assay of only the total hormone concentration will lead to a misdiagnosis of hyperthyroidism. Calculation of FT_3I or measurement of FT_3 by dialysis are both possible, although they have been less widely used than the FT_4I calculation.

A knowledge of the physiology of T_3 production is necessary for understanding of the alterations of T_3 levels in pathological states. Normally, only about 20% of circulating T_3 comes from direct thyroidal secretion of the hormone; the remainder is derived from circulating T_4 by removal of the 5' iodine atom. In both hypothyroidism and hyperthyroidism, the ratio of T_3 to T_4 in thyroid secretions increases, and there is also an increase in the peripheral conversion of T_4 to T_3. In nonthyroidal illness or stress, peripheral conversion of T_4 to T_3 is decreased. These observations lead to the following conclusions regarding the clinical use of T_4 measurements. First, the T_3 assay is not useful in the diagnosis of hypothyroidism since the absolute T_3 level is in the low-normal range in many patients with hypothyroidism. Second, T_3 levels are usually elevated in hyperthyroidism and, in fact, may be proportionately more elevated than T_4. Therefore, in patients with borderline high T_4 levels, a significant elevation of T_3 levels (taking into account changes in binding proteins) would strongly suggest a diagnosis of hyperthyroidism. In rare patients with hyperthyroid symptoms but normal T_4 levels, hyperthyroidism may be due solely to increased T_3 concentration. Third, in euthyroid patients with mild to moderate nonthyroidal illness, the FT_4I may be elevated, suggesting hyperthyroidism; T_3 levels, however, are low in this setting. Unfortunately, this does not completely rule out the diagnosis of hyperthyroidism since T_3 concentrations may drop from elevated to subnormal levels in hyperthyroid patients with superimposed nonthyroidal illness. A thyrotropin-releasing hormone (TRH) test could be useful in this differential diagnosis (see below). In severe nonthyroidal illness in euthyroid patients the FT_4I may decrease, suggesting a diagnosis of hypothyroidism. The T_3 level will also be low and the diagnosis may depend upon the results of a TRH test. Several drugs and radiologically useful compounds inhibit the peripheral conversion of T_4 to T_3. These include propylthiouracil, propranolol, glucocorticoids (high dose), the gallbladder "dyes," iopanoic acid (Telepaque) and sodium ipodate (Orogratin), and amiodarone.

TSH Level

TSH is a large glycoprotein hormone secreted by the pituitary gland; its production and secretion are regulated by the level of both FT_4 and FT_3, and the set point of this feedback inhibition is probably determined by TRH coming from the hypothalamus. There is some diurnal variation in serum levels of TSH, but this is not of sufficient magnitude to interefere with the diagnostic value of random samples. TSH is measured by specific RIAs which have little or no cross-reactivity with other glycoprotein hormones.

Serum TSH measurements are most important in the differential diagnosis of primary versus secondary hypothyroidism. In a patient with low FT_4I, an elevated basal TSH level confirms the diagnosis of thyroid disease. A low FT_4I with a "normal" TSH level would suggest the possibility of a pituitary or hypothalamic lesion and should lead to further testing (see Pituitary Disease, above). These test results can also be seen in patients with severe nonthyroidal illness or stress (see below). Since the evaluation and treatment of patients with primary hypothyroidism is different from those with other causes of hypothyroidism, a basal TSH measurement should be obtained in

298

all patients with a low FT$_4$I. The occasional patient with a low normal FT$_4$I and an increased TSH level has mild primary hypothyroidism.

Patients with hyperthyroidism have suppressed basal TSH levels. However, most TSH RIAs are designed to be most sensitive in the high-normal range and will not reliably distinguish low-normal from low TSH levels; many normal persons will have "nondetectable" TSH levels in commercial assays. Therefore, a low basal TSH level is not diagnostic of hyperthyroidism. A provocative test such as the TRH test would be required in this setting and can be useful in the diagnosis of borderline hyperthyroidism. Rarely, patients with TSH-producing pituitary lesions will have elevated TSH levels in the face of hyperthyroidism; such patients may also have elevations of the alpha subunit of TSH circulating in serum.

TRH Test (See Pituitary Section)
Antithyroid Antibody Levels (See Chapter 11)
Thyroglobulin Levels

Thyroglobulin is normally stored within thyroid follicles, but it can be detected by RIA in low concentrations (5–25 ng/mL) in the serum of normal persons. Levels may be elevated in a variety of conditions—hyperthyroidism multinodular goiter, and benign and malignant thyroid neoplasms—and thus are nonspecific. However, if preoperative thyroglobulin levels are elevated in a patient with a thyroid malignancy, sequential determinations may be useful in detecting recurrent disease, particularly if specimens are obtained during the period of thyroid hormone withdrawal before radioiodine scanning for metastases. The presence of antithyroglobulin antibodies in serum interferes with the assay for thyroglobulin.

CT Levels

Calcitonin (CT) is a polypeptide hormone secreted by the parafollicular C-cells within the thyroid gland. Its measurement, by RIA, is clinically useful as a marker for the tumor derived from these cells—medullary carcinoma of the thyroid (MCT). The tumors are occasionally familial, and CT levels are extremely useful in screening members of such families (see Multiple Endocrine Neoplasia Syndromes, below). In the routine evaluation of thyroid modules, measurement of CT is a low-yield procedure since MCT is relatively uncommon. If MCT is found at surgery, however, serial CT determinations are invaluable in long term follow-up of such patients.

rT$_3$ Levels

Reverse T$_3$ (rT$_3$) is an inactive thyroid hormone which is principally derived from circulating T$_4$ by removal of an iodine atom from the 5 position on the inner ring of the molecule. It is of physiological interest since it demonstrates the existence of two major routes of metabolism of T$_4$ one producing highly active T$_3$, and the other yielding inactive rT$_3$. In nonthyroidal illness, T$_3$ levels are low due to the inhibition of the 5′ deiodinase enzyme; rT$_3$ levels are increased, mainly due to decreased catabolism which depends upon the same 5′ deiodinase enzyme. An assay for rT$_3$ could help distinguish true hypothyroidism (low T$_3$, low rT$_3$) from nonthyroidal illness (low T$_3$, high rT$_3$). However, assays for rT$_3$ are not now widely available.

TSI

Thyroid-stimulating immunoglobulins (TSI) constitute a heterogeneous group of proteins of the immunoglobulin (IgG) class which play a major role in the pathogenesis of Graves' hyperthroidism. They can interact with the TSH receptor on thyroid cells, leading to the inappropriate stimulation of thyroid hormone secretion. There are several different assays for TSI based upon either binding properties or the stimulation of adenyl cyclase in thyroid slices. The methods are relatively complex, with variable sensitivity, and are generally reserved for research purposes. However, some investigators have claimed that serial measurement of TSI titers can result in early detection of a remission of Graves' disease and permit prompt discontinuation of antithyroid drug therapy. Further study is required before this test can become part of routine clinical management.

■ Nuclear Medicine and Echographic Techniques

Although not generally considered "clinical laboratory tests", these procedures will be discussed briefly since they form an integral part of the evaluation of thyroid disease.

Technetium Scans

Technetium pertechnetate ($^{99m}TcO_4^-$) is a radioactive anion which is handled like iodide (I^-) by the iodide pump in thyroid cells. There is rapid uptake and concentration of the radionuclide allowing visualization of functioning tissue within 10 to 20 minutes. $^{99m}TcO_4^-$ is not organified, however, so that it rapidly leaks out of the thyroid cells, resulting in minimal radiation exposure. The advantage of the technetium scan is that it is rapid and inexpensive and can be done even in a poorly functioning gland by using a large dose of radionuclide. The major disadvantage is the difficulty in performing a quantitative uptake measurement. In addition, occasional well-differentiated thyroid neoplasms have normal iodide pumping activity ("warm" on technetium scans), but have lost the ability to organify iodine ("cold" on ^{123}I scans). Interpretation of scan results is shown in Table 17-6.

^{123}I Uptake and Scan

^{123}I has generally replaced ^{131}I in thyroid imaging since the ^{123}I isotope exposes the gland to much less radiation. Radioactive iodine uptake (RAIU) involves both the iodide pump and the enzymatic organification of iodine; the radioactive RAIU test is thus a quantitative assessment of the functional activity of the gland. This test has been recommended as a routine part of the evaluation of hyperthyroidism, particularly in young patients, since some investigators have reported a high incidence of thyroiditis with transient hyperthyroidism (with 0% RAIU) in this group. However, basically the same information can also be obtained with a rapid $^{99m}TcO_4^-$ scan (demonstrating poor radionuclide uptake). The most common use of the ^{123}I uptake is in the calculation of the proper dose of ^{131}I to use in treating Graves' hyperthyroidism. The major problems with the use of ^{123}I are that (1) inorganic

Table 17-6
Practical Use of Laboratory Tests in the Diagnosis of Thyroid Disease

	TT_4	T_3RU	FT_4I	FT_4 dial	TT_3	rT_3	TSH	TSH response to TRH	Anti-TG Ab	Thyroid scan	RAIU
Hyperthyroidism Graves'	(↑)*	(↑)	(↑)	↑	(↑)	↑	ND	(ND)	−,↑	(Uniform uptake)	(↑)
Nodular goiter	↑	↑	(↑)	↑	(↑)	↑	ND	(ND)	−,↑	(Patchy)	↑,N
Primary hypothyroidism	↓	(↓)	(↓)	↓	↓,N	↓	(↑)	↑	−,↑	Decreased uptake Poor scan	↓,N
Subacute thyroiditis	↑	↑	(↑)	↑	↑	↑	ND	ND	−,↑	(Poor to absent image)	(↓↓)
Lymphocytic thyroiditis	(N,↓)	(N,↓)	(N,↓)	N,↓	N,↓	N,↓	(N,↑)	N,↑	(↑↑)	Patchy	N,↓,↑
Neoplasm (nodule)	N	N	(N)	N	N	N	N	N	−,↑	("Cold" area)	N
Nonthyroidal illness (stress) Mild-moderate	(N,↑)	(↑)	(↑)	↑	(↓)	↑	N	(N)	−	Normal	N
Severe	(↓)	(↑)	(↓)	N,↑,↓	↓	↑	N	(N,↓)	−	Normal	N

* ○, Clinically useful test (see text); ND, not detectable.

iodide will compete with the isotope for uptake so the RAIU cannot be performed in patients who have recently been exposed to iodinated contrast dyes, (2) the RAIU test takes 24 hours to complete, and (3) ^{123}I is expensive.

The ^{123}I scan is interpreted in the same way as the ^{99m}TcO$_4^-$ scan (Table 17-6). It has the same disadvantages as the ^{123}I uptake test.

Echography of the Thyroid

Use of ultrasound in visualizing the thyroid gland (B-mode scan) is helpful in distinguishing solid from cystic thyroid nodules. A purely cystic lesion is likely to be benign and may be treated by needle aspiration followed by cytological study of the fluid. A solid or mixed cystic and solid lesion suggests a neoplastic (benign or malignant) process.

■ Practical Use of Laboratory Tests in the Diagnosis of Thyroid Disease (Table 17-6)

Hypothyroidism

When a diagnosis of hypothyroidism is considered, the first laboratory tests to obtain are a TT$_4$ level and a T$_3$RU test from which can be calculated the FT$_4$I. A TT$_4$ alone is not sufficient due to the relative frequency of abnormalities of thyroid binding proteins. If the FT$_4$I is low, the diagnosis of hypothyroidism should always be confirmed by repeating the TT$_4$ and T$_3$RU tests and by obtaining a basal serum TSH level. This is necessary since a diagnosis of hypothyroidism generally commits the patient to lifelong thyroid hormone therapy. In addition, transient decreases in the FT$_4$I may be seen in patients with nonthyroidal illness and stress (see below). The TSH level, if elevated confirms the diagnosis of primary hypothyroidism, whereas a normal or low TSH level suggests pituitary or hypothalamic disease leading to more extensive testing (see Pituitary Disease, above). Measurement of T$_3$ by RIA and radionuclide studies are generally not necessary and may be misleading. Measuring antithyroid antibodies may help to define the etiology of the hypothyroidism, but will usually not alter subsequent therapy.

Hyperthyroidism

The usual screening laboratory tests are the TT$_4$ level and the T$_3$RU test, from which are calculated the FT$_4$I. Patients with moderate to severe hyperthyroid symptoms generally have TT$_4$ and FT$_4$I values at least 1.5 to 2 times the upper limit of normal for these tests. In the presence of exophthalmos, extraocular muscle palsy, or pretibial myxedema, the diagnosis of Graves' hyperthyroidism would be secure and no further diagnostic tests would be necessary. In the absence of those specific findings, a ^{99m}TcO$_4^-$ scan or a ^{123}I uptake and scan might be done to clearly distinguish Graves' hyperthyroidism, toxic nodular goiter, and thyroiditis with hyperthyroidism.

If the TT$_4$ and the FT$_4$I were only slightly elevated or in the high-normal range, two additional tests—the TT$_3$ by RIA and the TRH test—could provide additional diagnostic information (see above). Rare hyperthyroid patients have mid- or even low-normal TT_4 levels; clinical suspicion would lead to the measurement of T_3 by RIA resulting in the diagnosis of "T_3 toxicosis." Transient elevations of thyroid function tests in stressed patients are discussed below.

Subacute and Lymphocytic Thyroiditis

Routine thyroid function tests (TT_4, T_3RU, FT_4I) are usually mildly to moderately elevated during the early weeks of subacute thyroiditis; they may fall to hypothyroid levels before returning to normal. The erythrocyte sedimentation rate is usually elevated. Confirmation of the diagnosis requires a RAIU test or a $^{99m}TcO_4^-$ scan showing a near total absence of thyroid uptake.

Lymphocytic thyroiditis can be associated with low, normal, or high thyroid function tests. Radionuclide studies are equally variable. Laboratory confirmation of the diagnosis, short of thyroid biopsy, relies upon the demonstration of antithyroid antibodies in the serum.

Thyroid Nodules

In patients with solitary thyroid nodules, the major question is whether the neoplastic process is benign or malignant; routine thyroid function tests are usually normal. The role of serum calcitonin measurements was discussed above.

Nonthyroidal Illness and Stress

Major changes in thyroid function tests can occur in euthyroid patients undergoing a variety of medical, surgical, or psychiatric stresses. The type and magnitude of the alterations vary with the severity of the stress and the techniques used to measure the thyroid hormone levels. The changes, however, are transient and resolve rapidly (days to weeks) if the stress is removed.

Mild or moderate stress may cause an increase in the T_3RU test (decreased affinity of the binding proteins) with a normal or even a slight increase of the TT_4 level. The calculated FT_4I is therefore increased, suggesting the diagnosis of hyperthyroidism. However, the TT_3 by RIA is low, due to decreased peripheral conversion of T_4 to T_3, and the TRH test is normal in these patients. Moreover, if the stress is transient, the thyroid function tests rapidly revert to normal.

Severe stress, as seen in intensive care unit patients, may cause a major decrease in the TT_4. Despite an elevated T_3RU value, the FT_4I is often in the hypothyroid range. These patients also have a low TT_3 level by RIA. Basal TSH levels and TRH tests are usually normal, however, helping to rule out thyroid disease.

Parathyroid Disease and Calcium Metabolism

The successful evaluation and management of patients with abnormal serum calcium, phosphate, and magnesium values and with metabolic bone or kidney stone disease requires the appropriate selection and understanding of several laboratory tests.

Serum Calcium

Although the ionized serum calcium fraction is the biologically significant fraction of serum calcium, the determination of total serum calcium is generally adequate for clinical calcium disorders. Total serum calcium consists of the ionized fraction (50%), the fraction bound to protein (40% [90% to albumin and 10% to globulin]), and the fraction associated with citrate and phosphate (10%). Total serum calcium is regularly determined by the autoanalyzer technique, generally accurate but inferior to measurement by atomic absorption spectrophotometry. Total serum calcium values are misleading when compared to ionized serum calcium values in disease states in which the nonionized fractions of serum calcium are elevated. This occurs with changes in the concentration of serum albumin and serum globulin; total serum calcium rises with hyperalbuminemia and hyperglobulinemia and falls with hypoalbuminemia and hypoglobulinemia. Total serum calcium may be corrected for these changes in binding proteins by the following formulas: (1) For each 1-g increase in serum albumin, total serum calcium rises by 0.8 mg/dL; (2) total serum calcium mg/dL − albumin (g/dL) + 4 = corrected total serum calcium; and (3) for globulin, for each 1-g increase in serum globulin, total serum calcium rises by 0.16 mg/dL. Additionally, prolonged application of a tourniquet for venipuncture may, due to hemoconcentration, increase total serum calcium by as much as 10%. Serum ionized calcium may also be determined, but should be assayed only when the results of total serum calcium determinations are inconsistent with other laboratory values or with the clinical situation. Acute acidosis will increase the serum ionized calcium value by the following formula: for each 0.1 pH unit decrement, serum ionized calcium rises by 0.17 mg/dL. Acute alkalosis will have the opposite effect. Chronic acid-base disturbances do not alter the serum ionized calcium value. Measurement of ultrafilterable calcium (ionized calcium plus the calcium associated with citrate and phosphate) is, in general, an accurate reflection of the ionized serum calcium level and eliminates the diagnostic confusion caused by abnormalities in serum albumin and globulin levels. Serum calcium must be collected in the fasting state, as food may variably increase or decrease this value.

Urine Calcium

Urine for 24-hour calcium measurement must be collected in acid. Hypercalciuria is present when, on an ad libitum (normal) diet, calciuria exceeds 4 mg/kg in men and women or 250 mg in women and 300 mg in men in 24 hours. Calciuria will be increased by high sodium or protein intake and is affected by calcium intake. However, in normal persons each additional 100 mg of oral calcium intake increases calciuria by only 5–10 mg/24 hours. Diuretics, particularly thiazides, have a significant hypocalciuric effect and ideally should be discontinued for one to two weeks before calcium metabolism is evaluated. The fasting fractional excretion of calcium (FECa) is determined by obtaining, after an overnight fast, a simultaneous serum creatinine and a second-voided urine specimen in acid for calcium and creatinine. The FECa = (urine calcium/urine creatinine) × (serum creatinine) and is normally 0.03–0.16 mg of calcium per 100 mL of glomerular filtrate. This test should be performed after several days of a low-calcium diet. When abnormally high, the result indicates either increased bone resorption causing hypercalciuria or primary reduction in calcium reabsorption by the kidney.

Serum Phosphorus

Ninety percent of serum phosphorus is free, and 10% is protein-bound. Since serum phosphorus values are significantly higher in children than in adults, results must be interpreted according to age. Serum phosphorus may be significantly increased by food ingestion and should be measured in the fasting state. If whole blood samples remain unprocessed for prolonged periods of time, artifactual hypophosphatemia results from cellular uptake of serum phosphorus.

Urine Phosphorus

Urine phosphorus must be evaluated in terms of the tubular maximum for phosphate reabsorption (TmP/GFR), since simple 24-hour or spot urine measurements of phosphorus are largely indexes of dietary intake and give little diagnostic insight. Simultaneous serum and second-voided urine are obtained after an overnight fast, and phosphorus and creatinine are measured. The nomogram shown in Figure 17-1 is then employed to calculate the ratio of the renal clearances of phosphate and creatinine (serum creatinine × urine phosphorus)/(serum phosphorus × urine creatinine) and drawing a line between this value and the serum phosphorus value. This line is extended rightward to intersect with the vertical bar indicating the value for the TmP/GFR. Normal adult values are 2.5–4.2 mg/dL, except in post menopausal women not taking estrogen for whom the normal range is 2.8–4.5 mg/dL. (The TmP/GFR for children under the age of 15 is significantly higher.) The TmP/GFR is distinctly superior to the determination of the tubular reabsorption for phosphorus (TRP) value. As creatinine clearance falls below 30–40 mL/min, the calculation of TmP/GFR becomes invalid.

Serum Alkaline Phosphatase

Serum alkaline phosphatase has several sources, but the most important in normal adults are bone (60%) and liver (20%). Serum "bone" alkaline phosphatase, which reflects bone turnover, is distinguished from serum "liver" alkaline phosphatase by electrophoretic pattern, by heat lability, and by the fact that an elevation of this fraction is not paralleled by increases in the serum 5'-nucleotidase or gammaglutamyltranspeptidase enzymes which accompany increases in serum "liver" alkaline phosphatase. Serum alkaline phosphatase is two- to threefold higher in children than in adults. All references to serum alkaline phosphatase in this section are to the fraction originating from bone.

Magnesium

Magnesium determinations in serum and urine are uncomplicated processes important in the evaluation of hypocalcemia.

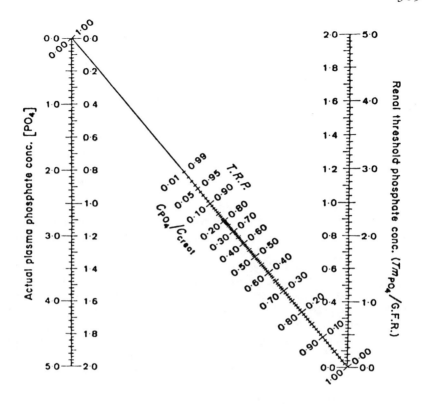

$$\frac{C_{PO_4}}{C_{creat}} = \frac{U_{PO_4} \times S_{creat}}{S_{PO_4} \times U_{creat}}$$

EXAMPLE: U_{PO_4} = 40 mg/dl

S_{creat} = 1.0 mg/dl

S_{PO_4} = 2.0 mg/dl

U_{creat} = 100 mg/dl

$$\frac{C_{PO_4}}{C_{creat}} = \frac{40 \times 1.0}{100 \times 20} = 0.2$$

TmP/GFR = 1.6

(Normal TmP/GFR = >2.5 mg/dl)

Figure 17-1 Determination of the tubular maximum for phosphate reabsorption (TmP/GRF).

PTH

Serum parathyroid hormone (PTH) is measured by radioimmunoassay (RIA). The interpretation of serum PTH values is complicated by the following factors:

(1) The immunoreactivity of PTH does not necessarily correlate with the biological activity of PTH. PTH circulates in the serum in three forms: the

1–84 amino acid (intact) molecule and the 1–34 amino acid (amino-terminal) fragment, which account for 20% of the immunoreactivity but all of the bioactivity of PTH, and the 35–84 amino acid (carboxy-terminal) fragment, which comprises 80% of the immunoreactivity but is biologically impotent. It is apparent that if the major component which is measured by RIA has little or no biological role, PTH determinations can be misleading. The inactive carboxy-terminal fragment is cleared from the circulation by the kidneys and rises to progressively higher levels with decreasing renal function.

(2) The antibody used in almost all PTH RIA techniques is raised against nonhuman PTH (usually porcine or bovine PTH). This leads to reduced sensitivity in PTH RIAs as complete cross-reactivity between human and animal PTH is not present.

(3) When the same samples from normal patients and patients with well-defined hyperparathyroidism or hypoparathyroidism are evaluated by several different laboratories, results are widely discrepant due to differences in both antisera and other aspects of RIA technique.

Thus, at present, the PTH RIA remains suboptimal, and physicians will encounter the hypercalcemic patient who has a normal serum PTH value by RIA, but is found at surgery to have primary hyperparathyroidism; the hypercalcemic patient with bony metastases in whom levels of PTH should be suppressed, but are normal or elevated; and the patient with surgical hypoparathyroidism and hypocalcemia in whom the PTH value is inappropriately normal. PTH samples are collected on ice and promptly centrifuged at $4\,°C$. Although a cytobiochemical assay of PTH very sensitively reflects the biological activity of PTH, this cumbersome technique is available only on a research basis.

To circumvent the problems posed by the RIA for PTH, some confirmation of the biological activity of PTH is sought. Since PTH directly depresses the renal reabsorption of phosphate and thus lowers the TmP/GFR, this measurement is a valid indicator of PTH activity. It is somewhat limited in its sensitivity and specificity, since not all patients with primary hyperparathyroidism have a depressed TmP/GFR, and there are other disorders not mediated by excess PTH in which the TmP/GFR is also depressed (see the discussion of hypophosphatemia below). PTH also directly influences and accounts for virtually all of the production of renal or nephrogenous cyclic AMP (cAMP) and the measurement of nephrogenous cAMP (NcAMP) is a highly specific and sensitive index of PTH biological activity. NcAMP is calculated by measuring the total urine cAMP (UcAMP), which reflects both the cAMP filtered (plasma or PcAMP) and secreted (NcAMP) by the kidney and subtracting PcAMP from UcAMP: NcAMP = UcAMP − PcAMP. Normally, 50% of UcAMP is derived from plasma and 50% is NcAMP. The measurement of UcAMP is relatively simple, whereas the measurement of PcAMP is complex. UcAMP is an accurate reflection of PTH biological activity, and little accuracy is lost in substituting the measurement of UcAMP for NcAMP. About 90% of patients with primary hyperparathyroidism will have increased UcAMP values, whereas UcAMP is low in almost all patients with hypoparathyroidism. UcAMP must be collected in acid (1 mL 6 N HCl for each estimated hour of urine collection) after an overnight fast, and the second-voided urine sample of the morning is used. It is preferable to measure UcAMP while the patient is on a low-calcium diet, as high calcium intake may suppress secretion to some degree and result in misleadingly normal UcAMP values in patients with primary hyperparathyroidism. This occurs because adenomatous or hyperplastic parathyroid tissue retains some degree of suppressibility by calcium loading. UcAMP must be expressed as nanomoles per 100 mL of glomerular filtrate; the determination of UcAMP is meaningless if expressed otherwise. A spot urine sample for UcAMP is as valid as a 24-hour urine sample.

Total UcAMP is calculated as follows:

$$\text{UcAMP} = \frac{\text{UcAMP (nmol/mL)}}{\text{Urine creatinine (mg/dL)}} \times \text{serum creatinine (mg/dL)}$$

UcAMP normally ranges from 1.8 to 4.3 nmol/100mL of glomerular filtrate.

Vitamin D Metabolites

Vitamins D_2 and D_3, 25-hydroxyvitamin D (25 OH D), and 1,25-dihydroxyvitamin D (1,25 OH2 D) may be measured in plasma by a variety of techniques. Samples are collected in heparinized tubes, centrifuged, and kept at 4 °C.

Other Tests

The serum chloride/phosphorus ratio, previously touted as diagnostically useful in evaluating hypercalcemia, is not an accurate test. Neither is the hydrocortisone suppression test, which is not specific for any one form of hypercalcemia. (Table 17-7).

Calcitonin

Serum for calcitonin is collected in heparinized tubes and analyzed by RIA; its value is primarily in the diagnosis of medullary carcinoma of the thyroid (see section on multiple endocrine neoplasia syndromes) and not in the diagnosis of disorders of calcium metabolism.

Hydroxyproline

Urinary hydroxyproline is collected over 24 hours in a jug containing 20 mL of 6 N HCl. To avoid the effect of diet, a low-gelatin diet is prescribed for the several days preceding the 24-hour urine collection (see Paget's Disease, below).

Uric Acid

Urine uric acid determinations are necessary for the evaluation of uric acid and calcium oxalate kidney stone disease. Urine uric acid excreted over 24 hours is measured in a jug which does not contain acid (acidification yields falsely low values), and the collection should not be performed within the few days after use of iodinated contrast material, particularly intravenous pyelogram dye, which causes spuriously high values. Obviously, the use of uricosuric drugs such as probenecid and sulfinpyrazone will elevate urine uric acid values. As purine ingestion directly influences uric acid exretion, the acutely ill patient with uric acid stone-induced renal colic and who is fasting may have a misleading normal value. The test is best performed when

Table 17-7
Differential Diagnosis of Hypercalcemia*

Disorder	Serum Ca	PTH	TmP GFR	FECa	UcAMP	Serum P	Alk Phos	1,25D	Urine Ca	Serum Ca Falls c̄ Steroid Therapy	Comments†
Primary hyper-parathyroidism	↑-↑↑	↑	↓	N/↑	↑	↓/N	N/↑	N/↑	↑/N	No	+ bone scan or bone biopsy, primary tumor often obvious
Cancer with metastases to bone	↑-↑↑	↓/N	↑/N	↑-↑↑	↓	N/↑	↑/N	↓	↑-↑↑	No, unless steroid-responsive tumor	See (A) below; − bone scan/biopsy
Cancer with humoral hypercalcemia	↑-↑↑	↓/N	↓	↑-↑↑	↑	↓/N	N/↑	↓	↑-↑↑		
Sarcoidosis	↑-↑↑	↓/N	↑/N	N	↓	N/↑	N/↑	↑	↑	Yes	Chest x-ray, tissue bi-opsy, serum ACE level
Tuberculosis	↑	↓/N	↑/N	N/↑	↓	N	N	?	N/↑	Some cases	Chest x-ray, skin test, cultures
Histoplasmosis	↑	↓/N	↑/N	N/↑	↓	N	N	?	N/↑	Some cases	Chest x-ray, cultures
Coccidioido-mycosis	↑	↓/N	↑/N	N/↑	↓	N	N	?	N/↑	Some cases	Chest x-ray, cultures
Berylliosis	↑	↓/N	↑/N	N/↑	↓	N	N	?	N/↑	Some cases	Tissue beryllium levels, work history
Myeloma	↑-↑↑	↓/N	↑/N	↑-↑↑	↓	N/↑	N/↑	↓	↑-↑↑	Yes	Protein electrophoresis, bone marrow
Vitamin D toxicity	↑-↑↑	↓/N	↑/N	N	↓	N/↑	N	N	↑/N	Yes	High serum 25-D levels; 1,25D high only with calcitriol use

Recovery from acute renal failure	↑	↑	↓	N/↑	↑	↓/N	↑	No	Blood urea nitrogen, creatinine, see (B) below
Immobilization	↑	↓/N	↑/N	↑-↑↑	↓	N	↑/N	No	Especially children or with primary bone disease (eg, Paget's)
Adrenal insufficiency	↑	?	?	?	?	?	?	Yes	ACTH stimulation test; rare and likely due to hemoconcentration c̄ normal ionized serum Ca2 +
Vitamin A toxicity	↑	↓/N	↑/N	↑	↓	N	N/↑	Yes	History, serum vitamin A levels
Milk-alkali syndrome	↑-↑↑	↓/N	↓/N	N	↓	N	N/↑	No	High serum HCO_3^- and urine pH; history

*↑ or ↓, Mild or moderate increase or decrease; ↑↑ or ↓↓, marked increase or decrease. When two possible results exist, the more likely finding is presented to the left of the shill. Abbreviations: Serum Ca, serum calcium; PTH, parathyroid hormone; TmP/GFR, tubular maximum for phosphorus reabsorption; FECa, fasting fractional excretion of calcium; UcAMP, urine cyclic AMP; Serum P, serum phosphorus; Alk Phos, alkaline phosphatase; 1,25D, 1,25(OH)2 Vitamin D; Urine Ca, urine calcium. PTH values are listed as if an "ideal" PTH RIA were employed producing the results expected due to the pathophysiology of the underlying disorder. Note that in any individual patient, PTH values may not correspond to the clinical expectation; other values, especially UcAMP and TmP/GFR, may be helpful. Most PTH RIAs do not distinguish between low and normal values; thus, the results indicate that normal values may be found in patients with disorders in which the PTH level is expected to be low.

†(A) The syndrome of humoral hypercalcemia of malignancy was formerly called the ectopic PTH syndrome or pseudohyperparathyroidism. Patients with this disorder produce a soluble factor distinct from PTH, but which, like PTH, causes an elevated serum calcium and urine calcium and UcAMP and a depressed TmP/GFR. Unlike primary hyperparathyroidism, it is associated with a decreased level of 1,25OH2 D. PTH levels are low or normal in such patients. Hypercalcemia is often more acute and severe, calciuria is of a greater degree, and a tumor is generally clinically evident (especially squamous cell tumors and hypernephromas). Hypercalcemia results from a profound increase in osteoclastic resorption of bone mediated by this humoral factor and is not due to tumor invasion of the bone.

(B) In the development of acute renal insufficiency, hyperphosphatemia causes hypocalcemia and secondary hyperparathyroidism. Phosphorus and calcium may be deposited in extraskeletal sites (especially when renal failure is due to rhabdomyolysis). In the diuretic recovery phase, persistent vigorous PTH secretion in combination with mobilization of extraskeletal calcium deposits may lead to transient hypercalcemia.

Table 17-7 (continued)

Table 17-7 (continued)

Disorder	Serum Ca	PTH	TmP GFR	FECa	UcAMP	Serum P	Alk Phos	1,25D	Urine Ca	Serum Ca Falls c̄ Steroid Therapy	Comments†
Thyrotoxicosis	↑	↓/N	↑/N	↑/N	↓	N/↑	N/↑	↓	↑/N	No	T₄, T₃
Familial hypocalciuric hypercalcemia	↑-↑↑	N/↑	↓/N	↓	N/↑	N/↓	N	N/↑	↓	No	See (C) below
Thiazides	↑				Results depend on underlying hypercalcemic disorder ↓						See (D) below
Iatrogenic	↑-↑↑				Changes too acute to measure other parameters ↑						Obvious history only with intravenous calcium, normal calcium afterwards

(C) Patients with familial hypocalciuric hypercalcemia may be distinguished from patients with primary hyperparathyroidism as familial hypocalciuric hypercalcemia is an autosomal dominant disorder which presents early in life, is not associated with other diseases present in patients with multiple endocrine neoplasia syndromes, is usually not associated with end organ damage due to hypercalcemia, and has disproportionately low values for PTH, UcAMP, FECa, and 24-hour urine calcium for the degree of hypercalcemia present. FECa and 24-hour urine calcium values best differentiate familial hypocalciuric hypercalcemia from primary hyperparathyroidism, but overlap may occur.

(D) Thiazides do not cause hypercalcemia in normal persons, but may do so in patients with underlying disorders of calcium metabolism, especially primary hyperparathyroidism.

the patient is eating regular meals. Urine uric acid is best determined by the uricase method, which is superior to the phosphotungstic acid method. Serum uric acid determinations are easily performed by the autoanalyzer technique. Patients with increased serum and urine uric acid, so-called "overproducers" of uric acid, are at increased risk for uric acid stone formation. Hyperuricemic patients who are normouricosuric are not at increased risk for uric acid stone formation. Normal women excrete less than 750 mg/24 hours, and normal men excrete less than 800 mg/24 hours.

Oxalate

Urinary oxalate measurements are quite difficult to perform, and commercial laboratories often report misleading results. Normal oxalate excretion is generally below 50 mg/24 hours, whereas patients with hyperoxaluric stone disease usually excrete more than 100 mg of oxalate per 24 hours. Urinary oxalate excretion is greatly affected by dietary oxalate, and more than one 24-hour urine sample should be collected while the patient is on a regular diet. This test need not be done for the patient with "garden variety" calcium oxalate stones and should be reserved for those patients with appropriate clinical settings for primary hyperoxaluric (severe recurrent stone disease in the first decade of life with oxalosis and renal failure) or enteric hyperoxaluria (particularly chronic inflammatory bowel disease of the small bowel but with preserved colonic function) or for patients with severe calcium oxalate stone disease not responding to appropriate treatment.

Cystine

Cystinuria is evaluated by microscopic examination of a cooled, concentrated, acidified urine sample which reveals diagnostic hexagonal or "benzene ring-shaped" crystals. A qualitative screen using cyanide-nitroprusside evaluation of a 24-hour urine sample collected in acid is performed and, if positive, is followed by a quantitative 24-hour urine cystine determination.

Stone Analysis

Key to the laboratory evaluation of kidney stones is the crystallographic analysis of the stone itself. The results of such analysis direct the nature of the associated laboratory evaluation.

Urine C&S

Urine culture and sensitivity (C&S) plays an important role in the diagnosis of magnesium ammonium phosphate or infection stones produced by urease-producing organisms. Urine C&S is done routinely in all stone patients, as infection may seriously complicate the course of stone disease.

Urine pH

Fasting AM urine pH determinations, best performed with nitrazine paper, are useful in the diagnosis of renal tubular acidosis (RTA) and the milk alkali syndrome, which are associated with calcium stone formation in uric acid stone disease in which persistently acid urine may cause uric acid stone formation in normouricosuric patients, and in patients with calcium phosphate softness in whom urine pH is usually above 5.5 (primary hyperparathyroidism, RTA, and the milk alkali syndrome).

Laboratory Evaluation of Hypercalcemia

The tests described above can be used to approach the diagnosis of hypercalcemia in a logical fashion (see Table 17-7).

Laboratory Evaluation of Hypocalcemia

Table 17-8 combines the tests described above to approach the laboratory evaluation of hypocalcemia.

Laboratory Evaluation of Hypophosphatemia and Hyperphosphatemia

The causes of hypophosphatemia (Table 17-9) and hyperphosphatemia (Table 17-10) are usually clinically apparent, and few ancillary laboratory values are needed.

Laboratory Evaluation of Magnesium Metabolism

Hypomagnesemia

Hypomagnesemia can be approached pathophysiologically by measuring urine magnesium, which normally falls to zero but rises when hypomagnesemia is due to urinary magnesium wasting. Thereafter, appropriate medical and drug history and other laboratory tests (particularly of renal function) allow identification of the specific cause of hypomagnesemia (Table 17-11).

Hypermagnesemia

Hypermagnesemia occurs only with renal failure or iatrogenically (eg, in the treatment of eclampsia). Clinical history and serum creatinine are sufficient to make the distinction.

Laboratory Evaluation of Osteopenia

Osteopenia refers to a state of reduced bone mass and can be subdivided into two large categories of disease: osteoporosis, in which there is a decreased mass of normally mineralized bone most often associated with normal laboratory values, and osteomalacia, in which there is defective mineralization of bone accompanied by abnormal laboratory values.

Osteoporosis

Most patients with osteoporosis have normal chemical findings. The clinical history and physical examination play a major role in identifying the etiologies of osteoporosis, such as premature menopause, hyperthyroidism, Cushing's syndrome, hypogonadism, malnutrition, diabetes mellitus, immobilization, multiple myeloma, leukemia, lymphoma, chronic (alcoholic) liver disease, and drug treatment with glucocorticoids, chronic heparin, and thyroid hormone. Twenty-four hour urine calcium, TmP/GFR, and FECa are simple tests to screen for evidence of excessive bone resorption as the cause of osteoporosis. Abnormal values for these studies and/or clinical suspicion of the disorders described above which may cause osteoporosis suggest evaluation of aspects of endocrine function—T_3, T_4, PTH, cortisol, estrogen, testosterone, and glucose—and testing for myeloma, lymphoma, leukemia, and chronic liver disease.

Osteomalacia
Table 17-12 indicates the laboratory evaluation of osteomalacia.

Laboratory Evaluation of Paget's Disease

Patients with active symptomatic Paget's disease have significantly elevated values of serum alkaline phosphatase (the easiest value to follow) and urinary hydroxyproline. Serum and urine calcium values are normal, except during immobilization when they may increase. Alkaline phosphatase and hydroxyproline fall after two or three months of therapy. A rapid and marked elevation in alkaline phosphatase suggests the possible development of an osteogenic sarcoma.

Laboratory Evaluation of Kidney Stone Disease

Many patients with a single kidney stone will later have another, and about four-fifths of patients with recurrent stones have an underlying metabolic disorder, most often hypercalciuria. Therefore, laboratory evaluation of these patients is essential to their proper management.

Crystallographic stone analysis of a previously passed stone will "streamline" the chemical evaluation of the stone patient; ie, a patient with previous calcium oxalate stones does not need a determination of urine cystine. A basic chemical evaluation as discussed below is useful in all patients with stones, as hypercalciuria and/or hyperuricosuria may serve as additional risk factors for stone formation in patients with less common causes of stone disease such as magnesium ammonium phosphate or cystine stones.

Radiographic studies (kidneys, ureters, and bladder or intravenous pyelogram) help to define the metabolic disorder since uric acid stones are radiolucent, whereas calcium, magnesium ammonium phospate, and cystine stones are radiopaque and magnesium ammonium phosphate stones often have a characteristic "staghorn" pattern. Nephrocalcinosis and medullary sponge kidney may be seen and help explain the cause for stone formation. Last, the number of residual stones may be identified.

A basic laboratory evaluation should include serum calcium, phosphorus, uric acid, creatinine, alkaline phosphatase, electrolytes, TmP/GFR, FECa, a 24-hour urine test for calcium (high oral calcium intake will increase the likelihood of observing hypercalciuria) and uric acid, urinalysis, urine pH, and urine culture and sensitivity. As calcium must be collected in acid and uric acid must not be collected in acid, two separate 24-hour urine collections are necessary. Although, ideally, diagnosis and treatment should not be based on just one 24-hour urine determination of calcium and uric acid, it is often unrealistic to ask patients to collect additional samples (unless values are equivocal). All 24-hour urine samples measure urine volume, which is important as a small subset of patients with recurrent kidney stones will have a very low urine volume as their only "laboratory abnormality." Twenty-four hour urine samples should include measurement of creatinine to assess the adequacy of the collection, which, when combined with the

Table 17-8
Evaluation of Hypocalcemia*

	Urine Ca	Serum P	TmP	Alk Phos	PTH	UcAMP	Comments†
Hypoparathyroidism	↓	↑	↑	N	↓	↓	hx parathyroid or thyroid surgery; other autoimmune endocrinopathy
Pseudohypoparathyroidism	↓	↑	↑	N	↑	↓	Characteristic phenotype (A)
Chronic renal failure	↓	↑	–	↑	↑	–	hx, creatinine, BUN ↑
Hypomagnesemia	↓	↑	↑	N	↓/N	↓/N	Serum Mg usually < 1.2 mg/dL, CA normal after MG therapy
Pancreatitis	↓	↓/N	↓	N	↑	↑	Amylase, lipase
Hungry bone syndrome	↓	↓	↓	N	↑	↑	hx parathyroid or thyroid surgery (B)
Interstitial nephritis c̄ renal Ca wasting, distal RTA	↑	↓	↓	N/↑	↑	↑	Renal tubular disorder (renal Na & K wasting, RTA, NDI)

Extensive osteoblastic metastases	↓	↓	↓	↑	↑	Bone scan, hx tumor
Osteomalacia	↓	↓/N	↓	↑	↑	Vitamin D metabolites, etc (Table 17-12) (C)
Rapid cell lysis as with chemoRx of lymphoma	↓	↑	↓	N	↑	
Excessive citrate (from transfusion) mithramycin toxicity	↓	↓/N	↓	N	↑	hx transfusion, drug use

*Abbreviations: RTA, renal tubular acidosis; NDI, nephrogenic diabetes insipidus; other abbreviations as in Table 17-7.

†(A) Although clinical history and PTH levels usually distinguish hypoparathyroidism from pseudohypoparathyroidism, occasionally a PTH infusion is needed. PTH (300 U) is given intravenously over 15 minutes, which normally increases UcAMP 20-fold and does so in patients with hypoparathyroidism, but only increases UcAMP 2- to 5-fold in patients with pseudohypoparathyroidism. Additionally, urine phosphorus rises 4- to 10-fold with PTH infusion in patients with hypoparathyroidism, but fails even to double in patients with pseudohypoparathyroidism.

(B) "Hungry bones" syndrome refers to patients with chronic bone resorption due to hyperparathyroidism and hyperthyroidism who undergo surgical correction of excess hormone production which is followed by a period of enhanced remineralization of bones "hungry" for calcium and phosphorus, causing low serum levels of both elements.

(C) Occurs in patients undergoing chemotherapy for lymphoma or leukemia or in patients with severe rhabdomyolysis in whom the release of large amounts of intracellular phosphorus is associated with hyperphosphatemia and hypocalcemia as well as hyperkalemia, hyperuricemia, and lactic acidosis.

Table 17-9
Evaluation of Hypophosphatemia*

	TmP/GFR	Urine P	Serum Ca	Urine Ca	PTH	UcAMP	Comments
Severe Hypophosphatemia (< 1 mg/dL)							
Parenteral hyperalimentation	↑	↓	N	N or ↑	↓ or N	↓ or N	Clinically obvious
Diabetic ketoacidosis	↑	↓	N	N or ↑	↓ or N	↓ or N	Serum glucose, ketones, and bicarbonate
Antacids which bind phosphorus	↑	↓	N	N or ↑	↓ or N	↓ or N	History of antacid use
Chronic alcoholism	↑	↓	N	N or ↑	↓ or N	↓ or N	Clinically obvious, alcohol level
Acute respiratory alkalosis	↑	↓	N	N or ↑	↓ or N	↓ or N	Arterial blood gas
Moderate Hypophosphatemia (1.0–2.4 mg/dL)							
Primary hyperparathyroidism	↓	↑	↑	↑	↑	↑	See Table 17-7
Secondary hyperparathyroidism	↓	↑	↓ or N	↓ or N	↑	↑	See below†
Primary renal phosphorus leak	↓	↑	N	N or ↑	N or ↓	↓ or N	Rickets and other proximal tubular defects may be present
Distal renal tubular acidosis	↓	↑	N or ↓	↑ or N	↑	↑	Low serum bicarbonate, high urine pH

*Abbreviations as in Table 17-7.
†Includes vitamin D deficiency states, malabsorption, primary renal calcium leak, and chronic hypocalcemia of other causes.

Table 17-10
Evaluation of Hyperphosphatemia*

	TmP/GFR	Urine P	Serum Ca	Urine Ca	PTH	UcAMP	Comments
Chronic renal failure	–	↓	↓	↓	↑	–	Creatinine, blood urea nitrogen
Hyperthyroidism	↑	↓	N or ↑	N or ↑	↓	↓	T_4, T_3
Hypoparathyroidism	↑	↓	↓	↓	↓	↓	See Table 17-8
Pseudohypoparathyroidism	↑	↓	↓	↓	↑	↑	See Table 17-8
Acute cell lysis as c̄ chemoRx of lymphoma	↓	↑	↓	↓	↑	↑	See Table 17-8
Excessive Rx with oral or intravenous phosphorus	↓	↑	↓	↓	↑	↑	History

*Abbreviations as in Table 17-7.

Table 17-11
Causes of Hypomagnesemia

Low/Absent Urine Magnesium	Inappropriately High Urine Magnesium
Starvation	Therapy with cisplatin, gentamicin,
Malabsorption	or diuretics
Prolonged diarrhea	1° or 2° hyperaldosteronism
Total parenteral nutrition lacking	Primary renal magnesium leak
magnesium supplementation	Interstitial nephritis
Primary hypomagnesemia	Chronic alcohol abuse
(selective magnesium malabsorption)	(combined decreased dietary magnesium intake and increased urine magnesium excretion)
	Renal tubular acidosis
	Acute tubular necrosis

values for serum creatinine and urine volume, allows the calculation of the creatinine clearance. If hypercalciuria or high-normal urine calcium values are present, measurements of UcAMP and PTH (after several days of a low-calcium diet), T_4, T_3, and protein electrophoresis are useful additional tests. When prior stone analysis is unavailable, a spot urine cystine screen test may be obtained. Urine oxalate is not measured routinely, but only under the conditions described above under the discussion of the laboratory evaluation of urine oxalate.

Table 17-13 details an approach to the laboratory evaluation of kidney stone disease.

Adrenal Gland

The proper laboratory evaluation of diseases of the adrenal gland depends upon whether the clinician suspects diseases of the adrenal cortex or the adrenal medulla. Diseases of the cortex may result from deficiency or excess of glucocorticoids and/or mineralocorticoids and congenital hyperplasia. Disorders of the medulla include pheochromocytoma and the hypoadrenergic states.

■ Disorders of Glucocorticoid Production

Basal Studies

Plasma or serum cortisol is most often determined by fluorimetric assay or radioimmunoassay (RIA) and less commonly by competitive binding radioassay. The fluorimetric method is generally quite accurate. However, cortisol values determined by this assay commonly exceed simultaneous RIA measurements by 2–3 μg/dL due to detection of nonspecific background fluorescence. Fluorescent drugs such as spironolactone, carbamazepine, quinacrine, niacin, quinidine, fusidic acid, and benzyl alcohol (used in some

Table 17-12
Evaluation of Osteomalacia*

	Serum Ca	Urine Ca	Serum P	TmP/GFR	PTH	UcAMP	Alk Phos	D	25D	1,25D	Urine pH	Comments[†]
Vitamin D deficiency and malabsorption	↓/N	↓	↓/N	↓	↑	↑	N/↑	↓	↓	↓/N		Other evidence of malabsorption
Impaired 25D production	↓/N	↓	↓/N	↓	↑	↑	N/↑	N	↓	↓/N		
Vitamin D-dependent rickets	↓/N	↓	↓/N	↓	↑	↑	N/↑	N	N	↓		
1,25 vitamin D resistance	↓/N	↓	↓/N	↓	↑	↑	N/↑	N	N	↑		
Chronic renal failure	↓	↓	↑	—	↑	—	N/↑	N	N	↓		Creatinine, blood urea nitrogen
Vitamin D-resistant rickets (occasionally associated with mesenchymal tumor)	N	N/↑	↓	↓	N	N	N/↑	N	N	N/↓		
Hypophosphatemia due to malnutrition, antacids, malabsorption	N	N/↑	↓	↑	N	N	N/↑	N	N	↑		See (A)
Hypophosphatasia	N	N	N	N	N	N	↓↓	N	N	N		See (B)
Distal RTA	N/↓	N/↑	↓/N	↓/N	↑	↑	N/↑	N	N	N/↓	↑	Distal RTA only
Chronic acidosis	N/↓	N/↑	↓/N	↓/N	↑	↑	N/↑	N	N	N/↓	↓	

*Abbreviations as in Table 17-7.
[†](A) Patients often have coexistent vitamin D deficiency and deficient oral calcium intake, giving a variable laboratory profile.
(B) Patients have increased serum and urine pyrophosphate and phosphoethanolamine.

Table 17-13
Laboratory Evaluation of Kidney Stone Disease*

	Serum Ca	24-hour Urine Ca	FECa	Tmp/GFR	PTH	UcAMP	Serum Uric Acid	24-hour Urine Uric Acid	Serum HCO₃⁻	KUB/IVP	24-hour Urine Volume	Urine pH	Urine C&S	Urine Oxalate	Urine Cystine	Stone Analysis: Ca Oxalate	Ca Oxalate + Phosphate	Ca Phosphate	Uric Acid	Cystine	MAP
Absorptive hypercalciuria (A)	N	↑ or N	N; rare ↑	N or ↓ or ↑	N or ↓ or ↑	N	N	N	N	Opaque stones	N	N	−	N	−	+	+	−	−	−	−
Primary hyperparathyroidism (A)	↑ or N	↑ or N	N/↑	↓/N	↑	↑	N	N	N	Opaque stones; rare nephrocalcinosis	N/↑	N	−	N	−	+	+	+	−	−	−
Renal leak hypercalciuria (A)	low ↑ or N/N	N	↑	↓/N	↑	↑	N	N	N	Opaque stones	N/↑	N	−	N	−	+	−	−	−	−	−
Distal RTA	low ↑ or N/N	N	↑	↓/N	N/↑	N/↑	N	N	↓	Opaque stones; occasional nephrocalcinosis	N	↑↑		N		+	+	+	−	−	−

Condition										Imaging / Stones											
Milk alkali syndrome	N/↑	N/↑	N	N/↑	↓/N	↓/N	N	N	↑	Opaque stones; nephrocalcinosis	N	↑↑	–	N	–	+	+	+	–	–	–
Sarcoidosis, vitamin D toxicity and other hypercalcemic disorders	↑ or N	↑ or N	N/↑	↑	↓/N	↓/N	N	N	N	Opaque stones	N	N	–	N	–	+	–	–	–	–	–
Hyperuricosuria	N	N	N	N	N	N/↑	↑	N	N	Lucent stones	N or ↓	N	–	N	–	+	–	+	–	–	–
Normocalciuric hyperuricosuria	N	N	N	N	N	N/↑	↑	N	N	Opaque stones	N/↓	N	–	N	–	+	–	–	–	–	–
MAP (magnesium ammonium phosphate) stones	N	N	N	N	N	N	N	N	N	Staghorn calculi	↑↑	N	+†	N	–	–	–	–	+	–	+
Cystinuria	N	N	N	N	N	N	N	N	N	Opaque stones	N	N	↑↑ (occasionally)	N	–	–	+	–	–	–	–
Enteric/primary hyperoxaluria	N	N	N	N	N	N	N	N	N	Opaque stones	N	↑/↑↑	–	N	–	+	–	–	–	–	–
Low urine output	N	N	N	N	N	N	N	N	N	Opaque stones	↓/↓↓	N	–	N	–	+	–	+	–	–	–
MSK (medullary sponge kidney)	N	N	N	N	N	N	N	N	N	MSK nephrocalcinosis	N	N	–	N	–	+	+	–	–	–	–

*Abbreviations as in Table 17-7.

†Urease producers. (A) One may differentiate further among these three entities with a formal calcium tolerance test (see Selected Readings). A more practical approach may be to observe the response to treatment with thiazide diuretics, as only patients with hyperparathyroidism will develop hypercalcemia when treated with this medication.

322

preparations of heparin) also give spuriously high values. The high serum levels of corticosterone and 21-deoxycortisol found in some patients with congenital adrenal hyperplasia (CAH) have the same effect. Prednisone, prednisolone, metamethasone, dexamethasone, and triamcinolone are not detected by this method. The competitive protein-binding radioassay employs transcortin (corticosteroid-binding globulin (CBG) as the ligand. CBG also binds significant amounts of cortiocosterone, deoxycortico-sterone, cortisone, 11-deoxycortisol, progesterone, and 17-hydroxypro-gesterone; therefore, conditions in which these compounds appear in greater than usual amounts (CAH, pregnancy, adrenal carcinoma) may cause spuriously high serum cortisol values by this method. Prednisolone treatment has the same effect.

Approximately 90% of cortisol is bound to carrier protein (80% to CBG and 10% to albumin). Although a more precise index of biologically active cortisol, the measurement of plasma-free cortisol is not now commercially available.

Repeatedly high basal levels of serum cortisol suggest the presence of adrenal hyperfunction (Cushing's syndrome), and low levels suggest adrenal insufficiency (Addison's disease). However, the normal fluctuations in cortisol levels throughout the day and the alterations caused by many factors make basal levels nondiagnostic and require the appropriate suppression and stimulation tests detailed below. Patients with intrinsically normal adrenal function may have elevated serum cortisol values for the following reasons: severe physical or emotional stress, alcoholic binge drinking, anorexia nervosa, chronic renal failure, endogenous unipolar depression, or conditions associated with CGB elevation (high total but normal free cortisol), oral contraceptives, pregnancy, estrogens, hyperthyroidism, familial CGB elevation. Decreased serum cortisol values may occur in patients whose adrenal function is intrinsically normal with conditions associated with low CGB levels (low but normal free cortisol): chronic liver disease, nephrotic syndrome, multiple myeloma, hypothyroidism, protein-losing enteropathy.

Serum adrenocorticotropic hormone (ACTH) values are commonly determined by RIA. Plasma must be collected in heparinized plastic (not glass) tubes, immediately placed on ice, and centrifuged while cold within 30 to 60 minutes. The serum is frozen until assayed. Basal serum ACTH levels are useful in the differential diagnosis of hypercortisolism (very high levels suggest the ectopic ACTH syndrome, whereas low or undetectable levels suggest the presence of an adrenal tumor) and hypocortisolism (high levels suggest primary adrenal insufficiency, whereas low levels suggest secondary adrenal insufficiency). The diurnal rhythm of ACTH and cortisol secretion accounts for higher serum levels of these hormones in the early and mid-morning periods with a progressive decline throughout the day; this phenomenon must be kept in mind when serum cortisol and ACTH levels are interpreted.

Urine Tests for Glucocorticoids

Urinary 17-hydroxycorticosteroids (17OHCS) reflect approximately one-third to one-half of all the metabolites of cortisol. 17OHCS levels are altered by a variety of factors which influence cortisol metabolism. These include hyperthyroidism, obesity, and severe endogenous unipolar depression. Certain drugs including phenytoin, phenobarbital, primidone, estrogens, meprobamate, phenylbutazone, and occasionally pentazocine and propoxyphene, may affect 17OHCS values by drug interference or by causing cortisol to be metabolized by the 6-betahydroxycortisol pathway, leading to a decrease in urinary 17OHCS and an increase in urinary 6-betahydroxycortisol. Other factors that may reduce urine 17OHCS are anorexia nervosa, starvation, hypothyroidism, pregnancy, renal failure and liver disease.

The determination of urinary ketogenic steroids has been largely replaced by the measurement of 17OHCS. Urinary 17-ketosteroids (17KS) primarily reflect adrenal androgen metabolism and account for less than 10% of cortisol metabolites.

Urine-free cortisol (UFC) rises in a linear fashion with serum cortisol once serum cortisol exceeds 20–25 μg/dL and fully saturates binding sites for cortisol on CBG and albumin. UFC is elevated in almost all patients with Cushing's syndrome (CS), whereas it is normal in obese patients with Cushingoid features, in 25% to 50% of whom 17OHCS may be elevated. UFC is elevated with severe physical or emotional illness (primarily endogenous unipolar depression) and is modestly elevated in pregnancy, acromegaly, and in patients using oral contraceptives. Unlike the determination of 17OHCS, the measurement of UFC is not invalidated by drug interference. UFC determinations cannot distinguish euadrenal patients from patients with adrenal insufficiency.

Stimulation Tests

Glucocorticoid stimulation tests are necessary to demonstrate inadequate cortisol reserve in patients with primary or secondary adrenal insufficiency. Commonly used tests involve direct adrenal stimulation (ACTH stimulation tests) and indirect adrenal stimulation via the stimulation of ACTH secretion (insulin hypoglycemia and metyrapone). Indirect tests do not distinguish primary from secondary adrenal insufficiency. Vasopressin stimulation testing is useful to differentiate hypothalamic from hypopituitary hypoadrenalism. Pyrogen stimulation tests are no longer performed. Stimulation tests by ACTH, synthetic ACTH (Cortrosyn), insulin, metyrapone, and vasopressin are described above (see Pituitary Disease).

■ Practical Use of Laboratory Tests in Diseases of Glucocorticoid Production

Hypercortisolism

The diagnosis of hypercortisolism begins with a baseline UFC measurement and/or a dexamethasone suppression test (DST). Random AM and PM serum cortisol levels are of little value since normal patients may have 6–10 AM serum cortisol levels as high as 35 μg/dL and 4 PM levels as high as 22 μg/dL. The evaluation of diurnal variation of serum cortisol is also not useful in the diagnosis of CS. Plasma ACTH levels as isolated values are not diagnostic of

CS, but help to differentiate among the three common forms of CS: (1) adrenal adenoma, in which ACTH levels are low and should be undetectable; (2) pituitary CS of Cushing's disease (CD), in which ACTH levels are in the mid- to high-normal range in 50% of patients and are moderately elevated in 50% of patients; and (3) ectopic ACTH syndrome, in which ACTH levels are usually twofold or more elevated. However, there is significant overlap of ACTH values in patients with CD and with the ectopic ACTH syndrome.

Basal 24-hour urine 17OHCS values are normal in 10% of patients with CS and are elevated in 30% of obese patients who do not have CS. Normal persons excrete 3–7 mg/day per g of creatinine, whereas patients with CS excrete at least 7 and usually more than 9 mg/day per g of creatinine. Basal UFC measurements are much more useful in the diagnosis of CS than are urine 17OHCS measurements. The use of basal UFC measurements results in only a 3% false-positive and a 5% false-negative rate in the diagnosis of CS.

Glucocorticoid stimulation tests such as insulin hypoglycemia, ACTH, and metyrapone are not helpful in the diagnosis of CS. Patients with CS do not in general show an increase in serum cortisol in response to hypoglycemia, but as many as 20% of patients in the subgroup with CD will have a normal rise in serum cortisol. Almost 100% of patients with CD will have a normal twofold increase in 24-hour urinary 17OHCS in response to metyrapone testing, but 50% of patients with the ectopic ACTH syndrome and 15% of patients with an adrenal tumor causing CS will also double their urine 17OHCS production. The ACTH test is similarly imprecise.

DST are most useful in establishing the diagnosis of CS and differentiating among the three forms of CS.

Overnight Single-Dose DST

The overnight single-dose DST ranks with the basal 24-hour UFC as the most practical and accurate test to diagnose CS. One milligram of dexamethasone is given orally at midnight, and serum cortisol is measured eight hours later. Normally serum cortisol is suppressed to less than 5 μg/dL. Only 2% of patients with CS will have normal cortisol suppression, whereas only 1% of healthy, nonobese normal persons will fail to suppress. However, false-positive results will occur in (1) 10% to 15% of obese patients, (2) 20% to 25% of hospitalized acutely ill patients, (3) a variable percentage of patients receiving either phenytoin or phenobarbital, (4) patients on high-dose estrogen treatment (in excess of 1.25 mg of Premarin a day), (5) many patients with chronic renal failure, (6) some alcoholic patients who are tested immediately after a period of "binge drinking," and (7) many patients with psychiatric illnesses such as anorexia nervosa and endogenous unipolar depression. With the exception of some patients with either chronic renal failure, treatment with phenytoin, or severe endogenous unipolar depression, patients with the above illnesses who have a false-positive response to the overnight DST can be separated from patients with CS when the low-dose, two-day DST is performed.

Low-Dose Two-Day DST

Baseline 24-hour urine 17OHCS are collected for two days and continued for an additional two days during which dexamethasone is given orally, 0.5

mg every 6 hours for 48 hours. The final 24-hour urine collection for 17OHCS will fall below 4 mg/day in almost 100% of patients without CS; in about 95% of patients with CS, 17OHCS remains above 4 mg/day on the second day of treatment with dexamethasone (5% false-negative tests). Occasional patients later found to have CS who suppressed with the low-dose DST may have impaired metabolism of dexamethasone which potentiates its suppressive effect or may have episodic cortisol secretion with reduced cortisol secretion during the study period. If UFC is measured, normal patients will suppress below 25 μg/day on the second day of the low-dose DST. There are inadequate data to define normal suppressibility of serum cortisol and plasma ACTH values during low- (or high)-dose DST.

High-Dose DST

The results of basal 24-hour UFC and low-dose DST establish the diagnosis of CS. The high-dose DST and plasma ACTH levels (plus radiological evaluation of the pituitary gland, adrenal glands, lungs, etc) differentiate among the forms of CS. The high-dose DST is often conducted as an uninterrupted continuation of the low-dose DST in which 2 mg of dexamethasone is given orally every 6 hours for 48 hours, and 24-hour urine samples for 17OHCS are collected. When compared with baseline values, 24-hour urine 17OHCS on the second day of the high-dose DST are suppressed by more than 40% to 50% in patients with CD. Patients with adrenal CS fail to suppress, whereas up to 25% of patients with the ectopic ACTH syndrome may suppress. (Although rarely the case, the high-dose DST is not needed if 40% to 50% suppression of urine 17OHCS occurs with values still in excess of 4 mg/day on day two of the low-dose DST, as this pattern is diagnostic of CD.) Some patients will require either a third day of the high-dose DST or a total daily dose of 16 or 32 mg of dexamethasone to achieve 40% to 50% suppression of 17OHCS. (The inital results of a single overnight 8-mg dose of DST to differentiate CD from other forms of CS are encouraging, but further confirmation of the validity of this method is needed: 8 AM plasma cortisol is measured on two consecutive mornings with 8 mg of dexamethasone given orally at 11 PM before the second plasma cortisol sampling; the subsequent 8 AM plasma cortisol falls by more than 50% in patients with CD, but not in patients with other forms of CS.) Basal plasma ACTH levels, when added to the results of the high-dose DST, give the following pattern of results: (1) patients with CD will suppress urine 17OHCS by 50% and have normal or modestly elevated ACTH levels; (2) patients with adrenal adenoma or carcinoma-causing CS will not suppress and will have low or undetectable ACTH levels; and (3) patients with the ectopic ACTH syndrome will not suppress and will have high ACTH levels. As 25% of patients with the ectopic ACTH syndrome will suppress and there is no precise separation of ACTH values in patients with CD compared with patients with the ectopic ACTH syndrome, additional factors such as clinical presentation (pronounced hyperpigmentation, myopathy, hypokalemic alkalosis, and absence of the characteristic Cushingoid habitus in patients with the ectopic ACTH syndrome), pituitary computed axial tomography scanning, a search for a nonpituitary nonadrenal tumor producing the ectopic ACTH syndrome (lung cancer, thymoma, islet cell tumor, bronchial carcinoid tumor, medullary thyroid carcinoma, pheochromocytoma, etc), metyrapone testing (100% of patients with CD will have a twofold increase in urinary 17OHCS whereas only 50% of patients with the ectopic ACTH syndrome will do so), and inferior petrosal sinus catheterization and ACTH sampling may be necessary. Since episodic cortisol secretion may occur in some patients with the various forms of CS, a negative laboratory evaluation warrants repeat studies at a later date if the clinical suspicion of CS remains high.

The tests discussed above can be employed to develop a protocol for the laboratory evaluation of hypercortisolism.

Hypocortisolism

The laboratory procedures listed above can be combined and used as shown in Table 17-14 to diagnose the different forms of adrenal insufficiency.

■ Disorders of Mineralocorticoid Production

Mineralocorticoid Excess States

Primary hyperaldosteronism (PH), the most common endocrine cause of mineralocorticoid excess, is due to aldosterone-producing adenomas (APA), idiopathic adrenocortical hyperplasia (IAH), or, rarely, to adrenocortical carcinoma or dexamethasone-suppressible adrenal hyperplasia (DSAH). Basal urine and serum aldosterone levels are elevated in patients with PH, and suppression tests lead to incomplete aldosterone suppression. Aldosterone excess causes extracellular fluid volume expansion and hypokalemia, both of which inhibit renin secretion. Low basal and stimulated peripheral renal activity (PRA) values are always present in PH. In contrast, elevated PRA values are seen in patients with secondary hyperaldosteronism. This occurs in states of extracellular fluid volume depletion due to renal and nonrenal sodium loss, abnormal body sodium distribution (congestive heart failure, nephrotic syndrome, and cirrhosis with ascites), diminished sodium intake and in patients with renovascular lesions. Determination of aldosterone and PRA values is central to the laboratory diagnosis of PH. Mineralocorticoid excess causes excessive distal renal sodium retention, resulting in high-normal or elevated serum sodium; sodium is reabsorbed in the distal tubule in exchange for potassium, and prodigious kaliuresis and accompanying hypokalemia in a hypertensive patient most often prompts the evaluation for PH.

Laboratory evaluation of these patients usually begins with measurement of serum and urine potassium. In euvolemic patients who have not taken diuretic agents in the preceding one or two weeks and are on a diet containing 120–150 mEq of Na+ per day, the finding of two low serum potassium values should be followed by urine potassium determination. If a spot urine potassium value in a hypokalemic patient who is hypertensive exceeds 20 mEq/L or if the 24-hour urine potassium excretion exceeds 30 mEq/L, it is then appropriate to obtain plasma renin and aldosterone levels. (Note that in patients with PH whose serum potassium is below 2.5 mEq/L or whose urine sodium is less than 10 mEq/L, urinary potassium values may fall below those listed above. Such patients should be reevaluated when serum potassium has

Table 17-14
Prolonged ACTH Stimulation Tests

Protocol 1
  ACTH Regimen: 250 μg intravenously over 8 hours daily for 3 days
  Results:

Urine 17OHCS	Serum Cortisol
2–3X increment by day 3 in normal persons	30–70 μg/dL at the end of the infusion in normal persons

Protocol 2
  ACTH Regimen: 250 μg intravenously over 12 hours for 48 hours
  Results:

Urine 17OHCS	Serum Cortisol
In normal persons:	(After 24 hours of ACTH infusion)
Day 1 = above 27 mg	In normal persons:
Day 2 = above 47 mg	65 ± 10 μg/dL
In secondary adrenal insufficiency:	In secondary adrenal insufficiency:
Day 1 = above 4 mg	20 ± 10 μg/dL
Day 2 = above 10 mg	In primary adrenal insufficiency:
In primary adrenal insufficiency:	usually below 10 μg/dL
fails to exceed 4 mg	

been raised to 3.0 mEq/L and extracellular fluid volume and sodium intake are normal.)

PRA levels must be determined to be certain that hyperaldosteronism is not secondary to hyperreninemia. Basal PRA is measured at 8 AM after overnight recumbency and before the patient arises. The sample is collected in a tube containing EDTA and immediately placed on ice. If this basal value is low and the plasma aldosterone value is elevated, no further evaluation of renin status is necessary. Conversely, if the basal PRA is elevated, secondary hyperaldosteronism is present. When the basal PRA is equivocal, a stimulated PRA value should be obtained. This is done either by restricting sodium intake to 10–20 mEq/day for five days and measuring PRA after the patient is erect and walking for two to four hours or, more conveniently, by administering 40 mg of furosemide orally the night before and the morning of PRA sampling. Blood is obtained after two to four hours of walking (or upright posture if the patient cannot walk). Normal values for basal and stimulated PRA will vary from assay to assay.

Both basal urine and plasma aldosterone determinations are central to the diagnosis of PH. Extracellular fluid volume status, diuretic therapy, serum potassium, posture, time of sampling, and certain pharmacological agents all affect aldosterone values (Table 17-15). Therefore, in patients in whom the diagnosis of PH is entertained, aldosterone values should be obtained (1) after diuretics and the other drugs listed in Table 17-18 have been discontinued for at least two weeks, (2) with patients on a high-normal or increased sodium diet (120–150 mEq of sodium per day) for the three to seven days before aldosterone sampling, (3) in patients whose serum postassium is at or above 3 mEq/L, and (4) in patients whose extracellular fluid volume is stable.

Table 17-15
Factors Affecting Aldosterone Values

Increased Aldosterone	Decreased Aldosterone
Extracellular fluid volume contraction	Extracellular fluid volume expansion
Diuretic therapy	Hypokalemia
Hyperkalemia	Supine position
Upright posture	Sampling plasma from 4 PM to midnight
Sampling plasma from midnight to 8 AM	ACTH deficiency
ACTH	Dopamine and dopaminergic drugs
Angiotensin 2	Mineralocorticoid consumption
Metaclopramide and other dopamine antagonists	(Florinef, deoxycorticosterone acetate, carbenoxolone, excessive licorice ingestion [glycyrrhizic acid])

Twenty-four-hour urine aldosterone values reflect selected metabolites of aldosterone. The most commonly employed technique measures the 18-glucuronide aldosterone metabolite, which accounts for only 5% to 15% of aldosterone production. The upper limit of normal is 17–20 μg/day, depending on the individual assay. Urinary tetrahydroaldosterone measures 25% to 40% of aldosterone production, but is not a widely available test; measurement of the 18-glucuronide metabolite is usually satisfactory. Unlike plasma aldosterone values, which do not readily differentiate patients with IAH from normal persons, 24-hour urine aldosterone values are almost invariably elevated in patients with IAH.

Samples for plasma aldosterone should be obtained after overnight recumbency. Heparin or EDTA must be present in the sampling tubes in which blood is collected, and the sample should be processed promptly. Under the conditions listed above, normal patients will have plasma aldosterone values below 13 ng/dL. Patients with APAs have aldosterone values above 20 ng/dL, whereas patients with IAH often have values within the normal range.

If basal urine or plasma aldosterone values are diagnostically elevated and basal or stimulated PRA is suppressed, then PH is present. Occasionally the diagnosis is equivocal, and attempts to suppress plasma aldosterone levels with deoxycorticosterone, Florinef, or intravenous saline are necessary. Patients are studied while on a diet of 120–150 mEq of sodium per day and are given either 10 mg of deoxycorticosterone intramuscularly every 12 hours for six doses, 0.3 mg of Florinef orally every 12 hours for six doses, or two liters of normal saline intravenously over 2 hours. Patients with APA or IAH have minimal or no suppression of plasma or urine aldosterone in response to these maneuvers.

Once the diagnosis of PH is established, APA must be differentiated from IAH, as APA responds well to surgery but IAH does not. Although radiographic procedures coupled with selective venous sampling (bilateral adrenal venography with selective adrenal venous plasma aldosterone determinations, computed axial tomography scanning, and iodocholesterol scanning) have a primary role in this process, laboratory testing is also of value. Patients with APA will have significantly higher plasma aldosterone values (almost always in excess of 20 ng/dL) than patients with IAH, although some overlap exists. If patients with PH remain erect from 8 AM to noon and plasma aldosterone values are sampled at both times, aldosterone values will increase in almost all patients with IAH, whereas almost all patients with APA will have either no change or a decrease in plasma aldosterone levels. Although not a widely available test, the plasma level of the aldosterone precursor 18-hydrodeooxycorticosterone is consistently much higher in patients with IAH; values may overlap with those of normal persons.

Dexamethasone testing using 1–2 mg orally per day for one to two weeks should be performed after the above evaluation is completed to exclude those rare patients with PH who have the familial disorder of DSAH. Although some patients with IAH and APA will have a fall in plasma aldosterone values with dexamethasone suppression, this effect is noted only during the first few days of dexamethasone therapy, and plasma aldosterone values then return to baseline. In constrast, patients with DSAH will have persistently normal plasma and urine aldosterone values as well as potassium and sodium balance and a significant improvement in blood pressure control with prolonged dexamethasone use. (Dexamethasone testing is obviously unnecessary if the patient has definitive radiographic confirmation of a unilateral adrenal mass.)

Throughout the laboratory evaluation of PH, serum potassium must be monitored and should be maintained above 3.0 mEq/L. Patients with PH are significantly potassium depleted (sometimes compounded by prior treatment with kaliuretic diuretic antihypertensive agents) and, with the diagnostic use of mineralocorticoid or saline treatment, are further subjected to hypokalemia. Significant hypokalemia can reduce aldosterone secretion, which may interfere with the diagnosis of PH.

Mineralocorticoid Deficiency
(See also chapter on acid-base balance)

Mineralocorticoid deficient patients may come to medical attention with the common finding of hyperkalemia with inappropriately low urinary potassium secretion. A few of these patients will have primary adrenal insufficiency, whereas others may be taking certain drugs (spironolactone, triamterene, amiloride, or indomethacin), but most of these patients will have a definable abnormality of renin and aldosterone production which has been called "hyporeninemic hypoaldosteronism." Plasma renin and aldosterone determinations are performed as described in the preceding section. In patients with significant orthostatic hypotension, volume-depleting maneuvers such as Lasix, a sodium-restricted diet, or prolonged ambulation are unnecessary and may be dangerous. In such patients, basal supine PRA and plasma aldosterone values combined with values obtained after short periods (30–60 minutes) of erect or sitting posture are often sufficient provocative maneuvers. Patients with isolated hyporeninemic hypoaldosteronism will have normal cortisol responses to ACTH testing.

■ CAH

Several enzyme deficiencies lead to the laboratory testing profiles diagnostic of the various forms of CAH. Measurements of several adrenal cortical products may be necessary to define each syndrome. Determinations of glucocorticoid and mineralocorticoid hormones have been described above. The major adrenal androgens are measured either directly as plasma dehydroepiandrosterone sulfate (DHEAS), dehydroepiandrosterone (DHEA), androstenedione, and testosterone or as the major urine metabolites which are collectively designated as the 17-ketosteroids (17KS). As adrenal androgen secretion is controlled by ACTH, diurnal changes in plasma androgen values occur in parallel to changes in ACTH secretion. Thus, plasma levels of DHEA and androstenedione are highest at 8 AM. DHEAS is metabolized more slowly, and sampling time is less crucial with this compound. Although testosterone has a diurnal pattern of secretion, the time of sampling is not as improtant as it is for DHEA and androstenedione. (The measurement and diagnostic value of testosterone are discussed in the section on hypogonadism.) DHEA and DHEAS are secreted in the largest quantities; therefore, their metabolites comprise the majority of urinary 17KS. Androstenedione contributes to 17KS to a lesser degree, and testosterone indirectly accounts for only about 1% of 17KS. 17KS values may be spuriously increased by chlorpromazine, meprobamate, spironolactone, nalidixic acid, and penicillin and decreased by propoxyphene, pentazocine, progestins, chlordiazepoxide, and reserpine. Specific plasma androgen assays are needed to identify the different forms of CAH. Urinary 17KS determinations nonspecifically reflect increased adrenal androgen production and are not useful in differentiating among the different forms of CAH. Table 17-16 indicates the laboratory testing profiles for the various forms of CAH. Most of these patients will have the 21-hydroxylase deficiency variant which is often easily distinguished clinically from the other forms of CAH. They are most easily recognized by their high serum levels of 17-hydroxyprogesterone and their tendency toward salt wasting with associated orthostatic hypotension and hyperkalemia. Patients with the more rare 17-hydroxylase deficiency variant may also have increased levels of 27-hydroxyprogesterone, but will have hypertension and hypokalemia.

■ Adrenal Medullary Disorders

Hyperadrenergic Disorders—Pheochromocytoma

The laboratory evaluation of pheochromocytoma is based largely upon urine and plasma determinations of catecholamines and catecholamine metabolites. Stimulation and suppression tests have a limited role. Traditionally, 24-hour urine collections for vanillylmandelic acid (VMA), total metanephrines, and free catecholamines, which may be reported as total catecholamines or as epinephrine and norepinephrine, are obtained. Fluorimetric assay methods are most widely used for catecholamines and spectrophotometric methods for VMA and metanephrines. All samples must be collected in jugs containing 10–20 mL of 6 N hydrochloric acid (pH below 3.0). Although less precise methods for VMA determination (upper limit of normal is usually 13

Table 17-16
Chemistry Profiles in CAH

Enzyme Deficiency	Pregnenolone	Progesterone	17-Hydroxyprogesterone	17-Hydroxypregnenolone	Dehydroepiandrosterone	Dehydroepiandrosterone Sulfate	Deoxycorticosterone	Corticosterone	11-Deoxycortisol	Cortisol	Aldosterone	Androstenedione	Adrenocorticotrophic Hormone	17KS	Peripheral Renin Activity	18-Hydroxycorticosterone
21-Hydroxylase	↑	↑	(↑*)	↑	↑	(↑)	(↓)	↓	(↓)	N/↓	N/↓	↑	↑	↑	↑	
11-Hydroxylase	↑	↑	(↑)	↑	↑	(↑)	(↑)	↓	(↑)	↓	↓	↑	↑	↑	↓	
17-Hydroxylase	↑	↑	(↓)	↓	↓	(↓)	(↑)	N/↑	(↓)	↓	↓	↓	↑	↓	↓	
Desmolase†	↓	↓	(↓)	(↓)	(↓)	(↓)	(↓)	↓	↓	↓	↓	↓	↑	↓	↑	
3-Betahydroxy-dehydrogenase	↑	↓	N	(↑)	↑	(↑)	↓	(↑)	N	(N)	(↓)	N	N	N	↑	
18-Hydroxylase	N/↑	N/↑	N	N	N	(N)	↑	↑	N	N	↓	N	N	N	↑	
Type I																(↓)
Type II																(↑)

*O, key differentiating measurements.
†Values for desmolase are predicted but not actually measured.

mg/24 hours) require that the patient follow a "VMA diet" which is free of bananas, tea, coffee, vanilla, chocolate, and some cereals, more accurate fluorimetric assay methods (upper limit of normal is usually 6.5–7.0 mg/24 hours) do not require any dietary restrictions. Since 24-hour urine catecholamines and catecholamine metabolites are elevated by any severe stress, false-positive results will occur when measurements are obtained during any severe intercurrent illness. A few patients with pheochromocytomas (generally less than 5% to 10%) may have normal values for any one of the three tests, but it is extremely rare (with the exception of patients with multiple endocrine neoplasia syndromes types 2 and 3) to have normal results for all three tests. Most authorities agree that total metanephrine and total catecholamine determinations are superior to the VMA test as a single screening study. Twenty-four-hour urine excretion of VMA is normally 2–7 mg, that of total metanephrines is 0.2–0.9 mg, and that of total catecholamines is 20–100 μg with 20–80 μg as norepinephrine and 0–20 μg as epinephrine. When 24-hour urine values are equivocal, spot urine samples may be obtained immediately after a symptomatic episode. If a pheochromocytoma is present, total metanephrines will exceed 2.2 mg/g of creatinine and VMA will exceed 5.0 mg/g of creatinine.

The interpretation of the results of tests for VMA, metanephrines, and catecholamines is confounded by a wide variety of drugs as indicated in Table 17-17.

When basal urine determinations are inconclusive, plasma epinephrine and norepinephrine may be measured. These determinations are performed radioenzymatically, and blood is collected in iced, heparinized tubes containing reduced glutathione. The sample is promptly centrifuged, and serum is kept frozen until assayed. Upright posture may increase plasma catecholamines two- to threefold, so plasma is sampled 30 minutes after an intravenous line is inserted at 8 AM while the patient is still supine. Physical exertion or emotional stress may also increase epinephrine and norepinephrine severalfold. Normal supine AM values are 220 ± 100 pg/mL for norepinephrine and 40 ± 20 pg/mL for epinephrine. Almost all patients with pheochromocytomas have total plasma catecholamines in excess of 1000 pg/mL, but only rare hypertensive patients without a pheochromocytoma have values in this range. False-positive results are almost invariably excluded by using a cutoff value for the diagnosis of pheochromocytoma of total plasma catecholamines in excess of 2000 pg/mL; this will result in occasional false-negative tests. False-positive catecholamine determinations may occur in patients taking L-Dopa, methyldopa, methylxanthines, isoproterenol, terbutaline, ephedrine, phenylephrine, amphetamine, nitroglycerine, diazoxide and hydralazine. Patients taking clonidine or receiving some iodine-containing contrast materials may have false-negative catecholamine determinations.

Plasma catecholamine sampling at venography may help to localize tumors, particularly extraadrenal tumors. However, adrenal venous effluent samples cannot be reliably interpreted since grossly false-positive results may occur leading to inaccurate tumor localization.

Conventional stimulation or suppression tests for pheochromocytoma using, respectively, intravenous glucagon, histamine, and tyramine or phentolamine are evaluated in terms of the effect on blood pressure and not on

Table 17-17
Drugs that Interfere with Tests for Pheochromocytoma

Increased VMA	Decreased VMA
Catecholamines	Monoamine oxidase inhibitors
Drugs which contain or release cate-cholamines or inhibit catecholamine metabolism, such as:	Clofibrate
	Mandelamine
	Alcohol
Amphetamines	Disulfiram
Methylxanthines	Chlorpromazine
L-Dopa	
Ephedrine	
Vasodilators	
Clonidine (rapid withdrawal)	
Nalidixic acid	
Lithium	
p-Aminosalicylic acid	
BSP	

Increased Metanephrines	Decreased Metanephrines
Catecholamines	Methylglucamine (present in various x-ray contrast media)
Drugs which contain or release cate-cholamines, as listed above for VMA	
Alcohol	
Chlorpromazine	
Monoamine oxidase inhibitors	

Increased Catecholamines	Decreased Catecholamines
Catecholamines	None
Drugs which contain or release catecholamines, as listed above for VMA	
Methyldopa	
(by fluorescent method)	
Tetracycline	
Erythromycin	
Chloral hydrate	
Quinidine	
Quinine	
BSP	
Nicotinic acid	
Bretylium	
Methenamine	
Mandelamine	

urine or plasma CAT or CAT metabolites. These potentially lethal tests have an unacceptably high incidence of false-negative and false-positive results, and they have little or no role in the diagnosis of pheochromocytomas. More recently, the effect of intravenous clonidine on plasma catecholamines has been reported. In patients with pheochromocytomas, clonidine does not alter plasma catecholamine levels, whereas these values fall significantly in normal persons and in hypertensive patients who do not have pheochromocytomas.

Hypoadrenergic States

Plasma catecholamines may be determined as described above to evaluate patients with autonomic insufficiency who are believed to have adrenergic hypofunction. When plasma norepinephrine is sampled first while the patient is supine and then after 10 minutes of standing, such patients will have an increase of less than 140 pg of norepinephrine per ml in association with an orthostatic fall of 20 mm Hg in the mean arterial blood pressure.

Gonadal Disease

Patients with gonadal disease may have symptoms of sex hormone deficiency or infertility due to disordered gamete production. Specific assays for testosterone, estradiol, gonadotropins, and prolactin have simplified the evaluation of the pituitary-gonadal-sex steroid axis. Semen analysis is the simplest and best test of fertility in male patients. Evaluation of female infertility is more complex.

■ Specific Laboratory Tests in the Evaluation of Gonadal Function and Gonadal Disease

Sex Steroids

Plasma Testosterone
The measurement of testosterone in plasma is complicated by its low concentration, structural similarity to other androgens, and binding to sex hormone-binding globulin (SHBG) and albumin. Technically, the assay is accomplished by solvent extraction, chromatography, and then either competitive protein binding or radioimmunoassay. The normal range for total testosterone in men is 350 to 1200 ng/dL; in women, the normal range is 20 to 80 ng/dL. Although a circadian pattern can be demonstrated in men with a peak in the early morning, this fluctuation will usually not affect the interpretation of random plasma testosterone determination.

The concept of the "free testosterone concentration" is clinically relevant since normally only about 2% of total testosterone is exchangeable with the intracellular space and therefore biologically active. The remainder is bound to serum proteins—60% to SHBG and 38% to albumin. However, variations in SHBG levels may affect the distribution so that the free hormone concentration may not always parallel the total testosterone level. Pregnancy, cirrhosis, hyperthyroidism, and estrogen therapy will raise SHBG levels and decrease the free fraction of testosterone; androgens, growth hormone excess, and hypothyroidism will decrease SHBG levels. The plasma concentration of free testosterone may be assayed by various methods including equilibrium dialysis, gel filtration, and charcoal absorption. Some laboratories report free testosterone levels, whereas others provide measurements of free plus loosely bound (albumin-bound) testosterone.

Plasma Dehydroepiandrosterone Sulfate
Dehydroepiandrosterone sulfate is a weak adrenal androgen, but its high plasma concentration (1500–2500 ng/mL) and minimal diurnal variation

make its measurement relatively easy. The assay can help to distinguish ovarian from adrenal pathology as the source of excess androgen in the hirsute female (see below).

Plasma Estrogens

Estradiol can be measured in random plasma specimens. Estradiol concentration fluctuates dramatically during the menstrual cycle with levels varying from 20–500 pg/mL. However, it is usually unnecessary to measure estradiol in menstruating women. In women with amenorrhea, the "normal" range for estradiol is that in the early follicular phase of the menstrual cycle (25–75 pg/mL); this measurement is essential for the proper interpretation of gonadotropin levels in these patients. Postmenopausal women have estradiol levels of approximately 10–20 pg/mL, most of which is derived from peripheral conversion of testosterone and estrone.

Progesterone

Progesterone can be measured in isolated plasma specimens. Its major clinical value in the workup of female infertility derives from the observation that a single luteal-phase progesterone level of 3 ng/mL or more is presumptive evidence for ovulation.

Gonadotropins and Other Peptide Hormones

LH and FSH

Gonadotropins were initially measured in urine via mouse bioassays with ovulation or uterine weight changes as end points. These have been replaced by relatively specific radioimmunoassays, although there are still some problems with cross-reactivity due to the similarity between subunits of the various glycoprotein hormones. The extreme homology of luteinizing hormone (LH) and human chorionic gonadotropin (hCG) required the development of a specific beta-hCG assay for certain clinical situations. LH radioimmunoassays may have considerable overlap with hCG, but this is usually not a clinical problem. The gonadotropins can be conveniently measured in random serum specimens, although the pulsatile nature of pituitary secretion must be kept in mind. Borderline high or low results can be clarified by obtaining several specimens 20 minutes apart and assaying them either individually or as a pooled single sample. An alternative is to measure gonadotropin in timed urine specimens.

The normal range for serum LH and follicle-stimulating hormone (FSH) varies with age and with the stage of the menstrual cycle in women (Table 17-18). Values may be expressed as either mIU of the 2nd International Reference Preparation of Human Menopausal Gonadotropins or as ng/mL of the National Pituitary Agency Reference Standard (LER 907). It is usually unnecessary to measure gonadotropin in menstruating women; in premenopausal women with amenorrhea, the "normal" range is that of the follicular phase of the menstrual cycle. Gonadotropin levels must always be interpreted in light of simultaneous plasma testosterone levels in men and estradiol levels in women.

hCG

Measurement of hCG in urine is the standard test for pregnancy. High concentrations allow use of a relatively insensitive latex precipitation

Table 17-18
Normal Serum Gonadotropin Levels (mIU/mL)

	FSH	LH
Adult man	4–13	6–23
Menstruating woman		
Follicular phase	4–17	5–30
Midcycle	13–25	30–150
Luteal phase	4–15	4–40
Postmenopausal woman	30–200	30–200

radioimmunoassay. Elevated levels in serum can be detected with a specific radioimmunoassay for the beta subunit of hCG, which has minimal cross-reactivity with LH. This test can detect very early stages of pregnancy but, more important, it is useful in screening for ectopic hCG production by various tumors. This is often applied in the workup of gynecomastia (see below).

Gonadotropin-Releasing Hormone
The use of gonadotropin-releasing hormone infusions in documenting secondary hypogonadism is discussed in detail above (see Pituitary Disease).

Serum Prolactin
The use of the prolactin level as a marker for the presence of a pituitary adenoma is discussed above (see Pituitary Disease). Of interest is the observation that up to 20% of all women with secondary amenorrhea have hyperprolactinemia, whereas 95% of those with both amenorrhea and galactorrhea have elevated prolactin levels. Although not all of these women have pituitary adenomas, obtaining a random prolactin level is clearly an effective screening procedure in this setting.

Genetic Analysis

Buccal Smear
The buccal smear, when properly done, is useful in confirming a diagnosis of Klinefelter's Syndrome (XXY genotype) in a hypogonadal man; this is the most common cause of primary hypogonadism in men. Epithelial cells are scraped from the buccal mucosa, spread thinly on a glass slide, fixed, and then stained with appropriate dyes (Giemsa). An experienced cytologist then examines the specimen for Barr bodies, representing the inactive X chromosome in the nucleus. A control slide from a normal woman should be processed simultaneously.

In normal women, 20% to 40% of buccal epithelial cells contain Barr bodies; acute systemic illnesses may lead to a decrease or disappearance of these chromatin clumps. The presence of Barr bodies in 15% or more of mucosal cells in a man confirms the presence of an extra X chromosome.

Karyotype
Chromosomal analysis of peripheral leukocytes or cultured fibroblasts is essential for evaluation of the woman with primary or secondary amenor-

rhea of gonadal origin (with high gonadotropin levels). The critical determination is whether a Y chromosome is present (eg, as in XY gonadal dysgenesis, or complete testicular feminization), which signifies a definite risk of malignant degeneration of the gonad requiring prophylactic surgery. In addition, the karyotype may be the only way to determine mosaic Klinefelter's or Turner's syndrome, although therapy may not be altered by these results.

Miscellaneous Tests of Testicular and Ovarian Function

Semen Analysis
Semen analysis is the single best test of male fertility. A specimen obtained by masturbation after two to three days of abstinence should be analyzed within one hour. Criteria for a normal ejaculate are (1) volume over 2 mL (2) over 20,000,000 sperm per mL, (3) over 50% motility, (4) over 50% normal size and shape sperm.

Vaginal Smear
Vaginal cytology can be a useful marker of estrogen effect. The cells can also be stained to demonstrate Barr bodies, which should be present in 50% to 80% of cells. In addition, microscopic analysis of cervical mucus may also provide an index of estrogen levels and of ovulation by changes in the "ferning" effect.

■ Practical Use of Laboratory Tests in the Diagnosis of Gonadal Disease

Incomplete Virilization/Eunuchoid Habitus

The key diagnostic maneuvers in this setting are (1) the documentation of low testosterone level (this may require assay of free testosterone since total testosterone levels may be in the low-normal range) and (2) measuring LH and FSH levels to distinguish patients with primary hypogonadism (with elevated gonadotropin levels) from those with pituitary or hypothalamic disease. Further evaluation of primary hypogonadism can frequently be limited to performing a buccal smear. Further evaluation of secondary (pituitary) hypogonadism requires a complete battery of screening tests as described above (see Pituitary Disease).

Incomplete Feminization/Primary Amenorrhea

Primary amenorrhea is the absence of menses and secondary sexual characteristics by age 14 or the absence of menses by age 16 regardless of the presence of secondary sexual characteristics. Abnormalities of vaginal and uterine development should be apparent at physical examination or from x-ray or ultrasonographic evaluation. Separation of ovarian from pituitary disease depends upon the measurement of estradiol, FSH, LH, and prolactin. A karyotype should be done in cases of primary ovarian failure (low estradiol, high gonadotropin) to search for the presence of a Y chromosome which would dictate gonadal resection.

Gynecomastia

The multiple causes of gynecomastia in men can be divided into five major categories: (1) drug induced—spironolactone, methyldopa, reserpine, diethylstilbestrol, cimetidine, digitalis, marihuana; (2) increased estradiol/testosterone ratio—primary hypogonadism, pituitary disease, hyperthyroidism, alcohol abuse; (3) excess hCG production—oat cell carcinoma of the lung, choriocarcinoma of the testis, other tumors; (4) normal puberty; (5) idiopathic. If the patient is not at puberty and there is no definite drug history, screening lab tests would include (1) plasma testosterone level, (2) serum prolactin, (3) thyroid function test, (4) beta hCG assay, and (5) chest x-ray.

Impotence

In most but not all patients, the etiology of impotence is psychogenic. Organic causes of impotence can be divided into four categories: (1) neurogenic, (2) vascular, (3) drug induced, and (4) endocrine. The first two types are usually suggested by the patient's history and physical examination—associated peripheral neuropathy and diabetes mellitus, severe peripheral vascular disease; libido is usually normal, at least at the onset. Impotence is a side effect of many commonly used drugs, particularly antihypertensive medications. Endocrinologic abnormalities may or may not be associated with decreased testicular size, altered hair pattern, or decreased libido. Screening laboratory tests would include plasma testosterone, serum LH and FSH, and serum prolactin levels. The results of these measurements should help pinpoint a testicular or pituitary cause of the impotence.

Hirsutism

If not familial, hirsutism in females generally means increased androgen levels. The diagnostic challenge is to determine the source—ovary versus adrenal. Initial screening can be limited to measuring plasma testosterone (total and free) and either urine 17 ketosteroids (17KS) or serum dehydroepiandrosterone sulfate levels. In addition, an overnight dexamethasone suppression test should be performed if Cushing's syndrome is suspected.

Over 70% of hirsute women have increased total testosterone levels (normal 20–80 ng/dL), and an even higher percentage have elevated free testosterone concentration. Total plasma testosterone levels over 200 ng/dL raise the strong possibility of a testosterone-producing ovarian tumor.

If the 24-hour urine 17KS excretion is less than 20 mg, adrenal disease is unlikely; the diagnosis of polycystic ovarian syndrome or a variant of it is suggested. If the 17KS excretion is over 20 mg per 24 hours, a dexamethasone suppression test is required (2 mg every six hours for five days). Results are interpreted as follows: (1) suppression of 17KS to less than 4 mg per day suggests congenital adrenal hyperplasia (2); partial suppression to 5–11 mg per 24 hours suggests polycystic ovarian syndrome; and (3) lack of suppression requires further workup for possible adrenal tumor. An alternative to measuring urine 17KS is the assay of serum dehydroepiandrosterone sulfate levels. Values within the normal range (1500–2500 ng/mL) rule out an adrenal source of excess androgen.

Male Infertility

The inital diagnostic test for male fertility is semen analysis, keeping in mind that the sperm count and motility may be adversely affected by any acute systemic illness or chronic heat exposure. Klinefelter's syndrome and other causes of primary hypogonadism should be apparent on physical examination. The presence of a normal size testis and azospermia should lead to a testicular biopsy to rule out ductal obstruction. Endocrine disorders are uncommon causes of male infertility, but it is worthwhile to measure testosterone, LH, FSH and prolactin levels. The presence of a varicocele should prompt referral to a urologist.

Female Infertility

With Secondary Amenorrhea or Oligomenorrhea

Workup of secondary amenorrhea generally begins with a urine hCG measurement to rule out pregnancy. If this test is negative, a medroxyprogesterone acetate (10 mg by mouth per day for five days) challenge should follow. Withdrawal bleeding within two to seven days confirms anovulation and strongly suggests polycystic ovarian syndrome. Serum prolactin level and thyroid function tests should be done to screen for pituitary and thyroid disease. Lack of withdrawal bleeding should lead to measurement of serum estradiol, LH, and FSH. Elevated gonadotropin levels, indicating primary ovarian failure, require a karyotype analysis to rule out the presence of a Y chromosome. Normal or decreased gonadotropins, in the face of low estradiol levels, suggest pituitary or hypothalamic disease. In this latter setting, an elevated prolactin level would provide evidence for a pituitary tumor, whereas a normal level coupled with a normal sella x-ray would suggest a hypothalamic lesion (eg, anorexia nervosa or its variants).

With Normal Menses

For the infertile woman with normal menses, the major question is whether ovulation is occuring normally. Ovulation can be documented by charting basal body temperatures over several menstrual cycles or by a serum progesterone level over 3 ng/mL during the luteal phase. If ovulation is occurring, then the differential diagnosis of the infertility includes (1) anatomic obstruction, (2) short luteal phase, (3) abnormal cervical mucus, and (4) immunologic factors.

Multiple Endocrine Neoplasia Syndromes

Three autosomally dominant transmitted disorders are referred to as the multiple endocrine neoplasia syndromes (MENs). Patients with MEN 1 have functional tumors or hyperplasia of the parathyroid glands, islet cell tissue of the pancreas, and pituitary gland. Patients with MEN 2 (also called MEN 2a) have medullary carcinoma of the thyroid (MCT), which may be preceded by c-cell hyperplasia (CCH), parathyroid gland hyperplasia, and pheochromocytomas which may be preceded by adrenal medullary hyperplasia

(AMH). Patients with MEN 3 (also called MEN 2b) have MCT or CCH and pheochromocytomas or AMH, but lack hyperparathyroidism. As a general rule, all members of the same family will have the same syndrome, and the endocrine glands affected in any one family member will conform to those specific for one of the three MENs described above. Rarely, "overlap" presentations will occur when, for example, a patient may have pheochromocytomas and insulinomas.

Several aspects of the laboratory evaluation for the MENs have been discussed earlier in this chapter, and no further mention will be made of the evaluation for pituitary tumors, hyperparathyroidism, and insulinomas. The diagnosis of any of the component endocrine disorders may be more difficult in patients with MEN as these patients are more often asymptomatic and may have more subtle clinical presentations than do patients with the sporadic form of these tumors. The diagnosis of CCH and AMH may also be difficult as these lesions are "precursor lesions" of more obvious endocrine tumors. Since these syndromes are transmitted in an autosomal dominant fashion with a high degree of penetrance and the endocrine tumors associated with them have a significant rate of morbidity and mortality, laboratory evaluation ideally should be sensitive enough to detect the asymptomatic patient with a tumor or a "precursor lesion" and to screen family members who are at risk for developing these syndromes.

MEN 1

The evaluation of hyperparathyroidism, pituitary tumors, and insulinomas has already been presented. The other common endocrine tumor in this syndrome is the gastrinoma (see Chapter 13). When basal gastrin levels are inconclusive, gastrin stimulation tests are performed using secretin, calcium, and a standard meal.

Other functional pancreatic islet cell tumors present in patients with MEN 1 are rare and will not be discussed in this chapter. They include tumors which produce glucagon and vasoactive intestinal polypeptide.

MEN 2 (2a)

Patients with MEN 2 may have MCT or CCH, pheochromocytomas or AMH, and primary hyperparathyroidism (the evaluation of this last disorder has already been discussed). Unlike patients with sporadic MCT, who usually have a thyroid nodule and in whom basal serum calcitonin (CT) is almost invariably elevated, patients with MEN 2 and 3 may have normal basal serum CT levels. This is especially likely when CCH is present or when early MCT is detected by the screening of kindred members at risk for MEN 2 or 3. If basal serum CT is not elevated, stimulation tests with intravenous pentagastrin or calcium gluconate are performed either alone or in combination. Pentagastrin is given as a bolus of 0.5 mg/kg of body weight, and calcium gluconate is given as 2 mg/kg of body weight intravenously over one minute. Patient with MCT or CCH will have significantly higher stimulated CT values (usually above 300 pg/mL) than will normal patients. Although other tumors may have elevated basal CT levels, with stimulation testing, the CT levels will almost invariably fall below those of patients with MCT or CCH.

Patients with MEN 2 or 3 and pheochromocytomas or AMH are often normotensive except during crises, and the laboratory evaluation may require repeated determinations of all of the urine and plasma studies discussed earlier in this chapter (see Adrenal Gland) including spot urine determinations after an attack. In some kindreds, the 24-hour urine epinephrine secretion is the most sensitive test, whereas in other kindreds 24-hour urine VMA has been more sensitive. When baseline values and noninvasive radiographic studies are negative but the diagnosis is still suspected, glucagon stimulation testing has been advocated.

MEN 3 (2b)

Patients with MEN 3 should have the laboratory evaluation discussed above for MCT or CCH and for pheochromocytoma or AMH. All patients with MEN 3 have characteristic mucosal neuromas which should allow clinical identification and lead to evaluation for endocrine tumors.

Patients with MEN 2 and 3 must have a negative laboratory evaluation for pheochromocytoma before surgery for other endocrine lesions to avoid intraoperative pheochromocytoma crisis should this lesion not be recognized preoperatively.

Screening tests for MEN are important to identify the presence of MEN in a patient found to have a tumor of just one component endocrine organ and to identify family members of a patient with MEN who may also have the disorder. Table 17-19 lists recommendations for screening for the MENs.

Table 17-19
Screening for MENs

Screening for MEN 1
A. Screening for patients with a lesion involving just one component endocrine organ (recommendations are based upon the frequency with which MEN 1 occurs with each endocrine tumor)
   Primary hyperparathyroidism—history and physical examination only
   Gastrinoma—serum calcium, prolactin (and "coned down" views of the sella turcica)
   Insulinoma—history and physical examination, serum calcium
   Pituitary tumor—history and physical examination, serum calcium
B. Screening for family members at risk for MEN 1—serum calcium prolactin, gastrin (and "coned down" views of the sella turcica)

Screening for MEN 2 and 3 (2a and 2b)
A. Screening for patients with a tumor of one component endocrine gland
   Primary hyperparathyroidism—history and physical examination only
   Pheochromocytoma—serum calcium and calcitonin unless pheochromocytoma is bilateral; then evaluate as in B
   MCT—serum calcium and urine metanephrines, VMA, and/or fractionated catecholamines unless MCT is bilateral; then evaluate as in B
B. Screening of family members at risk for MEN 2 or 3 and for patients with bilateral pheochromocytomas or MCT—basal and stimulated CT, serum calcium, urine metanephrines, VMA, and fractionated catecholamines

---

Carcinoid Syndrome

The carcinoid syndrome arises when a hormonally active carcinoid tumor secretes its vasoactive products into the systemic circulation bypassing the liver which contains monoamine oxidase which degrades serotonin, the major product of carcinoid tumors. This occurs most commonly when primary bowel tumor has metastasized to the liver. When clinical suspicion of the carcinoid syndrome exists, the first laboratory study ordered is the qualitative urine screen for 5 hydroxyindoleacetic acid (5 HIAA), a metabolite of serotonin. Normal values are less than 10 mg per day, whereas the qualitative test will be positive in patients excreting more than 30 mg per day. If the qualitative test is negative but the diagnosis still remains likely, a quantitative test may detect the unusual patient with carcinoid syndrome who excretes between 10 and 30 mg of 5 HIAA in 24 hours. Episodic hormone secretion may occur, and a single normal study may be insufficient. A spot urine sample obtained after a characteristic carcinoid attack may be assayed for 5 HIAA and creatinine and be interpreted by extrapolating the 5 HIAA excretion upward for normal 24-hour urine creatinine excretion.

False-positive 5 HIAA results occur in patients (1) with nontropical sprue who may excrete up to 25 mg per day; (2) who consume large amounts of bananas, avocados, red plums, pineapples, and eggplants; and (3) who receive glycerol guiacolate or reserpine. False-negative 5 HIAA results occur in patients (1) with small bowel obstruction; (2) with very recent small bowel surgery; (3) with malabsorption; (4) with limited oral intake of vitamin B_6 and tryptophan; and (5) receiving phenothiazines, methyldopa and Mandelamine. Urine must be collected in acid, and creatinine should be determined to assess the adequacy of the urine collection.

Patients with gastric carcinoid tumors may be unable to convert the serotonin precursor 5 hydroxytryptophan (5 HTP) to 5 hydroxytryptamine (5 HT or serotonin). Such patients have high serum and urine 5 HTP levels while urine 5 HIAA may be normal. Additionally, these patients may have increased serum and urine histamine levels. 5 HT levels can be measured in plasma, and platelets and are often increased in patients with the carcinoid syndrome unless the gastric carcinoid syndrome is present. Patients with functional bronchial carcinoid tumors may have elevated levels of 5 HIAA, 5 HTP, and 5 HT and may have associated ectopic hormone syndromes with high levels of a wide variety of polypeptides including, most notably, adrenocorticotropic hormone, calcitonin, and growth hormone.

■ Selected Readings

General

Alsever RN, Gotlin RW: *Handbook of Endocrine Tests in Adults and Children.* ed 2. Chicago, Year Book Medical Publishers, 1978.

Cryer PE: *Diagnostic Endocrinology.* ed 2. New York, Oxford University Press, 1979.

Felig P, Baxter JD, Broadus AE, et al (eds): *Endocrinology and Metabolism.* New York, McGraw-Hill Book Co, 1981.

Williams RH (ed): *Textbook of Endocrinology.* ed 6. Philadelphia, The W.B. Saunders Co, 1981.

Pituitary

Cohen KL: Metabolic, endocrine, and drug-induced interference with pituitary function tests: A review. *Metabolism.* 1977; 26:1165–1177.

Irie M, Tsushima P: Increase of serum growth hormone concentration following thyrotropin releasing hormone injection in patients with acromegaly or gigantism. *J Clin Endocrinol Metab* 1972;35:97–100.

Kleinberg DL, Noel GL, Frantz AG: Galactorrhea: A study of 235 cases, including 48 with pituitary tumors. *N Engl J Med* 1977;296: 589–600.

Lawrence AM, Goldfine ID, Kirsteins L: Growth hormone dynamics in acromegaly. *J Clin Endocrinol Metab* 1970;31:239–247.

Lin T, Tucci JR: Provocative tests of growth hormone release—a comparison of results with seven stimuli. *Ann Int Med* 1974;80:464– 469.

Lindholm J, Kehlet H, Blichert-Toft M, et al: Reliability of the 30 minute ACTH test in assessing hypothalamic-pituitary-adrenal function. *J Clin Endocrinol Metab* 1978;47:272–274.

Miller M, Dalakos T, Moses AM, et al: Recognition of partial defects in antidiuretic hormone secretion. *Ann Intern Med* 1970;73:721–729.

Staub JS, Noelpp B, Girard J, et al: The short metyrapone test: Comparison of the plasma ACTH response to metyrapone and insulin-induced hypoglycemia. *Clin Endocrinol* 1979;10: 595–601.

Zerbe RL, Robertson GL: Comparison of plasma vasopressin measurements with a standard indirect test in the differential diagnosis of polyuria. *N Engl J Med* 1981;305: 1539–1546.

Thyroid

Birkhauser M, Burer T, Busset R, et al: Diagnosis of hyperthyroidism when serum thyroxine alone is raised. *Lancet* 1977;2:53–56.

Chopra IJ, VanHerle AJ, Chua Teco GN, et al: Serum free thyroxine in thyroidal and nonthyroidal illnesses: A comparison of measurements by radioimmunoassay, equilibrium dialysis, and free thyroxine index. *J Clin Endocrinol Metab* 1980;51:135–143.

Schimmel M, Utiger RD: Thyroidal and peripheral production of thyroid hormones: review of recent findings and their clinical implications. *Ann Intern Med* 1977;87:760–768.

Parathyroids and Calcium Metabolism

Hypercalcemia

Bijvoet OLM: Kidney function in calcium and phosphate metabolism, in Avioli LV, Krane SM (eds): *Metabolic Bone Disease,* volume 1. New York, Academic Press Inc, 1977.

Broadus AE, Dominguez M, Bartter FC: Pathophysiologic studies in idiopathic hypercalciuria: Use of an oral calcium tolerance test to characterize distinctive subgroups. *J Clin Endocrinol Metab* 1978;47:751.

European PTH Study Group: Interlaboratory comparison of radioimunological parathyroid hormone determination. *Eur J Clin Invest* 1978;8:149.

Habener JF, Segre GV: Parathyroid hormone radioimmunoassay. *Ann Intern Med* 1979;91:782.

Raisz LG, Yajnik CH, Bockman RS, et al: Comparison of commercially available parathyroid hormone immunoassays in the differential diagnosis of hypercalcemia due to primary hyperparathyroidism or malignancy. *Ann Intern Med* 1979;91:739.

Hypocalcemia

Juan D: Hypocalcemia—differential diagnosis and mechanisms. *Arch Intern Med* 1979;139:1166.

Hypophosphatemia

Knochel JP: The pathophysiology and clinical characteristics of severe hypophosphatemia. *Arch Intern Med* 1977;137:203.

Hypomagnesemia and Hypermagnesemia

Massry SG, Seelig MS: Hypomagnesemia and hypermagnesemia. *Clin Nephrol* 1977;7:147.

Rude RK, Singer FR: Magnesium deficiency and excess. *Annu Rev Med* 1981; 32:245.

Metabolic Bone Disease
Frame B, Parfitt AM; Osteomalacia: Current concepts. *Ann Intern Med* 1978; 89:966.

Goldring SR, Krane SM: Metabolic bone disease: Osteoporosis and osteomalacia. *Disease-a-Month* 1981; 27:1.

Thomson DL, Frame B: Involutional osteopenia: Current concepts. *Ann Intern Med* 1976;85:789.

Paget's Disease
Wallach S, et al: *Paget's disease of bone.* Phoenix, Arizona, Armour Pharmaceutical co, 1979.

Nephrolithiasis
Broadus AE, Thier SO: Metabolic basis of renal stone disease. *N Engl J Med* 1979;300:839.

Coe FL, Favus MJ: Idiopathic hypercalciuria in calcium nephrolithiasis. *Disease-a-Month* 1980;26:1.

Adrenal Gland

Cushing's Syndrome
Crapo L: Cushing's syndrome: A review of diagnostic tests. *Metabolism* 1979;28:955.

Gold EM: The Cushing's syndromes: Changing views of diagnosis and treatment. *Ann Intern Med* 1979;90:829.

Hankin ME, Theile HM, Steinbeck AW: An evaluation of laboratory tests for the detection and differential diagnosis of Cushing's syndrome. *Clin Endocrinol* 1977;6:185.

Adrenal Insufficiency
Dluhy RG, Himathongkam T, Greenfield M: Rapid ACTH test with plasma aldosterone levels—improved diagnostic discrimination. *Ann Intern Med* 1974; 80:693.

Gwinup G, Johnson B: Clinical testing of hypothalamic-pituitary-adrenocortical system in states of hypo- and hypercortisolism. *Metabolism* 1975;24:777.

Rose LI, Williams GH, Jager PI, et al: The 48-hour adrenocorticotrophin infusion test for adrenocortical insufficiency. *Ann Intern Med* 1970;73:49.

Sheridan P, Mattingly D: Simultaneous investigation and treatment of suspected acute adrenal insufficiency. *Lancet* 1975; 2:676.

Hyperaldosteronism
Grim CE, Weinberger MH, Higgins JT, et al: Diagnosis of secondary forms of hypertension—a comprehensive protocol. *JAMA* 1977;237:1331.

Streeten DHP, Tomycz N, Anderson GH Jr: Reliability of screening methods for the diagnosis of primary aldosteronism. *Am J Med* 1979;67:403.

Weinberger MH, Grim CE, Hollifield JW, et al: Primary aldosteronism: Diagnosis, localization and treatment. *Ann Intern Med* 1979;90:386.

Hypoaldosteronism
DeFronzo RA: Hyperkalemia and hyporeninemic hypoaldosteronism. *Kidney Intern* 1980;17:118.

Phelps KR, Lieberman RL, Oh MS, et al: Pathophysiology of the syndrome of hyporeninemic hypoaldosteronism. *Metabolism* 1980;29:186.

Congenital Adrenal Hyperplasia
Kaplan SA: Diseases of the adrenal cortex II—congenital adrenal hyperplasia. *Pediatr Clin North Am* 1979;26:77.

Migeon CJ: Diagnosis and management of congenital adrenal hyperplasia. *Hosp Pract* 1977;12:75.

Pheochromocytoma
Bravo EL, Tarazi RC, Gifford RW, et al: Circulating and urinary catecholamines in pheochromocytoma—diagnostic and pathophysiologic implication. *N Engl J Med* 1979;301:682.

Kaplan NM, Kramer NJ, Holland OB, et al: Single-voided urine metanephrine assays in screening for pheochromocytoma. *Arch Intern Med* 1977;137:190.

Manger WM, Gifford RW: Current concepts of pheochromocytoma. *Cardiovascular Med* March 1978, p 289.

Plouin PF, Duclos JM, Menard J, et al: Biochemical tests for the diagnosis of phaeochromocytoma: Urinary versus plasma determinations. *Br Med J* 1981; 282:853.

Remine WH, Chong GC, VanHeerden JA, et al: Current management of pheochromocytoma. *Ann Surg* 1974;179: 740.

Gonads

Anderson DC: The role of sex hormone binding globulin in health and disease, in James VHT, Serio M, Giusti G (eds): *The Endocrine Function of the Human Ovary*. London, Academic Press Inc, 1976, pp 141–158.

Santner SJ, Murray FT, Davis B, et al: The integrated gonadotropin test. *Ann Intern Med* 1978;89:512–513.

Multiple Endocrine Neoplasia Syndromes

Ballard HS, Frame B, Harstock RJ: Familial multiple endocrine adenoma-peptic ulcer complex. *Medicine* 1964;43: 481.

Deveney CW, Deveney KS, Way LW: The Zollinger-Ellison syndrome—23 years later. *Ann Surg* 1978;188:384.

Khairi MRA, Dexter RN, Burzynski NJ, et al: Mucosal neuroma, pheochromocytoma and medullary thyroid carcinoma: MEN type III. *Medicine* 1973;54:89.

Rude RK, Singer FR: Comparison of serum levels after a one-minute calcium injection and after pentagastrin injection in the diagnosis of medullary thyroid cancer. *J Clin Endocrinol Metab* 1977; 44:980.

Samaan NA, Castillo S, Schultz PN, et al: Serum calcitonin after pentagastrin stimulation in patients with broncho-genic and breast carcinoma compared to that in patients with medullary thyroid carcinoma. *J Clin Endocrinol Metab* 1980;51:237.

Steiner AL, Goodman AD, Powers SR: Study of a kindred with pheochromocytoma, medullary thyroid carcinoma, hyperparathyroidism, and Cushing's disease: MEN, type II. *Medicine* 1968; 47:371.

Carcinoid

Grahame-Smith DG: Natural history and diagnosis of the carcinoid syndrome. *Clin Gastroenterol* 1974;3:575.

The practice of oncology depends upon the practice of good internal medicine with its required knowledge of general laboratory evaluation. Nonetheless, several tests, primarily useful for management of patients with cancer, may help in diagnosis, prognosis, therapy, response to therapy, and prediction of recurrence. We classify these tests as biologic tumor markers, enzymes, hormonal receptors, and routine tests useful in the appropriate metastatic workup.

CEA

Serum carcinoembryonic antigen (CEA) levels are elevated in 70% to 90% of patients with disseminated gastrointestinal adenocarcinomas. CEA is also elevated in other advanced neoplastic conditions such as breast cancer, neuroblastoma, and all cell types of lung cancer. Nonneoplastic conditions such as inflammatory bowel disease, alcoholic cirrhosis, pancreatitis, and diverticulitis are also associated with an elevated CEA, and smokers have a slight increase. Thus, the sensitivity and specificity are inadequate for screening purposes. At present, the use of CEA is standard only in the diagnosis, the prognosis, and the follow-up of colorectal carcinoma. Preoperative CEA levels have been shown to correlate directly with stage of disease (Dukes' C and D), size of the primary tumor, and grade of the tumor. A postoperative CEA level is helpful prognostically, and, if all the malignant tissue has been removed, the CEA level should be normal by six weeks after the operation. If the CEA does not fall to a normal level, nearly all of these patients will show a subsequent rise of titer and later have clinical tumor relapse. If the CEA levels become normal postoperatively, the patients should then be followed clinically and with serial CEA levels. Many studies have shown that there may be a progressive rise in CEA levels which precedes clinical relapse by 4 to 10 months. In one study, 97% of patients with recurrent colorectal carcinoma had elevated CEA levels, and in 75% of these the rising levels preceded the clinical symptoms of recurrent tumor by 5 to 6 months. The same study showed that a slow rise in which concentrations remained under 75 μg/L for 12 months was associated with local recurrence and a better prognosis, whereas a rapid rise to over 100 μg/L in 6 months was more commonly associated with metastatic spread and a poorer prognosis. A decrease in CEA level correlates with an objective partial response in colorectal patients treated with chemotherapy and the survival of these patients is significantly increased over those with no change or increasing CEA levels. In summary, the CEA level is most valuable in colorectal carcinoma in predicting prognosis and in follow-up evaluation.

18

The Laboratory in Oncology

Arthur P. Staddon

hCG

Human chorionic gonadotropin (hCG) is the ideal biologic tumor marker, since its levels rise with the development of malignant disease and disappear with curative treatment. In women with the diagnosis of hydatidiform mole, weekly hCG assays are followed. If the levels become undetectable at eight weeks, the prognosis is excellent. Rising levels of hCG predict malignant sequelae, and the patient should be evaluated. If the disease is confined to the pelvis or is metastatic only to the lung, single-agent chemotherapy is given at two-week intervals, and therapy is evaluated by following weekly hCG levels. Therapy should be continued until the hCG level is undetectable for three consecutive weeks. Curability using this approach should be nearly 100%. Patients who have hCG titers of greater than 100,000 per 24-hour urine collection often have liver and brain metastases and are at high risk for failing single-agent chemotherapy. These patients should be treated with combination chemotherapy. This is an example of quantitative titers predicting prognosis and directing therapy.

A second area in oncology where the measurement of hCG is valuable is testicular cancer. Until recently, the assays for hCG were insensitive and nonspecific as luteinizing hormone and follicle-stimulating hormone both have alpha subunits which are immunologically similar to the alpha subunit of hCG. The beta subunit of hCG is unique to each of these peptides, so that sensitive radioimmunoassays for the beta subunit of hCG are now available. This enables one to use the beta-hCG assay in testicular cancer where levels may be much lower than those seen in gestational trophoblastic disease, as discussed above. Many studies have shown that 40% to 60% of patients with nonseminomatous germ cell tumors will have a positive beta subunit hCG. The hCG has been localized to the syncytiotrophoblastic cells of choriocarcinoma and in tumor giant cells seen in association with embryonic carcinoma. Between 5% and 20% of patients with pure seminoma will have an elevated beta hCG level, and the prognosis of these patients does not appear to differ from the prognosis of pure seminoma patients without elevated hCG levels. As the biologic half-life of hCG is 18–24 hours, serial levels can be followed soon after orchiectomy. Patients with persistent elevations of beta hCG have stage II or stage III disease. If the beta hCG continues to be elevated after a lymphadenectomy when no tumor was identified, then the patient has stage III disease. In essence, the evaluation of testicular cancer by markers improves the accuracy of our clinical staging. The response to therapy can be most effectively monitored by serially measuring serum beta hCG. When therapy is effective there is a rapid decrease of the hCG, which will become undetectable with continued response. Recurrence can be detected by rising hCG levels often months before recurrence is otherwise clinically detectable. In summary, assay of beta hCG in testicular cancer is valuable in diagnosis, in staging, in evaluation of response to therapy, and in detection of recurrence.

Alpha Feto Protein

Alpha feto protein is a serum alpha-1-globulin with a biologic half-life of five days that is synthesized in fetal life in the yolk sac, the liver, and the gastrointestinal tract. With a sensitive radioimmunoassay, alpha feto protein is present in low levels in normal persons. Elevated levels of alpha feto protein are found in patients with hepatoma, in nonseminomatous germ cell malignancies, and, to a lesser extent, in malignancies of the gastrointestinal tract, pancreas, lung, and breast. Alpha feto protein levels may also be elevated in conditions associated with liver regeneration such as hepatitis, cirrhosis, and metastatic liver disease. Elevated levels of alpha feto protein may also be found transiently during a normal pregnancy as it crosses the placenta. Alpha feto protein has become useful as a biological marker in patients with hepatoma and nonseminomatous testicular carcinoma as a direct result of the development of a sensitive radioimmunoassay. In nonseminomatous testicular carcinoma, 70% of patients had elevated levels of serum alpha feto protein; the majority of these were under 3000 ng/mL, not detectable by previous methods. There have been no cases of pure seminoma with elevated serum alpha feto protein, and an elevation of alpha feto protein in this setting suggests nonseminomatous elements and a poorer prognosis. About 90% of nonseminomatous testicular tumors will have an elevated level of beta hCG and/or alpha feto protein. An elevated serum alpha feto protein in testicular carcinoma has clinical significance similar to that of an elevated beta hCG as noted above. One must remember that the biologic half-life of alpha feto protein is five days, and postorchiectomy serum to follow alpha feto protein levels should not be drawn at intervals of less than a week. Persistent elevation implies stage II or stage III disease, and persistent elevation after a pathologically negative lymphadenectomy implies stage III disease. Effective therapy causes the alpha feto protein levels to fall to normal levels, and recurrence can be detected by rising levels.

In patients with primary hepatocellular carcinoma, 81% have elevated levels of alpha feto protein, and 62% have levels greater than 1200 ng/mL. In contrast, only 15% of patients with metastatic liver carcinoma have elevated levels, with all but one patient having levels below 1200 ng/mL. The same study noted higher levels of alpha feto protein in patients with hepatoma who were hepatitis B surface antigen positive. The serum level falls to normal after the successful surgical resection of a hepatoma and rises with recurrence. In summary, serum alpha feto protein is helpful in diagnosis, in following response to therapy, and in detecting recurrence in both primary hepatocellular carcinoma and nonseminomatous testicular carcinoma.

Acid Phosphatase

Serum acid phosphatase has been a part of the evaluation of patients with prostatic cancer, and its elevation is associated with disseminated disease. Serum acid phosphatase is a measurement of a group of enzymes located in the prostate gland, liver, spleen, bone, kidney, leukocytes, and erythrocytes which have phosphatase activity at an acid pH. As each enzyme is immunologically unique, several new techniques including radioimmunoassay and counterimmunoelectrophoresis have been developed that specifically measure prostatic acid phosphatase. These techniques provide vastly improved sensitivity and reveal elevation in a fair percentage of patients with early stages of the disease, when the tumor is still localized and potentially curable. Only a small number of surgically staged patients have prostatic acid phosphatase levels, but these results suggest that 50% of stage B patients (tumor confined to the prostate by clinical staging) to 90% of stage D patients (distant dissemination of tumor) have elevated prostatic acid phosphatase levels. Thus, the prostatic acid phosphatase is a much more sensitive test, especially in the early stages of the disease. Most studies have shown that the prostatic acid phosphatase is also extremely specific. There have been some suggestions that the prostatic acid phosphatase may be a screening test for prostatic carcinoma, enabling disease to be detected at an earlier, potentially curable stage. However, as the incidence of the disease is low, the positive predictive value (the probability that a person with a positive test actually has the disease) of the new assays is low; therefore, prostatic acid phosphatase is not a good screening test. Since the prostatic acid phosphatase is elevated in many patients with local disease, it is not a reliable predictor of metastatic disease. If the prostatic acid phosphatase is elevated, further evaluation to determine the extent of disease is indicated and would usually include diagnostic imaging techniques. Acid phosphatase and prostatic acid phosphatase have been used to follow the response to therapy in advanced prostatic carcinoma, but it has been shown that the levels may fluctuate without treatment and therefore serial levels are not reliable in following disease. As there is no easy way to follow response in advanced prostate carcinoma, evaluation of new chemotherapeutic protocols is difficult. In summary, the value of prostatic acid phosphatase is in predicting malignant disease of the prostate, without accurately predicting metastatic disease, or indicating reliably the response to therapy.

Receptors in Breast Cancer

Endocrine therapy can cause objective remission and prolongation of life in approximately one-third of patients with advanced breast cancer, but until the recent availability of assays specific for estrogen and progesterone receptors, it was difficult to predict who would respond. These assays now allow more accurate prediction of both response to hormonal manipulation and prognosis. The steroid hormones, including estrogens and progestins, diffuse into the cells of responsive tissues (uterus, vagina, and some breast cancers) and bind with the receptor protein. The steroid receptor complex enters the nucleus and interacts to stimulate the production of messenger RNA that codes for the synthesis of new protein. It is thought that cells with estrogen receptor in the presence of estrogen allow for the production of the progesterone receptor. McGuire feels that the presence of a progesterone receptor in a tumor shows that the tumor cells are able to synthesize a biologic end product under estrogen stimulation, and this suggests that endocrine responses are still intact. In contrast, tumor cells with estrogen receptors that lack progesterone receptors may have lost some or all of their biologic endocrine responsiveness and may be less responsive to endocrine manipulation. In clinical practice, patients with positive estrogen receptors and positive progesterone receptors have a 67% to 80% response to endocrine therapy as opposed to a response of about 30% for estrogen receptor-positive, progesterone receptor-negative patients. Estrogen receptors have been measured routinely on breast cancer tissue for the past seven years, and progesterone receptors have been measured more recently. The receptors are measured by homogenizing the cells and incubating them with radioactively labeled estrogen or progesterone and then measuring the concentration of label in the cytosol directly. It has been shown that the response to endocrine therapy is directly related to the amount of estrogen receptor present in the breast cancer. If the estrogen receptor is present in amounts greater than 100 fmol/mg protein, then the response rate is about 80%. If the receptor is absent or is less than 3 fmol/mg, the response rate is under 12%. Values between 3–100 fmol/mg give about 45% objective response, although some laboratories consider 3–10 fmol/mg as borderline positive. Overall, there is about a 50% objective response in estrogen receptor-positive patients. As discussed above, patients who have both positive estrogen receptors and progesterone receptors have about an 80% objective response, with up to 90% getting benefit from endocrine therapy. In estrogen receptor-positive, progesterone receptor-negative patients the response is about 27%, and in estrogen receptor-negative patients the response is under 10%.

Endocrine therapy includes adding hormones (estrogen, progestins, and androgens) as well as ablative therapy (oophorectomy, adrenalectomy, and antiestrogens). The specific choice of endocrine therapy chosen for patients with positive receptors depends on the menopausal status, the sites of metastatic disease, and the associated side effects. In summary, the most important aspect of endocrine receptors in breast cancer is in more accurately predicting response to hormonal therapy. To do this most accurately, the assays should be done on tumor from a metastatic site at the time of treatment, if the tissue is easily available, as the tumor may dedifferentiate at the time of metastases. If new tissue is not readily available, then the results of prior receptor assays are used in choosing therapy.

Estrogen receptors also have significance as a prognostic indicator. When patients are comparably matched for tumor size, location, nodal status, age, and menopausal status, the patients who are estrogen receptor positive have a better prognosis than those who are estrogen receptor negative. In several large studies, 20% of estrogen receptor-positive patients developed metastatic disease at 36 months, as opposed to 55% of a comparable group of estrogen receptor-negative patients. In other words, the patients who are estrogen receptor negative have more aggressive disease with an associated poorer prognosis. As estrogen receptor-negative patients have such an appreciably higher risk of metastatic disease, they should be more aggressively treated with adjuvant chemotherapy. It is clear that premenopausal women with positive axillary nodes benefit from one year of adjuvant chemotherapy with a prolonged, disease-free survival. There is strong evidence that postmenopausal women with positive nodes have prolonged disease-free survival if the adjuvant chemotherapy is given in greater than 85% of the ideal doses. In estrogen receptor-negative patients who have breast cancer that has spread to the nodes, the maximum doses of adjuvant chemotherapy should be used, if possible. There is some feeling that estrogen receptor-negative, stage I patients (small tumors without involved nodes) and stage II patients (large tumors) who have negative nodes might benefit from adjuvant chemotherapy. This is currently being studied. In addition, estrogen receptor-positive patients with a high risk of recurrence may benefit from the addition of hormonal therapy to the adjuvant chemotherapy, and this approach is also undergoing study. One early report showed a benefit from the addition of tamoxifen to L-phenylalanine mustard and 5-fluorouracil in postmenopausal women with positive estrogen receptors. Other studies are in progress using cyclophosphamide, methotrexate, 5-fluorouracil, and tamoxifen. There are some early data suggesting there may be benefits from the addition of a second hormone (such as an androgen). The use of estrogen receptors as a predictor of response to chemotherapy is an area of controversy. Initial studies suggested that estrogen receptor-negative patients had a significantly greater response to chemotherapy. There are now several studies, and estrogen receptor status does not seem to be a clear predictor of response to chemotherapy. In summary, steroid receptors are helpful in predicting response to hormones, and they are an independent prognostic indicator.

■ Selected Readings

Holyoke ED, Block GE, Jensen E, et al: Biologic markers in cancer diagnosis and treatment. *Curr Probl Cancer* 1981; 6:1–42.

Javadpour N: The role of biologic markers in testicular cancer. *Cancer* 1980;45:1755–1761.

McGuire WL: Steroid receptors and breast cancer. *Hosp Pract* 1980;15: 83–88.

Perez CA, Knapp RC, Young RC: Gynecologic tumors, in DeVita VT, Hellman S, Rosenberg SA (eds): *Cancer: Principles and Practice of Oncology.* Philadelphia, J.B. Lippincott, 1982, pp 872–874.

Sugarbaker PH, Dunnick NR, Sugarbaker EV: Diagnosis and staging, in DeVita VT, Hellman S, Rosenberg SA (eds): *Cancer: Principles and Practice of Oncology.* Philadelphia, J.B. Lippincott, 1982, pp 248–254.

Wood CB, Ratcliffe JG, Burt RW, et al: The clinical significance of the pattern of elevated serum carcinoembryonic antigen (CEA) levels in recurrent colorectal cancer. *Br J Surg* 1980;67:46–48.

19

■ Pregnancy Testing

Pregnancy tests measure the concentration, or detect the presence, in a woman's serum or urine, of a specific product of the syncytiotrophoblast of the placenta. In theory, any such specific product, such as estriol or placental lactogen, could be used, but in practice all currently used pregnancy tests detect human chorionic gonadotropin (hCG).

The earliest pregnancy tests were bioassays, based on the effects of hCG on the ovaries of various animal species. These have been supplanted by the cheaper, more convenient immunoassays. Two types of immunoassays are commonly used: the rapid, qualitative agglutination inhibition assays and the radioimmunoassays, which are potentially quantitative and which now approach some agglutination inhibition assays in speed.

Agglutination inhibition assays are most often used with urine specimens. hCG is readily excreted in urine, and its concentration in a first morning urine is generally of the same order of magnitude as the serum concentration. The assay is based on the ability of free hCG in urine to compete with hCG irreversibly bound to latex particles for binding sites on an antibody to hCG. The amounts of antibody and latex-bound hCG are held constant. If no free hCG is present in the urine, the antigen-antibody reaction will cause the latex particles to agglutinate or form clumps. If enough free hCG is present in the urine, it will occupy the binding sites on the antibody and prevent agglutination of latex particles; hence, *agglutination inhibition*. The minimum concentration of hCG in the urine necessary to inhibit agglutination is the *analytic sensitivity* of the test and varies widely among test kits.

A typical slide test kit has an analytic sensitivity of 2000 U/L, corresponding to the levels of hCG usually present six to seven weeks after the last menstrual period. Results are available within a few minutes. These tests are easily interpreted with some experience and are satisfactory for office use. A typical tube test kit has an analytic sensitivity of 250 U/L, corresponding to five to six weeks after the last menstrual period. Results are available within two hours.

Specificity can limit the usefulness of some agglutination inhibition assays. Antibodies to hCG can often cross-react with pituitary hormones, especially luteinizing hormone (LH) and thyrotropin (TSH). This can lead to false-positive results during the midcycle LH surge, in perimenopausal women with high LH levels, and in some thyroid disorders with high TSH levels. In case of doubt, a more specific test should be used.

Antibodies to the beta subunit of hCG (β-hCG) are generally more specific than antibodies to the whole hCG molecule. Radioimmunoassay kits generally use these antibodies, as do

Donald R. Coustan
Richard D. Plotz

some agglutination inhibition assay kits. Thus, radioimmunoassays can detect much lower levels of hCG, typically 5–10 U/L, without danger of false-positive results from LH or TSH. The principle of the radioimmunoassay is similar to that of the agglutination inhibition assay: β-hCG in the serum or urine to be tested competes with a constant amount of radioactively labeled β-hCG for a constant number of antibody binding sites. Antigen-antibody complexes are isolated, usually by centrifugation, and the amount of radioactivity is measured in a gamma counter. The less radioactivity present, the more unlabeled β-hCG was present in the serum or urine tested. A series of standards with known β-hCG concentrations can be tested along with patient specimens, and the concentration of β-hCG in the patient specimens can be determined. When a radioimmunoassay is used for serum pregnancy testing, a cutoff level of 25–30 U/L is usually used as the criterion for a positive test. This corresponds to about the time of the missed menstrual period.

Radioimmunoassays require a gamma counter, which is usually present only in hospital or commercial laboratories, and they are therefore less readily available than the less sensitive agglutination inhibition assays. The one to three weeks saved in diagnosis of pregnancy can be important, however, especially for women with a history of spontaneous abortions or ectopic pregnancies, or for women who desire an elective abortion.

The quantitative determination of β-hCG is useful also in monitoring trophoblastic disease and in diagnosis of ectopic pregnancy. After diagnosis of hydatidiform mole, serial determinations of β-hCG are the best single prognostic indicator, with a steady decrease to undetectable levels within a few months a favorable sign. Similar criteria can be used to monitor the response to chemotherapy for choriocarcinoma or invasive mole.

Kadar et al (1981) applied hCG measurements to the diagnosis of ectopic pregnancy in conjunction with sonographic findings. In the presence of an intrauterine sac on sonography, 43 of 43 patients with intrauterine pregnancies had serum hCG levels > 6500 U/L, whereas 2 of 2 patients with ectopic pregnancies had levels < 6000 U/L. If no sac was present, higher hCG levels were associated with a *greater* likelihood of ectopic pregnancy, but this association was statistically insignificant.

■ Hematology in Pregnancy

Volume Changes (Figure 19-1)

Plasma volume in the nonpregnant woman approximates 2500 mL, or about 40 mL/kg of body weight. During pregnancy this volume increases dramatically, reaching approximately 3600 mL (58 mL/kg) by term. This approximately 45% increase begins as early as the 10th week of pregnancy and reaches its maximum by 30–34 weeks. Patients with hypertensive complications of pregnancy may increase their plasma volume less than normal healthy pregnant women. On the other hand, patients with multiple pregnancies may have startlingly increased plasma volume compared with single pregnancies.

Red Cell Mass

Red cell mass also increases during pregnancy, but not as dramatically as plasma volume. The normal healthy nonpregnant subject has a red cell mass of approximately 1350 mL. This rises by approximately 250 mL by the third trimester, rising progressively without a plateau. Thus, the increment is approximately 18%. If iron supplements are given to the pregnant woman, the increase in red cell mass almost doubles to about 400 mL. By adding the plasma volume to the red cell mass it can be seen that the total blood volume increases by approximately 38% in the course of pregnancy.

Hemoglobin and Hematocrit

The hematocrit and hemoglobin change predictably with the changes in plasma volume and red cell mass. If the average nonpregnant woman's hematocrit is approximately 39%, a progressive fall occurs until at 30 weeks the hematocrit averages 34%. Hemoglobin levels decline similarly. From an

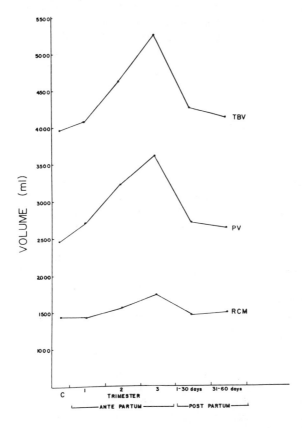

Figure 19-1 Changes in total blood volume (TBV), plasma volume (PV), and red cell mass (RCM) during and after pregnancy. Figures are the composite value derived from studies of several investigators. Reprinted with permission from Lange and Dynesius: *Clin Hematol* 1973;2:437.

average of approximately 13.5 g/dL before pregnancy hemoglobin progressively declines to an average of 11.5 g/dL at the 30th week with a possible slight rise during the last 10 weeks. Criteria used to trigger an anemia
workup will differ from center to center, but usually, a hemoglobin of 11
g/dL or a hematocrit of 30% or less would be grounds for further evaluation.

Anemia Evaluation

The reticulocyte count is often used to distinguish abnormal destruction of
red cells (elevated reticulocyte count) from subnormal production (low or
normal reticulocyte count) in the face of anemia. Since approximately 1% of
the total circulating red cells are replaced daily, the expected reticulocyte
count is 1%. This does not change drastically during pregnancy.

Iron deficiency anemia accounts for approximately two-thirds of the cases
of anemia diagnosed during pregnancy. The typical nonpregnant normal
serum iron level of 120 μg/dL declines as pregnancy progresses to an average
of 80 μg/dL in the third trimester. Some of this fall can be prevented with
iron supplementation. However, individual values as low as 40 μg/dL have
been reported in normal pregnancy. These fluctuations may be related to the
previously mentioned changes in plasma volume as well as the presence of
iron deficiency. In addition, it should be cautioned that serum iron can be
transiently elevated for several hours after the ingestion of iron-containing
medications. Therefore, measurement is best in the morning with no recent
oral iron intake. Transferrin, measured as total iron-binding capacity, normally varies between 250–400 μg/dL. Serum transferrin usually increases by
about 15% in normal pregnant women who are not iron deficient. Iron deficiency is diagnosed when the percentage of saturation of transferrin (iron
divided by total iron-binding capacity) falls below 20%, iron sufficiency
usually being accompanied by ratios of 25% to 35%. Caution should be ex-
ercised in interpreting low iron/total iron-binding capacity ratios in the
presence of total iron-binding capacity levels in the low or low normal
range. Such values may be found in chronic infection, chronic inflammatory
disease, or malignancy. The total iron-binding capacity may also be depressed by poor protein nutrition, but the serum iron level is usually normal
or elevated in such cases. Although the definitive diagnosis of iron deficiency is based upon the demonstration of absent bone marrow iron stores,
such histologic confirmation is rarely justified in the pregnant woman. A
therapeutic trial of oral iron therapy would be a more reasonable approach.
Serum ferritin concentration has been assessed as an index of the status of
iron stores. In general, high serum ferritin correlates with high iron stores. A
cross-sectional study of 80 patients at various stages of pregnancy suggests
that average serum ferritin rises by approximately 50% in the first trimester
(from 63 ng/mL in the nonpregnant state to approximately 97 ng/mL), but
then falls dramatically to approximately 22 ng/mL in the second trimester
and 15 ng/mL in the third trimester. This suggests that in the normal pregnant woman iron stores are depleted as pregnancy progresses.

Red blood cell indexes do not appear to change significantly during
pregnancy, but osmotic fragility increases progressively. When megaloblastic anemia occurs during pregnancy, it is generally due to folic acid deficiency, pernicious anemia being exceedingly rare in the gravid woman. In

the development of folate deficiency, decrease in serum folate is the first measureable manifestation. Although serum folate has been shown to fall during pregnancy, it is not clear that such a fall is "normal," unless one considers a folate deficiency to be normal for pregnancy. Since the fall in serum folate occurs long before anemia develops, diminished serum folate in the presence of anemia is not diagnostic for folate deficiency anemia. Because of the frequent coexistence of iron deficiency and folate deficiency anemias, reliance on red blood cell indexes is inappropriate in differentiating macrocytic from microcytic states. A look at the peripheral smear may reveal the mixed population of red cells characteristic of combined deficiencies. The appearance of hypersegmented neutrophils remains a valid sign of folic acid deficiency in pregnancy. The measurement of red cell folic acid may be the most accurate biochemical test of folate deficiency anemia, and red cell folate levels are probably not changed by pregnancy in the presence of adequate folate intake. Because a fall in red cell folate levels is a late consequence of folate deficiency, normal values do not rule out the presence of an evolving deficiency state. With universal prenatal vitamin use (400 μg or more per day), folate deficiency anemia is unusual. Exceptions include states of increased red cell turnover, such as hemoglobinopathies.

Hemoglobin electrophoresis, a standard diagnostic test for hemoglobinopathies, is unaffected by pregnancy. However, it is important to be aware that women with thalassemia minor may become quite anemic during pregnancy, perhaps due to folate deficiency.

Leukocytes

Leukocyte counts appear to rise from an average of 6,000–7,000 mm³/mL to approximately 10,000/mL at term, with a normal range from 5,000–17,000/mL at this time. This mostly reflects an elevated neutrophil number, although monocytes have also been reported to rise (Figure 19-2).

Platelets

Platelet counts, on the other hand, tend to fall throughout the course of pregnancy, averaging 278 ± 75/mL $\times 10^{-3}$ by term. The explanation for this is most likely the previously mentioned gestational increase in blood volume.

■ Amniotic Fluid Bilirubin

Bilirubin in amniotic fluid may reflect fetal hemolysis, as occurs with maternal isoimmunization. The usual measurement is of the net absorbance of amniotic fluid at a wavelength of 450 nm measured by drawing a straight baseline on a spectrophotometric tracing between the points at 365 and 550 nm and subtracting the baseline from the height of the actual curve at 450 nm (Figure 19-3). The difference is reported as change in absorbance at 450 nm. Liley (1961) determined the points at which vigilance and aggressive intervention (immediate delivery or intrauterine transfusion) are indicated. These points vary with the length of gestation, generally decreasing toward term (Figure 19-4). Both the position of a point on the graph and the trend of

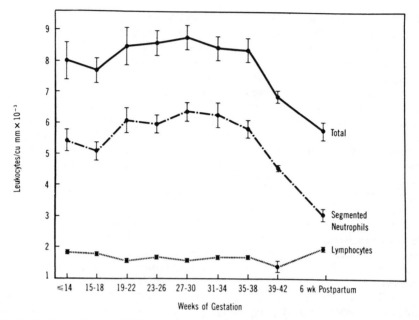

Figure 19-2 Mean (± SEM) total leukocyte, neutrophil, and lymphocyte counts in 23 women during normal pregnancy and at six weeks postpartum. Reprinted with permission from Pitkin and Witte: *JAMA* 1979;242:2697. Copyright 1979, American Medical Association.

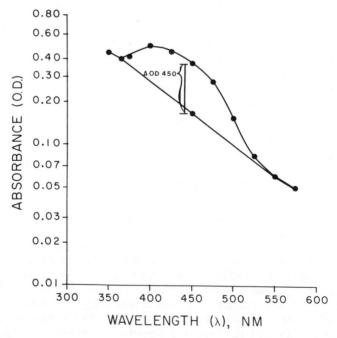

Figure 19-3 Spectrophotometric scan of amniotic fluid showing change in absorbance at 450 nm, replotted on semilog paper according to Liley (1961).

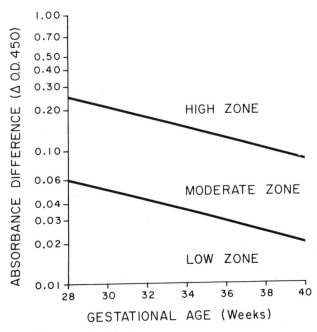

Figure 19-4 Liley's graph of change in absorbance at 450 nm versus gestational age showing zones of low, moderate, and high risk (adapted from Liley 1961).

successive determinations are important in management of the pregnancy. Values in the low zone indicate little risk from fetal hemolytic disease. Values in the high zone require prompt intervention. Intermediate values require continued vigilance, with the risk roughly indicated by the position within the moderate zone; high-moderate values tend to worsen with time, whereas low-moderate values tend to improve.

Liley's data begin at 28 weeks of gestation. It is incorrect to extrapolate the lines on Liley's graph to evaluate fluids obtained before the 28th week. Bishop and Brown (1972) have prepared a graph valid from 20 weeks on, based on their own data (Figure 19-5). Interpretation of values plotted on this graph is similar to that for Liley's graph. As intrauterine transfusion is possible well before the 28th week, our laboratory often receives specimens that can be evaluated only by reference to Bishop and Brown's graph, and we use this graph routinely.

■ Amniotic Karyotyping

Any chromosomal abnormality that can be detected by routine Giemsa staining techniques (G-banding) can be diagnosed by examination of cells shed into amniotic fluid. These include abnormal deletions, trisomies, and translocations, as well as bizarre forms such as ring chromosomes. In our laboratory, the most common indications for amniotic karyotyping are advanced maternal age (to detect Down's syndrome and other aneuploidies) and previous chromosomal abnormality in the family. It is generally

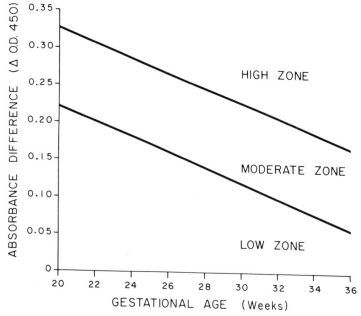

Figure 19-5 Bishop and Brown's graph of change of absorbance at 450 nm versus gestational age showing zones of low, moderate, and high risk (adapted from Bishop and Brown 1972).

considered unethical to use amniotic karyotyping to ensure that only babies of a specific sex will be born. If the mother is known to be heterozygous for an X-linked deleterious gene, such as hemophilia A or B or Duchenne muscular dystrophy, however, it may be legitimate to use amniotic karyotyping to determine the sex of the fetus and to provide this information to the parents, who may wish to abort male fetuses selectively.

Amniotic karyotyping requires growing, dividing cells. It cannot be performed directly or rapidly on the cells shed into the amniotic fluid. These cells can usually be cultured easily, with a failure rate of only about 5%, but they grow slowly, taking two to three weeks to reach the stage at which a karyotype can be made. Therefore, if abortion is contemplated, the amniocentesis must be performed as early as possible, ideally at 14 to 16 weeks of gestation. There is then adequate time to repeat the amniocentesis if the cells from the first specimen do not grow and still obtain a result before the 20-week limit on elective abortions imposed in some jurisdictions.

Rarely, only cells of maternal origin grow in the tissue culture. These cells cannot be routinely distinguished from amniotic cells of fetal origin. When this occurs, a male fetus may be falsely identified as female or an abnormal fetus as chromosomally normal. Parents must be informed that such an error may occur and cannot be prevented by the most careful technique.

■ Amylase

Serum amylase (automated saccharogenic method) gradually rises during the first half of pregnancy, reaching an average of nearly 120 mg of glucose per dL at 21–25 weeks and then falling to an average of approximately 85 mg of glucose per dL at term (Figure 19-6). Although values above 100 mg of glucose per dL are abnormal in nonpregnant women and in the first trimester of pregnancy, 64% of 28 normal women at 21–25 weeks had values above 100. By term only 12% remained above that level. Isoenzyme studies have suggested that much of the increase in amylase activity may be in the salivary fraction.

The amylase/creatinine clearance ratio (Cam/Ccr) has been suggested as a more reliable index of pancreatitis than serum amylase alone, since renal tubular reabsorption of amylase may be decreased during acute pancreatitis, and this change may outlast the elevated serum amylase value. The ratio is calculated as follows:

$$Cam/Ccr = \frac{urine\ amylase}{serum\ amylase} \times \frac{serum\ creat}{urine\ creat} \times 100$$

It may be done on spot urine and serum samples, with normal nonpregnant values being between 1 and 4% and values in pancreatitis ranging from 6.6 to 14.5% in one series. DeVore et al (1980) measured the Cam/Ccr on a cross section of 70 patients at various times in pregnancy. They found that the Cam/Ccr fell from a mean of 3.3% in the nonpregnant woman to 2.3% in the first trimester, 2.0% by the end of the second trimester, and back to about 3.0% in the third trimester. The fall was attributed to changes in

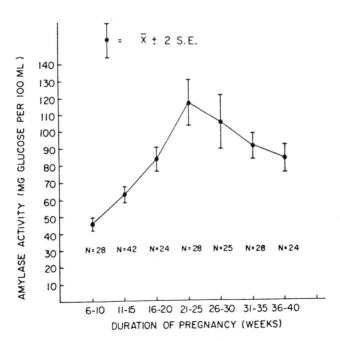

Figure 19-6 Mean ± SE values for serum amylase activity during pregnancy. (N refers to number of patients studied in each five-week period). Reprinted with permission from Kaiser et al: *Am J Obstet Gynecol* 1975;122:283.

creatinine clearance occurring during pregnancy. In four patients with clinically evident pancreatitis, Cam/Ccr was elevated (3.8% to 7.5%) for the stage of gestation, and the change in Cam/Ccr outlasted the elevated serum amylase. Eight patients with toxemia of pregnancy *and* epigastric pain had elevated Cam/Ccr (4% to 12%), whereas only one of six with toxemia without epigastric pain had an elevated Cam/Ccr (4%). Additionally, two of four patients with the diagnosis of hyperemesis gravidarum had elevated Cam/Ccr. Thus, measurement of Cam/Ccr may be a useful means of diagnosing pancreatitis in the pregnant woman.

■ Carbohydrate Metabolism

Carbohydrate metabolism is changed during pregnancy because of a number of factors. The presence of a fetal-placental unit, which acts as a "glucose sink," is believed to be responsible for the lower fasting plasma glucose values observed in pregnant women (averaging about 75 ± 3 mg/dL). On the other hand, postprandial glucose levels measured in the third trimester are higher than in nonpregnant women. A primary factor in the elevation of postprandial glucose is felt to be the presence of large quantities of human chorionic somatomammotropin, also known as human placental lactogen. This placentally produced polypeptide is believed to be responsible for the relative insulin resistance occurring in pregnancy. Thus, relative hyperglycemia occurs postprandially despite markedly increased serum insulin levels. Nevertheless, plasma glucose throughout the day in normal pregnant women is maintained in the rather narrow range of 60 to 120 mg/dL.

Glucose tolerance testing for the diagnosis of gestational diabetes remains somewhat controversial. Because the diagnosis carries with it prognostic and therapeutic implications, accuracy is essential. The most thoroughly validated set of criteria are those of O'Sullivan and Mahan (1964). After three days of carbohydrate loading, pregnant women are given a 100-g oral glucose challenge. Blood is drawn before and one, two, and three hours after the challenge. Whole blood glucose is determined on each sample by the Somogyi-Nelson method of analysis. If any two of the four thresholds are met or exceeded, gestational diabetes is diagnosed. At present, virtually all clinical laboratories have abandoned the Somogyi-Nelson method and have adopted more specific glucose oxidase methods for measuring glucose. This necessitates a lowering of O'Sullivan and Mahan's threshold values by approximately 5 mg/dL each. In addition, most laboratories have switched from whole blood to plasma or serum samples. This necessitates increasing each threshold value by approximately 14%. Although the revised thresholds were originally reported as 95, 180, 160, and 135 mg/dL at fasting, one, two, and three hours, respectively, the original (O'Sullivan and Mahan) numbers on which these revisions were based had been rounded off. If the unrounded thresholds are used, the revised thresholds are as depicted in Table 19-1. The National Diabetes Data Group has recently proposed a new set of thresholds for the glucose tolerance test on plasma or serum in pregnancy. These are derived from O'Sullivan and Mahan's whole blood values, but do not include a correction for the change in method from Somogyi-Nelson to glucose oxidase. Thus, they are slightly higher than the values we have proposed. To avoid administering a 100-g three-hour glucose tolerance test to all pregnant women, a screening test has been proposed. For this test, 50 g of glucose is administered orally, and a plasma glucose measurement is made one hour later. If the value is 135 mg/dL or greater, a full 100-g three hour oral glucose tolerance test (as described above) is given. The screening test is generally performed at 26 to 28 weeks of gestation.

■ Coagulation Studies

Fibrinogen

Plasma fibrinogen concentration normally begins to rise by the second month of pregnancy from a nonpregnant mean of approximately 250 mg/dL to a mean near 400 mg/dL at term. Fibrinogen levels in a pregnant woman must be interpreted with this fact in mind, since a value of 200 mg/dL is not normal in the third trimester and may reflect an ongoing consumptive process.

Other Procoagulant Factors

Most procoagulant factors increase during pregnancy, exceptions being XI and XIII (fibrin-stabilizing factor). Factors XI and XIII, in fact, decrease by as much as 50% at term. Factor VIII levels (measured as antigen or as procoagulant) increase during pregnancy.

Coagulation Assays

The Quick prothrombin time, which measures factors V, VII, X, II (prothrombin) and I (fibrinogen), is not changed by pregnancy. Neither is the activated partial thromboplastin time, which measures factors I, II, V, VIII.

Fibrinolysis

The presence of fibrin degradation products in the serum of a pregnant woman, as measured by commercially available semiquantitative techniques, is abnormal. The presence of increased amounts of fibrinogen during pregnancy and the finding that intravascular fibrin deposition normally occurs, and is accompanied by compensatory fibrinolysis, would seem to be

Table 19-1
Criteria Used for Glucose Tolerance Test in Pregnancy

	Whole Blood Somogyi-Nelson (mg/dL)	Plasma or Serum Glucose-Oxidase (mg/dL)	Plasma or Serum National Diabetes Data Group (mg/dL)
Fasting	90	95	105
1 hour	165	180	190
2 hour	145	155	165
3 hour	125	140	145

inconsistent with the absence of fibrin degradation products. This inconsistency might be due to the relative insensitivity of tests used to measure fibrinogen-fibrin degradation products.

■ Electrolytes

Sodium

During the course of pregnancy, sodium retention (as measured by an increase in total body sodium) is more than offset by a relatively greater increase in total body water. As early as the first trimester, serum sodium falls by an average of 4 mEq/L, and this decrease is maintained throughout pregnancy. Newman (1957) found a range of serum sodium from 131.0 to 144.5 mEq/L in 27 pregnant women as opposed to 136.5 to 150.0 mEq/L in nonpregnant control women. Average serum sodium was 139.2 mEq/L in pregnancy versus 143.3 in the nonpregnant state.

Potassium

Like sodium, serum potassium falls slightly but significantly during pregnancy. Pregnant women averaged 4.01 mEq/L, as compared with nonpregnant women who averaged 4.25 mEq/L. The range for pregnancy was reported as 3.15 to 5.2 mEq/L (Newman, 1957).

Calcium

The effect of pregnancy upon serum calcium remains somewhat controversial. Total serum calcium clearly falls from approximately 9.5 mg/dL in the nonpregnant state to approximately 8.6 mg/dL in the third trimester. This fall, however, is related to falling serum albumin values with 1 g of albumin binding 0.7 mg of calcium. Thus, the fall is in the bound fraction of serum calcium. Various investigators have measured free (ionized) calcium in pregnancy, and conflicting results have been reported. Measurement of ionized calcium has been difficult in the past, and many of the earlier studies were cross-sectional. Pitkin et al (1979) used modern methods of measurement and longitudinally followed 30 normal women throughout pregnancy, beginning in the first trimester and continuing to six weeks postpartum. No significant change in ionized calcium occurred; mean values were 2.33 ± 0.07 mEq/L in the first trimester, 2.25 ± 0.09 mEq/L in the second trimester, and 2.27 ± 0.11 mEq/L in the third trimester. The average value at six weeks postpartum was 2.31 ± 0.10 mEq/L. It is thus likely that serum ionized calcium is maintained within a very narrow range in pregnancy as well as in the nonpregnant state.

Magnesium

Serum magnesium is generally 1.5 to 2.0 mEq/L in nonpregnant women. Pitkin et al (1979) found a mean value of 1.44 ± 0.16 mEq/L in the second trimester of pregnancy, significantly lower than the mean of 1.55 ± 0.13 at six weeks postpartum in the same women.

Chloride

Serum chloride changes little, if at all. Newman (1957) reported an average of 104.7 mEq/L in nonpregnant women, with an average of 103.5 mEq/L in pregnant women. The range in nonpregnant women was 100.5 to 109.5 mEq/L, whereas in pregnancy it was 96.0 to 108.0 mEq/L.

Bicarbonate

Because of the sustained respiratory alkalosis present in pregnancy, maternal arterial PCO_2 values average 27 to 32 mm Hg. This is most likely a result of progesterone-induced hyperventilation. Renal bicarbonate excretion is increased in an attempt to maintain a normal pH in the blood. Arterial plasma bicarbonate levels averaging 19.5 mEq/L have been reported in normal pregnant women (Anderson et al, 1969). More recently, Fadel et al (1979) compared 59 normal healthy pregnant women in the third trimester with healthy nonpregnant women and found plasma bicarbonate levels of 19.0 ± 2.8 mEq/L in pregnancy, as opposed to 23.6 ± 0.99 mEq/L in the nonpregnant state. Base excess in the pregnant women averaged − 4.2 ± 2.2 mEq/L, as opposed to − 1.0 ± 1.44 mEq/L in nonpregnant controls.

Phosphorus

Serum inorganic phosphorus levels decline slightly, being 4.13 ± 0.95 mg/dL in the third trimester versus 4.66 ± 0.74 mg/dL at six weeks postpartum (Pitkin et al, 1979). Since the traditionally accepted normal range is 3.0 to 4.5 mg/dL (1.0 to 1.5 mmol/L), it appears that values during pregnancy are within the normal range.

Osmolality

Serum osmalality, about 290 mmol/kg in the nonpregnant woman, decreases to about 280 mmol/kg by the third trimester of pregnancy. This has been attributed to the fall in electrolytes and serum proteins occurring during gestation.

■ Infectious Disease

A number of infectious diseases have implications which are peculiar to pregnancy. Some of these, such as toxoplasmosis, cytomegalovirus, and syphilis, are discussed thoroughly in other chapters in this book. Rubella will be discussed here, because the major sequelae of this disease are related to its occurrence in the pregnant woman. An understanding of the laboratory tests involved in the diagnosis of rubella infection is essential for anyone caring for pregnant women and their newborns.

Rubella is an RNA virus, spread mainly by aerosol dissemination, and inoculated into the upper respiratory tract. The incubation period (using appearance of the rash as the endpoint) is 11–14 days. Because the virus is not routinely isolated in most laboratories, the diagnosis of maternal rubella infection is generally based on the demonstration of an appropriate rise in titers of the specific hemagglutination inhibition (HAI) antibody at the appropriate time. The HAI antibody begins to appear at about the time of the rash, and reaches its peak about 10–14 days later. There is some variation in techniques for measuring HAI titers. There is also, in general, a twofold titer range of variability if two samples of the same specimen are tested simultaneously. Thus, most experts would insist that there be a greater than fourfold increase in titer to diagnose rubella. It is important to emphasize that the acute and convalescent specimens, drawn 7–10 days apart, be run simultaneously. Otherwise, interassay variability increases the possibility of error. In actual practice, many laboratories run the acute specimen when it arrives, but save the serum to reanalyze (in triplicate) with the convalescent specimen. Figure 19-7 illustrates the sequence of appearance of HAI, complement fixation (CF), and IgM antibodies in rubella infection. It should be noted that CF antibodies appear later than the HAI type, and their presence may be useful in diagnosing recent rubella infections if specimens are obtained too late to detect the rise in HAI titers. IgM antibodies are present only transiently (half-life of five days), and are a useful diagnostic test *only* if they are present. Their absence does not rule out recent infection. It should be pointed out that the likelihood of full-blown congenital rubella syndrome varies with the timing in gestation of maternal rubella. If exposure occurs in the first month, the risk is approximately 50%. In the second and third months, it is approximately 25% and 10%, respectively. By the fifth month of pregnancy, the likelihood of rubella syndrome occurring is probably not increased. However, other forms of morbidity due to later exposure or persistent viral infection in the fetus have been postulated.

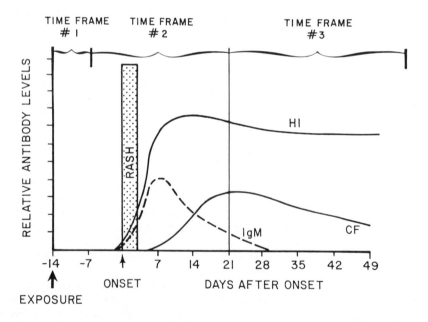

Figure 19-7 Times of appearance and disappearance of hemagglutination inhibition (HI), compliment fixation (CF), and specific IGM antibody responses in acute rubella infection. Reprinted with permission from *JAMA* 1981;245(16):1647–1652. Copyright 1981, American Medical Association.

Figures 19-8 through 19-10 represent the suggestions of Centers for Disease Control experts (Mann et al, 1981) for the evaluation of pregnant women seen within one week, from one to five weeks, and greater than five weeks of exposure to a possible case of rubella.

One area of difficulty is the interpretation of low titers of rubella antibody. Most laboratories report a threshold of 1:10 to be indicative of true immunity. Harris et al (1978) reported that 17% of 90 patients with rubella titers of 1:10 responded to immunization with an eightfold or greater rise in titer, suggesting that a titer of 1:10 did *not* necessarily indicate immunity and that such patients should be vaccinated. Additionally, these investigators reported three pregnant women with titers of 1:10 who developed documented rubella during pregnancy!

■ Lipids in Serum

Plasma cholesterol begins to rise at the end of the first trimester of pregnancy (Figure 19-11). From normal nonpregnant levels of approximately 200 mg/dL, cholesterol reaches a mean of approximately 300 mg/dL in the third trimester. It is of interest that, at least in one study, cholesterol was still elevated at six weeks postpartum, although levels were normal at one year postpartum (the next time testing was done).

Plasma triglyceride levels rise from approximately 100 mg/dL in nonpregnant women to approximately 300 mg/dL by term. Levels are almost down to normal by six weeks postpartum (approximately 120 mg/dL).

Lipoprotein changes are most likely responsible for the above increases in cholesterol and triglyceride. Very low density lipoprotein cholesterol and triglyceride start to increase in the second trimester, reaching levels three to four times normal by term. Low density lipoprotein triglyceride increases somewhat more than low density lipoprotein cholesterol. High density lipoprotein triglyceride increases by about 50% in the first trimester and by another 50% in the second trimester. High density lipoprotein cholesterol, on the other hand, increases only during the first trimester and then remains at about 21% above means of nonpregnant women for the rest of pregnancy.

■ Liver Function Tests

Serum Protein

Serum albumin falls rapidly during the first trimester, then continues to fall more slowly throughout the remainder of gestation. The total fall is in the range of 1 g/dL, or about 22%. As a result, total serum proteins fall by approximately 20%. Other serum proteins, such as ceruloplasmin, transferrin, and various binding proteins, increase during pregnancy. Haptoglobin concentration is not changed by pregnancy.

BSP Removal

Bromsulphthalein (BSP) removal is a standard test of hepatic function. This anionic phthalein dye is bound to plasma protein after its intravenous administration. Most is then cleared by the liver, where it is conjugated and

368

Figure 19-8

Time Frame No. 1: Within 1 week after exposure to rash illness

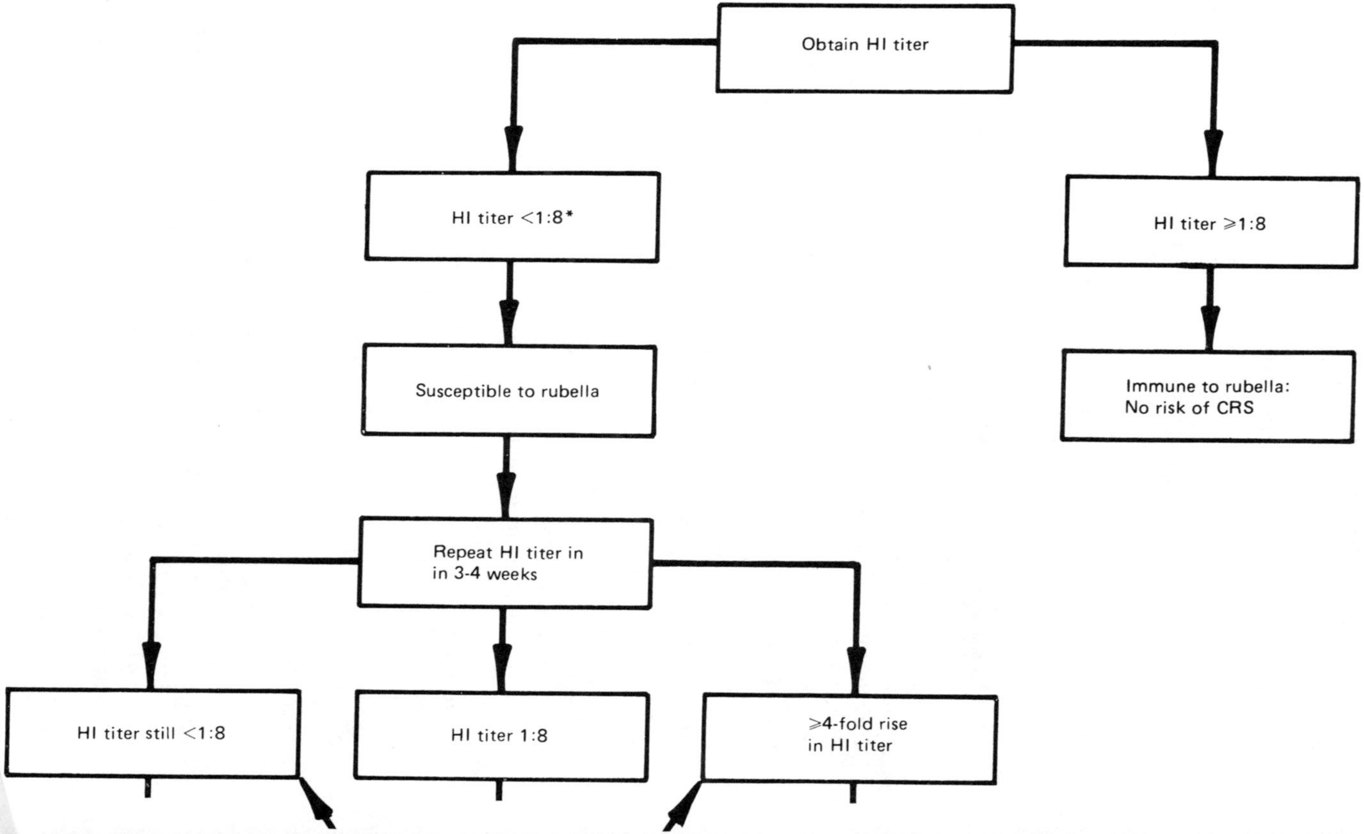

Obtain HI titer

HI titer ≥1:8 → Immune to rubella: No risk of CRS

HI titer <1:8* → Susceptible to rubella → Repeat HI titer in 3-4 weeks

HI titer 1:8

HI titer still <1:8

≥4-fold rise in HI titer

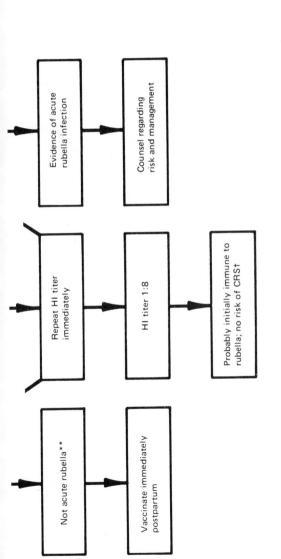

*An HI titer of <1:8 is used to indicate susceptibility. The actual susceptibility cut-off level may vary in different laboratories (e.g., <1:10).

**The patient should be followed closely during the first trimester for rash illness or exposure to rubella. Another HI titer at the end of the first trimester is advisable especially if rubella is present in the community.

†Over 99% of acute rubella infections will result in development and maintenance of HI titers >1:32 for at least 6 months after onset. Original HI titer <1:8 is suspect.

370

Time Frame No. 2: 1-5 weeks after exposure to rash illness OR if rash illness, up to 3 weeks after rash onset

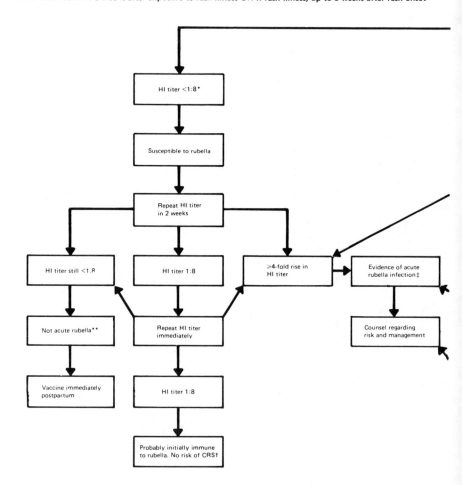

* An acute titer of <1:8 is used to indicate susceptibility. The actual susceptibility cut-off level may vary in different laboratories (e.g., <1:10)
** The patient should be followed closely during the first trimester for rash illness or exposure to rubella. Another HI titer at the end of the first trimester is advisable especially if rubella is present in the community.
† Over 99% of acute rubella infections will develop and maintain HI titers >1:32 for at least 6 months after onset. Original HI titer <1:8 is suspect
‡ In the absence of rash illness, if reinfection is a major consideration, a properly timed IgM antibody assay may help to differentiate primary from secondary infection
¶ Absence of rubella-specific IgM may not exclude recent rubella infection
¶¶ The physician may elect to proceed as with a titer of 1:8-1:32

Reproduced with the permission of JAMA, April 24, 1981, Vol. 245, No. 16,
"Assessing Risks of Rubella Infection During Pregnancy" pp. 1647-1652.
Copyright 1981, American Medical Association.

Figure 19-9

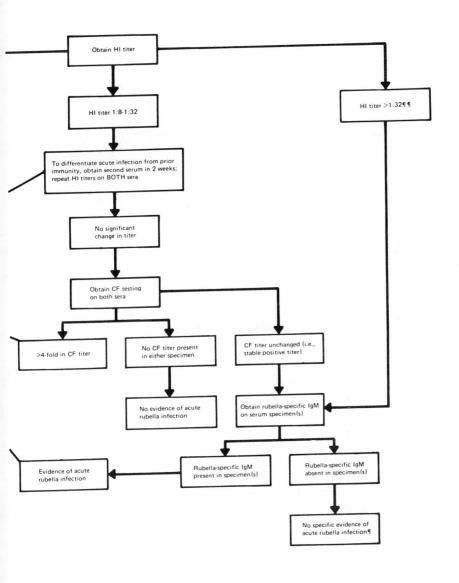

372

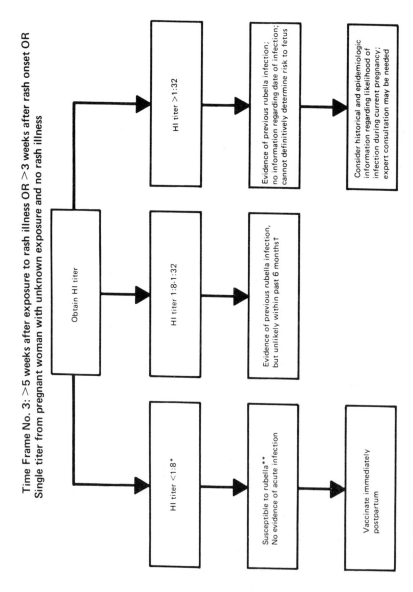

Time Frame No. 3: >5 weeks after exposure to rash illness OR >3 weeks after rash onset OR Single titer from pregnant woman with unknown exposure and no rash illness

Obtain HI titer

HI titer <1:8*

HI titer 1:8-1:32

HI titer >1:32

Susceptible to rubella**
No evidence of acute infection

Evidence of previous rubella infection, but unlikely within past 6 months†

Evidence of previous rubella infection; no information regarding date of infection; cannot definitively determine risk to fetus

Vaccinate immediately postpartum

Consider historical and epidemiologic information regarding likelihood of infection during current pregnancy; expert consultation may be needed

*An HI titer of <1:8 is used to indicate susceptibility. The actual susceptibility cut-off level may vary in different laboratories (e.g., <1:10).

**The patient should be followed closely during the first trimester for rash illness or exposure to rubella. Another HI titer at the end of the first trimester is advisable, especially if rubella is present in the community.

†Over 99% of acute rubella infections will result in development and maintenance of HI titers of >1:32 for at least 6 months after onset.

Figure 19-10

373

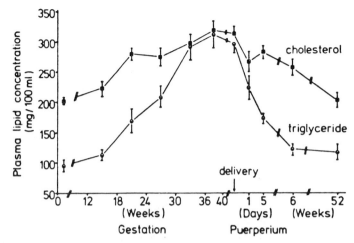

Figure 19-11 The changes in plasma cholesterol and triglyceride concentrations during pregnancy and in the puerperium. Fasting lipid concentrations were measured serially throughout pregnancy, at delivery, and in the puerperium, and at 12 months. The results are the mean ± SEM, and include normal and complicated pregnancies. Reprinted with permission from Potter and Nestel: *Am J Obstet Gynecol* 1979;133:167.

secreted into the bile. A number of changes in BSP metabolism occur during pregnancy. These include increased hepatic storage capacity, decreased rate of excretion into bile, and increased protein binding in the bloodstream. The net effect is a slight increase in BSP retention at 45 minutes, the upper limit of normal being 8% rather than the 5% described for nonpregnant women.

Bilirubin

Serum bilirubin levels are not changed by pregnancy. Mild elevation in total bilirubin (generally less than 3 mg/dL) may be seen in some, but not all, patients with cholestasis of pregnancy.

Enzymes

Alkaline phosphatase increases throughout pregnancy, reaching levels two to four times normal by the third trimester. This increase is due to the placental production of heat-stable alkaline phosphatase, as opposed to hepatic alkaline phosphatase which is heat labile, being inactivated by heating to 65 °C. Thus, unless fractionation is done, alkaline phosphatase is not a reliable liver function test in pregnancy.

Serum glutamic-oxaloacetic transaminase and serum glutamic-pyruvic transaminase are unaltered by pregnancy and are reliable tests of hepatocellular damage during pregnancy. Slight increases in both of these enzymes have been reported by some investigators, but they generally remain within the normal range. Both of these enzymes become elevated in most patients with cholestasis of pregnancy.

Lactic dehydrogenase rises slightly as pregnancy progresses, but does not generally exceed the normal range.

Serum gamma glutamyl transpeptidase is unchanged during the first two trimesters of pregnancy and is a reliable test at those times. However, some controversy exists about the levels obtained in the third trimester, and an increase may normally occur.

Bile acids are not changed in normal pregnancy. Measurement of bile acids has recently become a useful diagnostic test from cholestasis of pregnancy, in which bile acid elevation (cholic acid in particular) is often the earliest liver function change. Cholestasis of pregnancy occurs in less than 1% of patients in the United States, but is much more common in Scandinavia and Chile, where as many as 2.5% of pregnancies may be affected. The major clinical sign of this syndrome is pruritus. Although some controversy exists, it is generally agreed that an increased perinatal mortality rate is associated with cholestasis. Bile acid levels ranging from slightly elevated to more than 100 times normal have been reported. Thus, frequent measurement of serum bile acids during pregnancy is worthwhile in patients with a past history of family history of cholestasis or in patients complaining of pruritus.

■ Pituitary Hormones

Prolactin, an anterior pituitary hormone, rises dramatically even in the first trimester of pregnancy (Figure 19-12), reaching levels at or above 100 ng/mL. By the third trimester, the mean prolactin level is above 200 ng/mL. These high prolactin levels are a re³ection of hyperplasia of the lactotroph cells in the pituitary gland; pituitary gland weight increases by about 15% during pregnancy. Prolactin is not useful for diagnosing pituitary adenomas during pregnancy unless its level is extremely elevated. Jovanovic et al (1978) described a group of patients experiencing spontaneous abortion, none of whom showed the normal prolactin rise seen in pregnancy. This same group went on to show that in 10 poorly controlled diabetics evaluated before 12 weeks of gestation, prolactin was well below the levels seen in normal pregnancy. Once excellent diabetic control was attained, all patients manifested appropriate prolactin levels for the duration of pregnancy. Thus, the measurement of prolactin shows some promise as a test of fetal well being in the first trimester. Unfortunately, another study (Riss et al, 1981) has failed to corroborate these findings.

The pituitary gonadotrophic hormones, follicle-stimulating hormone and luteinizing hormone, are undetectable during pregnancy. Growth hormone is generally undetectable, but cross-reactivity with human placental lactogen (hPL) makes this assay difficult in pregnancy. The effect of pregnancy upon maternal ACTH levels remains controversial, with reported pregnant means ranging from normal levels to two to three times normal. There is evidence that the ACTH response to metyrapone inhibition of 11B-hydroxylase is stunted during pregnancy, perhaps because of increased maternal cortisol levels.

Serum thyrotropin (TSH), measured by immunoassay, may increase in the first and second trimesters (Table 19-2), but return to normal values in the third trimester. Some studies suggest that TSH does not change during pregnancy.

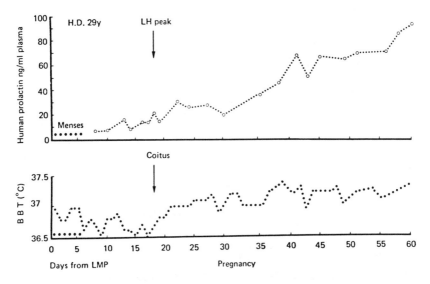

Figure 19-12 Plasma prolactin levels during first trimester of pregnancy in a 29-year-old subject. Reprinted with permission from Saxena BJ: in Fuchs, Klopper (eds): *Endocrinology of Pregnancy*. ed 2. New York, Harper & Row, 1977, p 235.

Table 19-2
Serum TSH Levels during Pregnancy*

Subjects	No.	Serum TSH (μU/mL) Mean	SE	Range
Euthyroid women	15	8.3	1.0	2.8–15.3
Progestogen-treated women	8	6.2	0.6	4.8–10.1
Pregnant women				
First trimester	33	12.8	0.6	2.7–18.2
Second trimester	10	11.1	1.2	5.9–18.2
At delivery	17	7.6	0.6	4.1–11.5
Postpartum women				
5 days	15	8.5	0.7	4.8–14.5
Neonates	18	9.9	1.0	5.0–23.3

*Reprinted with permission from Malkasian and Mayberry: *Am J Obstet Gynecol* 1970; 108(8):1236.

The posterior pituitary hormones, oxytocin and vasopressin, are difficult to measure. Oxytocin, for example, is released in spurts from the neurohypophysis. Because it has a relatively short half-life, serum levels are constantly fluctuating. Reports on its value in pregnant women are conflicting; most likely it is not changed throughout pregnancy. Likewise, diabetes insipidus does not appear to be uniformly affected by pregnancy.

■ Renal Function

Renal Plasma Flow

By the 12th week of pregnancy, renal plasma flow increases by 50% to 75% over normal nonpregnant values. Although early studies suggested a decline in renal plasma flow as term approached, later investigations reported that the increase was sustained to term as long as studies were done with subjects in the lateral recumbent, rather than supine, position. This difference is attributed to the fact that, in the supine woman near term, the gravid uterus can compress the vena cava, diminishing venous return, and perhaps also compress the renal arteries.

Even more recent studies now suggest some fall in renal plasma flow during the last month of pregnancy no matter what position the patient is in. This has been attributed to increased vascular resistance, as manifested by the rise in blood pressure observed in late pregnancy.

Glomerular Filtration Rate

Like renal plasma flow, glomerular filtration increases by 30% to 50% by the beginning of the second trimester of pregnancy. This increase is sustained to term and does not decrease during the last month. As a result of the increased glomerular filtration rate, many solutes are presented to the kidney in amounts higher than normal. If the amount presented exceeds the ability of the kidney to reabsorb a particular solute, it may appear in the urine in seemingly abnormal amounts. Glucose is an example of such a solute.

Serum Creatinine and Creatinine Clearance

Creatinine is filtered, but not reabsorbed, although it is secreted by the tubules to a small extent. Thus, creatinine clearance is somewhat in excess of true glomerular filtration rate as measured by insulin clearance. Creatinine clearance increases as pregnancy progresses, with values of 150–200 mL/min usually attained. Probably as a result of this increased clearance, without a measurable change in creatinine production, serum creatinine falls from a mean of 0.67 ± 0.14 mg/dL in nonpregnant subjects to a mean of 0.46 ± 0.13 mg/dL in pregnant women. A serum creatinine exceeding 0.8 mg/dL is not normal in a pregnant woman!

Serum Urea Nitrogen

In the same way that creatinine falls during pregnancy, serum urea nitrogen falls from a nonpregnant mean of 13 ± 3.0 mg/dL to a mean of 8.7 ± 1.5 mg/dL in pregnancy. Thus, values above 12 mg/dL are abnormally high.

Uric Acid

Uric acid is freely filtered, actively reabsorbed, and secreted into the tubule. Uric acid levels fall during the first half of pregnancy, averaging 3.2 to 3.5 mg/dL. Some increase toward prepregnancy levels occurs during the last trimester, but values above 4.5 mg/dL are distinctly unusual. In hypertensive disorders in pregnancy, high uric acid levels may be an early sign of the development of toxemia. The elevation of uric acid in toxemia is probably a reflection of hypovolemia with diminished renal blood flow. Women taking diuretic agents may manifest elevated uric acid levels, even in the absence of toxemia.

■ Adrenal Function

Glucocorticoids

Measurement of cortisol levels in pregnancy is confounded by the fact that corticosteroid-binding globulin levels have practically doubled by midgestation. Thus, serum cortisol levels are markedly increased. However, the normal diurnal variation in cortisol is maintained. Doe et al (1980) found that evening (9 PM) plasma 17-hydroxycorticosteroids (17-OHCS) averaged 7.4 μg/dL in nonpregnant women and increased to 24 μg/dL in pregnancy. Morning levels (9 AM) increased from 19 μg/dL to 43 μg/dL. However, all of the increase in cortisol cannot be accounted for by increased protein binding. The same authors found that free cortisol, measured in the evening, increased from 0.4 μg/dL in nonpregnant women to 1.0 μg/mL in pregnancy. Morning cortisol went from an average of 1.4 μg/dL to 2.6 μg/dL. Likewise, urinary free cortisol increases during pregnancy. However, 24-hour urine 17-OHCS decreases from an average of 5.34 mg/day in nonpregnant women to 1.99 mg/day in midpregnancy. This apparent inconsistency may be related to a change in cortisol metabolism during pregnancy, with a decrease in excretion of the tetrahydro metabolites of cortisol. Because progesterone competes with cortisol for intracellular binding sites, it has been speculated that the increased free cortisol levels seen in pregnancy are secondary to decreased intracellular cortisol binding in the hypothalamus and pituitary gland, with a compensatory readjustment in the hypothalamic-pituitary-adrenal axis.

The usual test for integrity of the pituitary-adrenal axis is the administration of metyrapone, a blocker of 11-B hydroxylation in the adrenal gland. The normal rise in 17-OHCS is blunted during pregnancy, and so this test loses validity. Addison's disease is more difficult to diagnose during pregnancy because of the elevated serum cortisol levels normally occurring. That is, a patient with Addison's disease may have cortisol levels in the normal nonpregnant range. For this reason, the adrenocorticotropic hormone (ACTH) infusion test is most reliable for making the diagnosis. The lack of an increase in serum cortisol and urinary 17-OHCS levels is a reliable index of adrenal inability to respond. Similarly, the diagnosis of Cushing's syndrome is more difficult in pregnancy. In addition to manifesting elevated cortisol levels, normal pregnant women exhibit increased cortisol release after ACTH stimulation. Thus, dexamethasone suppression is the key to diagnosing Cushing's syndrome in pregnancy. Both low-dose and high-dose dexamethasone suppression should be utilized and are valid in the pregant woman.

Adrenal Androgens

Levels of testosterone and androstenedione increase progressively during pregnancy. Bammann et al (1980) found that nonpregnant women had serum total testosterone levels of 20 to 80 ng/dL, with a mean of 48.3 ± 1.66 ng/dL. In the third trimester a mean testosterone level of 416 ± 27 ng/dL was found, with all levels well above 80 ng/dL. Even in the first two trimesters, the mean value for total testosterone was 187 ± 15 ng/dL. Of 61 women tested during the first two trimesters, only 3 had testosterone levels in the normal range, and all 3 were tested in the first trimester. Free testosterone does not appear to rise until the third trimester. Levels in the first two trimesters averaged 1.15 ± 0.09 ng/dL (nonpregnant mean was 0.96 mg/dL). In the third trimester it averaged 3.04 ± 0.24 ng/dL. It has been speculated that the initial rise in total testosterone is related to an increase in sex hormone-binding globulin, since free testosterone is not changed. However, the third trimester increase, which includes both free and bound forms of the hormone, may be due to a contribution from the fetoplacental unit. It should be mentioned that some researchers have found, in early pregnancy, a significant difference in testosterone levels between mothers carrying a male fetus and those carrying a female fetus. Others have been unable to corroborate this, so that determination of maternal testosterone levels is not a commonly employed method of fetal sex determination.

Urine 17-ketosteroids do not appear to change in normal pregnancy. Measurement of testosterone levels in blood and urine 17-ketosteroids finds its greatest application in pregnancy when maternal virilization is noted. Table 19-3 depicts steroid levels found in a range of pathologic conditions of the ovary causing virilization in pregnant women.

Amniotic Fluid

The diagnosis of congenital adrenal hyperplasia, of the 21-hydroxylase deficiency form, has been made by measurement of the 17-hydroxyprogesterone level in amniotic fluid. In the case described, the amniotic fluid level was 33 nmol/L at 17 weeks of gestation as compared with a mean of 7.6 nmol/L and a range of 4 to 11.5 nmol/L in 31 normal pregnant women at 15–21 weeks of gestation. Similarly, the less common 11B-hydroxylase deficiency has been diagnosed in utero.

■ Alpha Feto Protein

Alpha feto protein (AFP) is produced by the fetal liver and yolk sac. It is a major constituent of first- and second-trimester fetal serum, with a peak concentration of 2–3 ng/mL at 14 weeks of gestation. It normally reaches the amniotic cavity in much smaller amounts, mainly in fetal urine. Amniotic fluid AFP levels are typically about 10 μg/mL at 16 weeks. AFP also reaches maternal serum by an unknown route in even smaller amounts. Levels of 40 μg/mL are typical at 16 weeks, compared with normal nonpregnant levels of < 10 μg/mL.

If the fetal microcirculation or cerebrospinal fluid is directly exposed to the amniotic cavity, as in open neural tube defects or ventral wall defects, AFP levels rise dramatically both in amniotic fluid and in maternal serum. This has led to the use of AFP measurements as a screening tool for antenatal diagnosis of fetal anomalies.

Table 19-3
Ovarian Pathology and Range of Steroid Levels
Reported with Virilization in Pregnancy

Ovarian Pathology	Testosterone (ng/dL plasma)	17-Ketosteroids (mg/24-hour urine)
Neoplasms		
Arrhenoblastoma	4000	18–158
Leydig cell tumor		46–203
Hilus cell tumor	3530	
Brenner tumor		Normal
Lipoid cell tumor		158
(adrenal rest cell tumor)		
Granulosa theca cell tumor		170
Krukenberg tumor		119–238
Dermoid cyst		9–272
Mucinous cystadenoma	240	33–97
Papillary mucinous cystadenoma	5320	
Mucinous cystadenocarcinoma		62
Hyperplasias		
Luteoma of pregnancy	470–3510	9–230
Hyperreactio luteinalis	1000–15,000	82–267

From Hensleigh and Fainstat (1980) with permission.

Because of wide biological variability of amniotic fluid and maternal serum AFP levels in normal pregnancies and incomplete standardization of AFP preparations, the results of AFP determinations are usually reported, not as concentrations, but in terms of the distribution of values in specimens from normal pregnant women analyzed in the same laboratory.

Amniocentesis is used in diagnosis of neural tube defects when the risk of these malformations is known to be elevated. Where a screening program for maternal serum AFP exists, amniocentesis is also used to evaluate persistently high maternal serum AFP levels. Maternal serum AFP is usually reported as a multiple of the median normal value. Levels greater than 2.0 times the normal median should be repeated on a new specimen before further evaluation is undertaken. Amniotic fluid AFP is usually reported as a number of standard deviations above the mean, with +5.0 a typical value requiring sonographic evaluation.

Care must be taken during amniocentesis not to puncture the placental disk, as contamination with even a small amount of fetal serum can lead to falsely elevated amniotic fluid AFP measurements. Some laboratories measure acetylcholinesterase, produced by neural tissue, in the amniotic fluid specimen to increase specificity for neural tube defects. The accurate assessment of gestational age is also essential, since AFP levels in both amniotic fluid and maternal serum change markedly during pregnancy.

The great majority of "positive" (greater than 2.0 times the median normal level) maternal serum AFP levels are associated with normal pregnancies. In order to prevent undue anxiety, it is therefore essential that screening of maternal serum for AFP be conducted in conjunction with a well-organized counseling and follow-up program, preferably organized regionally. Such programs are in operation in many areas.

■ Thyroid Function Tests

An understanding of the interpretation of thyroid function tests during pregnancy requires appreciation of the following principles. (1) Thyroid-binding proteins are increased during pregnancy. (2) Normal pregnant women have normal circulating levels of unbound thyroid hormone. Using these principles, we can accurately predict what will happen to the clinical test results during pregnancy.

Serum thyroxine (T_4), whether determined by radioimmunoassay, competitive protein binding, or displacement, increases because of the increase in thyroid-binding protein. This increase occurs within two weeks of conception and may be of such a degree that the T_4 result is in the hyperthyroid range. If the free T_4 were measured, it would be in the normal range. However, measurement of *free* T_4 is generally not practical.

Measurement of thyroid-binding protein is usually by means of the T_3 *uptake*. This is a measurement of the unoccupied binding sites present in the patient's serum, but is usually reported in an inverse manner. That is, a hypothyroid individual generally has an *increased* number of unoccupied binding sites. The T_3 uptake is reported as *lower* than normal. Although this method of reporting may appear to be illogical, it is justified because of the way the test is performed, and it has the salutary effect of making it easier to remember (ie, a *hypo*thyroid patient has a *low* T_3 uptake). Because the pregnant woman has an increased number of unoccupied binding sites, she will have a *low* T_3 uptake, often in the hypothyroid range.

When both of the above tests are performed, as they usually are, we may have the paradoxical finding (in the pregnant woman) of a hyperthyroid T_4 and a hypothyroid T_3 uptake. How are we to resolve this apparent enigma? One way would be to measure free T_4. When this is done, pregnant women generally exhibit values within the normal range. However, determination of this value (using equilibrium dialysis of labeled T_4) is not universally performed, is expensive, and may be less reliable in the face of the large amounts of thyroid-binding protein seen in pregnancy. Instead, a value derived from the T_4 and T_3 uptake measurements, the *free T_4 index,* is widely used. In some places, this is referred to as the "T_7" or "estimated free T_4." It is obtained by multiplying the T_4 by the T_3 uptake, and dividing the product by the normal mean for T_3 uptake. The result is an indirect estimate of free T_4 and should be normal in a pregnant woman.

When hypothyroidism is suspected TSH is often measured. Although some disagreement exists as to normal TSH levels in pregnancy, a low TSH value effectively excludes primary hypothyroidism; depending upon the T_4 and T_3 uptake values, hypothalamic or pituitary hypothyroidism may be suspected.

■ Erythroblastosis Fetalis and Hemolytic Disease of the Newborn

Because the fetus contains genetic material of paternal origin, fetal tissues are potentially immunogenic to the mother. This is usually of no importance, since the placenta acts as a barrier to the passage of fetal antigens into the maternal circulation. Occasionally during gestation, however, and often at delivery, fetal blood may enter the maternal circulation and elicit antibody formation against fetal red blood cell antigens. During subsequent pregnancies, maternal antibodies can cross the placenta and destroy fetal red blood cells. If this occurs early in gestation, it may cause fetal edema or even fetal death. If it occurs near the time of delivery, hemolytic disease of the newborn may result.

Any red blood cell antigen expressed in the fetus can theoretically cause fetal or neonatal hemolysis. In practice, there are wide differences in the frequency and severity of hemolytic disease caused by the various red blood cell antigens. The main causes of these differences are the degree of genetic polymorphism in the blood group system, the class and subclass of antibody most often produced in response to the antigen, the strength of the antigen on fetal red blood cells, and the immunogenicity of the antigen.

The most polymorphic blood group system is the ABO system. The A and B antigens are quite immunogenic, and most people with blood group O have circulating antibodies to them as a result of exposure to similar environmental antigens. But the A and B antigens are weakly expressed on fetal cells, and most antibodies to the A and B antigens are of the immunoglobulin M (IgM) class and therefore do not cross the placenta. Thus, fetal and neonatal hemolysis due to ABO incompatibility, although fairly common, is rarely severe. The major Rh antigen (D), on the other hand, although less polymorphic than ABO, is extremely immunogenic, is strongly expressed on fetal cells, and usually elicits IgG antibodies, which cross the placenta. Furthermore, the antibodies are nearly always of the IgG_1 and IgG_3 subclasses, which are strongly hemolytic. Thus, Rh hemolytic disease, when it occurs, often affects the fetus early and severely. Other antigens are much less frequent causes of fetal and neonatal hemolytic disease. They are the minor Rh antigens (C, c, E, and e), Kell, Duffy, Kidd, Lutheran, and the MNSsU system antigens. Lewis and I antigens are not expressed on fetal cells and never cause fetal or neonatal hemolytic disease.

All pregnant women should have a blood typing (ABO and Rh) and antibody screen performed, preferably at the first prenatal visit. If an antibody is detected, it should be identified. Ideally, the father should be tested for the corresponding antigen, and a cross-match should be performed with maternal serum and paternal cells. The antibody titer should be measured. If this is the first affected pregnancy of the mother, a titer of 1:32 or higher is associated with increased risk to the fetus. In subsequent pregnancies, any rise in antibody titer requires further evaluation. The earlier the rise, the greater the risk to the fetus. The clinical correlation of antibody titers is not strong, however.

It may be useful to determine the hemolytic potential of a maternal serum antibody. Monocytes and tissue macrophages have surface immunoglobulin receptors that bind at the same site as complement. Increased macrophage binding of an antibody correlates with increased hemolytic potential. An assay ("mac assay") that measures macrophage binding is performed commercially at some centers. When fetal hemolysis is suspected, amniocentesis may be performed to assess the severity. The interpretation of these results is discussed in the section on amniotic fluid bilirubin.

Hemolytic disease of the newborn is best assessed by hemoglobin and bilirubin measurements. Neonatal hemoglobin concentrations below 16.0 g/dL may represent a hemolytic anemia, the value correlating with the severity of hemolysis. Bilirubin levels greater than 10.0 mg/dL are abnormal. Depending on the gestational age and clinical condition of the infant, phototherapy or exchange transfusion should be performed at some bilirubin concentration between 10.0 and 20.0 mg/dL. The precise level warranting therapy varies among institutions. In very early premature infants, exchange transfusion may be required at a bilirubin level as low as 5.0 mg/dL to prevent kernicterus.

■ Fetal Lung Maturity

Because fetal respiratory movements expel lung surfactant into the amniotic cavity, amniotic fluid reflects the amount and type of surfactant being produced in the fetal lung. Gluck et al (1974) showed that measurements of surfactant in amniotic fluid could predict the occurrence of respiratory distress syndrome in the newborn infant. Two major types of amniotic fluid analysis are currently widely used to assess fetal lung maturity and the likelihood of respiratory distress syndrome: chromatographic methods, such as the lecithin/sphingomyelin (L/S) ratio of Gluck et al, and foam stability methods, such as the "shake test" of Clements (1972).

The chromatographic methods require centrifugation of the amniotic fluid specimen, followed by precipitation with methanol, extraction with chloroform, concentration with cold acetone, spotting on a thin-layer silica gel plate, and chromatographic development. This process has not been satisfactorily automated. The spots representing surfactant are visualized either by a variety of stains or by charring and are scanned in a densitometer. The density of the spots corresponding to lecithin and sphingomyelin is determined, and the result is reported as a ratio of these two values.

Gluck et al found that an L/S ratio greater than 2.0:1 almost invariably predicted fetal lung maturity. The exceptions were usually in infants of diabetic mothers delivered before 38 weeks of gestation. The value of 3.0:1 is sometimes used as an indicator of fetal lung maturity in such cases.

In an effort to increase the power of the L/S ratio, Gluck et al have proposed that phosphatidyl glycerol (PG) be determined in cases where the L/S ratio result is inconclusive. He found that the presence of PG in amniotic fluid *always* predicted mature fetal lungs. Unfortunately, his method for PG determination requires two-dimensional chromatography, and it is therefore beyond the capacity of most laboratories to perform more than an occasional PG determination.

The foam stability methods are based on the ability of surfactant to decrease surface tension in the face of the surface tension-raising influence of ethanol. In Clements' original method, equal volumes of amniotic fluid and 95% ethanol were shaken in a test tube. The persistence of an unbroken ring of foam around the meniscus (positive result) indicated the presence of an amount of surfactant indicative of fetal lung maturity. This test, although easy to perform, had too many false-positive results to replace the L/S ratio where the latter test was available. It has been useful, however, as a rapid or bedside test when the L/S ratio cannot be performed. Recently, Sher et al (1978) proposed a modification of the shake test. Various volumes of ethanol are added to 0.5-mL aliquots of amniotic fluid and shaken. The foam stability index (FSI) is the greatest volume fraction of ethanol that allows foam to persist for 15 seconds. Values of 0.48 or greater indicate fetal lung maturity, whereas values of 0.45 or less indicate a high likelihood of respiratory distress syndrome. A cassette with premeasured amounts of ethanol in several tubes, to which amniotic fluid is to be added, is now commercially available. Amenta and Silverman (1982), using a titration procedure to determine the FSI, found this test to be equal to the combination of L/S ratio and lecithin concentration in predicting respiratory distress syndrome. In their laboratory, the LS ratio is not ordinarily performed when the FSI is 0.48 or greater.

The simplicity and availability of the FSI test suggests its use initially in predicting fetal lung maturity. The FSI cannot be used in the presence of blood or meconium contamination or with specimens from a vaginal pool of amniotic fluid, however. In these cases, or when the FSI is indeterminate, (0.46–0.47), the L/S ratio should be determined. As described by Gluck et al, this should be regarded as the definitive test. PG should be used only when delivery is considered urgent in the presence of a borderline L/S ratio or when the L/S ratio is between 2.0 and 3.0 as measured by a method other than that of Gluck et al, as the determination of PG is a cumbersome, time-consuming procedure.

■ Selected Readings

Adrenal Function

Bammann BL, Coulam CB, Jiang NS: Total and free testosterone during pregnancy. *Am J Obstet Gynecol* 1980;137: 293–298.

Beck P, Eaton CJ, Young IS, et al: Metyrapone response in pregnancy. *Am J Obstet Gynecol* 1968;100:327–330.

Doe RP, Dickinson P, Zinneman HH, et al: Elevated nonprotein-bound cortisol (NPC) in pregnancy, during estrogen administration and in carcinoma of the prostate. *J Clin Endocrinol Metab* 1969; 29:757.

Hensleigh PA, Fainstat T: How to diagnose and manage virilization in pregnant patients. *Contemp OB/GYN* 1980;15: 219–225.

Hughes IA, Laurence KM: Antenatal diagnosis of congenital adrenal hyperplasia. *Lancet* 1979;ii:7–9.

Migeon CJ, Kenny FM, Taylor FH: Cortisol production. VIII. Pregnancy. *J Clin Endocrinol Metab* 1968;28:661.

Mishell DR, Thorneycroft IH, Nagata Y, et al: Serum gonadotropin and steroid patterns in early human gestation. *Am J Obstet Gynecol* 1973;117:631–642.

Nagamani M, McDonough PG, Ellegood JO, et al: Maternal and amniotic fluid 17 a-hydroxyprogesterone levels during pregnancy: Diagnosis of congenital adrenal hyperplasia in utero. *Am J Obstet Gynecol* 1978;130:791–794.

Rosenthal HE, Slaunwhite WR, Sandberg AA: Transcortin: A corticosteroid-binding protein of plasma. X. Cortisol and progesterone interplay and unbound levels of these steroids in pregnancy. *J Clin Endocrinol Metab* 1969;29:352.

Sippell WG, Dorr HG, Becker H, et al: Simultaneous determination of seven unconjugated steroids in maternal venous and umbilical arterial and venous serum in elective and emergency cesarean section at term. *Am J Obstet Gynecol* 1979;135:530.

384

Alpha Feto Protein

Maternal Serum Alpha-Fetoprotein: Issues in the Prenatal Screening and Diagnosis of Neural Tube Defects. Proceedings of a conference held by the National Center for Health Care Technology and the Food and Drug Administration, 28–30, July 1980. U.S. Govt. Doc. HE 20:2:M41.

Amniotic Fluid Bilirubin

Bishop E, Brown T: Management of erythroblastosis. *ACOG Tech Bull* 1972;17:1–8.

Liley AW: Liquor amnii analysis in management of pregnancy complicated by rhesus sensitization. *Am J Obstet Gynecol* 1961;82:1359–1370.

Amniotic Karyotyping

Milunski A: *The Prevention of Genetic Disease and Mental Retardation.* Philadelphia, The W.B. Saunders Co, 1975.

Amylase

DeVore GR, Bracken M, Berkowitz RL: The amylase/creatinine clearance ratio in normal pregnancy and pregnancies complicated by pancreatitis, hyperemesis gravidarum, and toxemia. *Am J Obstet Gynecol* 1980;136:747–754.

Kaiser R, Berk JE, Fridhandler L: Serum amylase changes during pregnancy. *Am J Obstet Gynecol* 1975;122: 283–286.

Carbohydrate Metabolism

Carpenter MW, Coustan DR: Criteria for screening tests for gestational diabetes. *Am J Obstet Gynecol* 1982; 144:768–773.

Cousins L, Rigg L, Hollinsworth D, et al: The 24-hour excursion and diurnal rhythm of glucose, insulin, and C-peptide in normal pregnancy. *Am J Obstet Gynecol* 1980;136:483–488.

Jovanovic L, Peterson CM, Saxena BB, et al: Feasibility of maintaining normal glucose profiles in insulin-dependent pregnant diabetic women. *Am J Med* 1980;68:105–111.

Lewis SB, Wallin JD, Kuzuya H, et al: Circadian variation of serum glucose, C-peptide immmunoreactivity and free insulin in normal and insulin-treated diabetic subjects. *Diabetologia* 1976;12: 343–350.

O'Sullivan J, Mahan C: Criteria for the oral glucose tolerance test in pregnancy. *Diabetes* 1964;13:278–285.

Coagulation Studies

Fletcher AP, Alkjaersig NK, Burstein R: The influence of pregnancy upon blood coagulation and plasma fibrinolytic enzyme function. *Am J Obstet Gynecol* 1979;134:743.

Lavery JP: When coagulopathy threatens the pregnant patient. *Contemp OB/GYN* 1982;20:191–199.

Electrolytes

Andersen GJ, James GB, Mathers NP, et al: The maternal oxygen tension and acid-base status during pregnancy. *J Obstet Gynaecol Brit Cwlth* 1969;77: 16–19.

Fadel HE, Northrop H, Misenheimer R, et al: Normal pregnancy: A model of sustained respiratory alkalosis. *J Perinat Med* 1979;7:195–201.

Newman RL: Serum electrolytes in pregnancy, parturition, and puerperium. *Obstet Gynecol* 1957;10:51–55.

Pitkin RM, Reynolds WA, Williams GA, et al: Calcium metabolism in normal pregnancy: A longitudinal study. *Am J Obstet Gynecol* 1979;133:781.

Erythroblastosis Fetalis and Hemolytic Disease of the Newborn

Ball CA (ed): *A Seminar on Perinatal Blood Banking.* American Association of Blood Banks, 1978.

Schanfield MS: Human immunoglobulin (IgG) subclasses and their biological properties, in *Blood Bank Immunology,* American Association of Blood Banks workshop, 1980.

Sherwood WC, Cohen A (eds): *Transfusion Therapy: The Fetus, Infant and Child.* New York, Masson, 1980.

Fetal Lung Maturity

Amenta JS, Silverman JA: Amniotic fluid lecithin, phosphatidylglycerol, L/S ratio, and foam stability test in predicting respiratory distress in the newborn. *Am J Clin Pathol* 1983;9:52–64.

Clements J, Platzker A, Tierner D, et al: Assessment of the risk of the respiratory-distress syndrome by a rapid test for surfactant in amniotic fluid. *N Engl J Med* 1972;286:1077– 1081.

Gluck L, Kulovich MV, Borer MC, et al: The interpretation and significance of the lecithin/sphingomyelin ratio in amniotic fluid. *Am J Obstet Gynecol* 1974; 120:142–154.

Sher G, Statland BE, Freer DE, et al: Assessing fetal lung maturation by the foam stability index test. *Obstet Gynecol* 1978;52:673–677.

Hematology in Pregnancy

Carr MC: The diagnosis of iron deficiency in pregnancy. *Obstet Gynecol* 1974;43:15–21.

Fenton V, Saunders K, Cavill I: The platelet count in pregnancy. *J Clin Path* 1977;30:68–69.

Griffin JFT, Beck I: Changes in maternal peripheral leucocytes around delivery. *Br J Obstet Gynaecol* 1980;87:402– 407.

Kaneshige E: Serum ferritin as an assessment of iron stores and other hematologic parameters during pregnancy. *Obstet Gynecol* 1981;57: 238–242.

Lange R, Dynesius R: Blood volume changes during normal pregnancy. *Clin Hematol* 1973;2:437.

Pitkin RM, Witte DL: Platelet and leukocyte counts in pregnancy. *JAMA* 1979;242:2696–2698.

Scott JR, Cruikshank DP, Kochenour NK, et al: Fetal platelet counts in the obstetric management of immunologic thrombocytopenic purpura. *Am J Obstet Gynecol* 1980;136:495–499.

Sejeny SA, Easthan RD, Baker SR: Platelet counts during normal pregnancy. *J Clin Pathol* 1975;28:812–813.

Taylor DJ, Phillips P, Lind T: Puerperal haematological indices. *Br J Obstet Gynaecol* 1981:88:601–606.

Infectious Disease

Harris RE, Jordan PA, Monif GRG: Rubella antibody titer: The significance of low-titered rubella antibodies. *Obstet Gynecol* 1978;52: 243–245.

Horstmann DM: Rubella: Still a problem for obstetricians. *Contemp OB/GYN* 1979;13:67–83.

Mann JM, Preblud SR, Hoffman RE, et al: Assessing risks of rubella infection during pregnancy. *JAMA* 1981;245: 1647–1652.

Monif GRG: Rubella virus, in *Infectious Diseases in Obstetrics and Gynecology.* ed 2. Philadelphia, Harper & Row, 1982, pp 89–102.

Preblud SR, Herrman KL, Mann JM, et al: Rubella . . . a clinical update. *ACOG Tech Bull* 1981;62:1–8.

Lipids in Serum

Potter JM, Nestel PJ: The hyperlipidemia of pregnancy in normal and complicated pregnancies. *Am J Obstet Gynecol* 1979;133:165–170.

Liver Function Tests

Fallon HJ: Liver diseases, in Burrow GN, Ferris TF (eds): *Medical Complications During Pregnancy.* Philadelphia, The W.B. Saunders Co, 1982, pp 278–301.

Laatikainen T, Ikonen E: Serum bile acids in cholestasis of pregnancy. *Obstet Gynecol* 1977;50:313–318.

Samuelson K, Thomassen PA: Radioimmunoassay of serum bile acids in normal pregnancy and in recurrent cholestasis of pregnancy. *Acta Obstet Gynecol Scand* 1980;59:417–420.

Scholtes G: Liver function and liver diseases during pregnancy. *J Perinat Med* 1979;7:55–68.

Shaw D, Frohlich J, Wittman BAK, et al: A prospective study of 18 patients with cholestasis of pregnancy. *Am J Obstet Gynecol* 1982;142:621–625.

Walker FB, Hoblit DL, Cunningham FG, et al: Gamma glutamyl transpeptidase in normal pregnancy. *Obstet Gynecol* 1974;43:745–749.

Pituitary Hormones

Barberia JM, Abu-Fadil S, Kletzky OA, et al: Serum prolactin patterns in early human gestation. *Am J Obstet Gynecol* 1975;121:1107–1110.

Jovanovic L, Dawood MY, Landesman R, et al: Hormonal profile as a prognostic index of early threatened abortion. *Am J Obstet Gynecol* 1978;130:274.

Marrs RP, Kletzky OA, Mishell DR: Functional capacity of the gonadotrophs during pregnancy and the puerperium. *Am J Obstet Gynecol* 1981;141:658–661.

Sadovsky E, Weinstein D, Ben-David M, et al: Serum prolactin in normal and pathologic pregnancy. *Obstet Gynecol* 1977;50:559–561.

Riss P, Mick R, Spona J: First trimester serum prolactin levels in normal and complicated pregnancies. *Gynecol Obstet Inves* 1980;11: 113–118.

Pregnancy Testing

Braunstein DG, Rasor J, Adler W, et al: Serum human chorionic gonadotropin levels throughout normal pregnancy. *Am J Obstet Gynecol* 1976;126:678–681.

Dawood MY, Saxena BB, Landesman R: Human chorionic gonadotropin and its subunits in hydatidiform mole and choriocarcinomas. *Obstet Gynecol* 1977; 50:172–181.

Kadar N, DeVore G, Romero R: Discriminatory hCG zone: its use in the sonographic evaluation for ectopic pregnancy. *Obstet Gynecol* 1981;58: 156–161.

Renal Function

Lindheimer MD, Katz AI: The kidney in pregnancy. *N Engl J Med* 1970;283: 1095–1097.

Sims EAH, Krantz KE: Serial studies of renal function during pregnancy and the puerperium in normal women. *J Clin Invest* 1958;37:1764–1774.

Thyroid Function

Malkasian GD, Mayberry WE: Serum total and free thyroxine and thyrotropin in normal and pregnant women, neonates, and women receiving progestogens. *Am J Obstet Gynecol* 1970;108: 1234–1238.

Abetalipoproteinemia, 47
Abnormal range of values in laboratory tests
  in apparently healthy patients, 6
  determination of, 1, 2, 4
  indexes of test proficiency and, 6, 7
  problems with use of, 4, 6
  sensitivity and specificity and, 15
ABO system, 381
Abortion, therapeutic, 360
Abscess, 145
Absorption tests, 223
Acanthrocytes, 44, 46
Accuracy for negative prediction, 1, 6, 9–13
  calculation of, 10–13
  pretest disease likelihood and, 12–13
  proportion of tested population with disease
    and, 10
  screening tests and, 14
  sensitivity and specificity and, 10
Accuracy for positive prediction, 1, 6, 9–13
  calculation of, 10–13
  confirmation tests and, 14
  pretest disease likelihood and, 12–13
  proportion of tested population with disease
    and, 10
  sensitivity and specificity and, 10
Acetazolamide, 98
Acetylcholinesterase, 379
N-acetylprocainamide (NAPA), 72
Achlorhydria, 212, 213, 228
Acid-base disturbances, 77–83
  blood gas value analysis in, 77–78
  calcium measurements and, 303
  clinical approach to, 81, 82–83
  metabolic acidosis in, 79–80
  metabolic alkalosis in, 81
  mixed, 77, 78, 81, 82
  potassium levels in, 87
  respiratory acidosis in, 80–81
  respiratory alkalosis in, 81
  simple, 77, 78
Acidemia, 77
  blood gases and, 77
  metabolic acidosis with, 79–80
Acidosis, 77
  calcium measurements and, 303
  hyperkalemia with, 82, 88
  osteomalacia with, 319
  see also Metabolic acidosis; Respiratory
    acidosis
Acid phosphatase, as oncology marker, 349–350
Acromegaly
  cortisol in, 323
  growth hormone in, 281, 286, 287, 288
ACTH, see Adrenocorticotropic hormone
    (ACTH)
Activated partial prothrombin time, in preg-
    nancy, 363
Acute-phase reactants, 193–195
Acute tubular necrosis, 92, 93, 267
Addison's disease, 98, 188, 322, 377
Adenomatous goiter, 188
Adenovirus, 256
ADH, see Antidiuretic hormone (ADH)
ADP, 55
Adrenal function
  laboratory evaluation of, 318–334
  pregnancy and, 377–378

Adrenal hyperplasia
  congenital, see Congenital adrenal hyperplasia
    (CAH)
  dexamethasone-suppressible (DSAH), 326,
    329
Adrenal insufficiency
  adrenocorticotropic hormone (ACTH) and,
    282, 322
  cortisol and, 322
  glucocorticoid stimulation tests in, 323
  hypercalcemia differential diagnosis and, 309
  hypoglycemia and, 276
  laboratory tests in, 326, 327
  mineralocorticoid deficiency in, 329
Adrenalitis, 189
Adrenal medullary disorders, 330–334
Adrenal medullary hyperplasia (AMH),
    330–340, 341
Adrenal tumors, 115, 322
Adrenocortical carcinoma, 326
Adrenocorticotropic hormone (ACTH)
  aldosterone and, 328
  antidiuretic hormone (ADH) and deficiency
    of, 284, 290
  carcinoid tumors and, 342
  congenital adrenal hyperplasia (CAH) and,
    330, 331
  cortisol response to, 281–282, 329
  cosyntropin injection test of, 282–283, 323
  Cushing's syndrome (CS) with, 281, 324
  hypercortisolism with, 323–324
  insulin tolerance test (ITT) in, 283–284, 323
  measurement of, 322
  metyrapone test with, 284, 323
  pregnancy and, 374
  radioimmunoassay of, 282
  stimulation tests of, 282–284, 323
Aerobic sputum culture, 138
Agammaglobulinemia, 176
Agglutination tests, 166
  latex particles in, 166, 168, 169, 170, 171
  pregnancy testing with, 353
Airflow measurements in, 126–130
Alanine aminotransferase (ALT), 233; see also
    Serum glutamic-pyruvate transaminase
    (SGPT)
Albumin
  acute glomerulonephritis with, 108
  alkaline phosphatase and, 242
  calcium measurements with, 303
  cerebrospinal fluid (CSF) IgG index with, 265
  drug binding to, 63
  electrolyte analysis with, 78
  liver function tests with, 233, 234–235, 249
  nephrotic syndrome with, 106, 107
  proteinuria with, 93
  testosterone binding to, 334
  thyroxine (T_4) binding to, 295
Albuminuria, 105
Alcohol and alcoholism
  cortisol and, 322
  dexamethasone suppression test (DST) and,
    324
  glucose tolerance and, 270
  gynecomastia and, 338
  hypophosphatemia and, 316
  liver disease induced by, 233, 247, 248
  liver function tests and, 232, 233, 244

Index

387

platelet counts and, 55
SGOT and SGPT and, 249
Alcoholic cirrhosis, 9, 239, 248, 347
Alcoholic hypoglycemia, 276
Alcoholic ketoacidosis (AKA), 274
Alcoholic pancreatitis, 217
Aldolase, 267
Aldosterone
  adenomas producing (APA), 326, 328–329
  factors affecting, 328
  hyperaldosteronism with, 326, 327–328
  potassium and, 101
  renovascular hypertension with, 117
Alkalemia, 77
  blood gases in, 77
  metabolic and respiratory alkalosis with, 81
Alkaline phosphatase
  bone turnover of, 304
  hypercalcemia with, 308–310
  hypocalcemia with, 314–315
  kidney stone disease and, 313
  King-Armstrong unit for, 22
  liver function with, 239, 241–242, 243, 245,
    249, 304
  measurement of, 304
  osteomalacia with, 319
  Paget's disease with, 313
  pregnancy and, 373
  primary "thrombocythemia" and, 49
  pulmonary disease with, 142
Alkalosis, 77
  calcium measurements and, 303
  hypokalemia with, 82
  see also Metabolic alkalosis; Respiratory
    alkalosis
Allergy
  eosinophilia with, 40, 41
  food, 179, 224
  immunoglobulins in, 177, 178
Allopurinol, 108, 208
Alpha-1-antitrypsin, 142, 193
Alpha feto protein (AFP), 348–349, 378–379
Alpha methyldopa, 114
Alveolar-capillary block syndrome, 135
Alveolar-arterial oxygen gradient (A-adO$_2$),
    132–133
Alveolar macrophages
  infectious disease with, 146
  sputum examination with, 137
Amebiasis, 227
Amenorrhea
  estradiol in, 335
  female infertility with, 339
  karyotype in, 336–337
  laboratory tests in, 337–338
  prolactin in, 281, 289, 336
Amenorrhea-galactorrhea syndrome, 281
Amikacin, 66, 68
Amiloride, 329
Amino acids, in Fanconi syndrome, 97, 98
Aminoglycosides, 98, 152
  combination therapy with, 156, 158
  therapeutic range of, 61
δ-aminolevulinic acid (ALA), 257, 258, 260
δ-aminolevulinic acid (ALA) synthetase, 259
Aminophylline, 75
Amniotic fluid
  adrenal function deficiencies with, 378
  bilirubin in, 357–359, 381–382

foam stability index (FSI) in, 383
  hemolytic diseases in, 381–382
  karyotyping with, 359–360
  lecithin/sphingomyelin (L/S) ratio with, 382–383
  phosphatidyl glycerol (PG) in, 382, 383
Amphotericin B, 100
Ampicillin, 151, 158
Amylase
  acute pancreatitis with, 214–216, 275
  diabetic ketoacidosis (DKA) with, 275
  diseases with elevation of, 215
  hyperglycemic nonketonic coma with, 275
  pleural fluid, 141
  pregnancy and, 360–362
  Somogyi unit for, 22
Amyloidosis, 100, 107, 117, 185, 209
Anaerobic infections
  blood cultures of, 150
  colony counts in, 148
  Gram stain for, 146
  sputum examination of, 138
Analgesics, 98, 100
Androgens
  breast cancer receptors and, 352
  factors affecting, 334
  hirsutism and, 338
  pregnancy and, 377–378
Androstenedione
  congenital adrenal hyperplasia (CAH) and, 330,
    331
  pregnancy and, 377
Anemia, 25–31
  antibodies in, 189, 191, 192
  causes of, 25, 27
  of chronic disease, 25, 26, 29
  chronic lymphocytic leukemia with, 39
  dimorphic, 31
  erythrocyte sedimentation rate (ESR) and, 194
  iron deficiency and, 27–28
  neonatal, 382
  pregnancy and, 356–357
  race and, 28
  renal function in, 30–31
  see also specific types of anemia
Aneuploidies, 359
Angiography, pulmonary, 122, 123
Angioneurotic edema, 183–184
Angiotensin II, 117, 328
Anisocytosis, 41, 43
Ankylosing spondylitis, 207
Anion gap, 78–79, 82, 83
  hyperkalemia with, 88
  metabolic acidosis with, 79–80, 82
Anions, 78
Anorexia nervosa, 286, 288, 322, 323, 324
Anoxemia, 33
Antacids, 316
Antibiotics
  bacterial tolerance of, 155–156
  combinations of, 156–159
  eosinophilia induced by, 40
  minimal bactericidal concentration (MBC) of,
    151, 153–154
  minimal inhibitory concentration (MIC) of, 151,
    153–154
  serum levels of, 152, 154
  synergy studies of, 156–159
Antibodies
  acute-phase reactants with, 193–195

detection of, 185–187
measurement of, 166–168
to tissue antigens, 187–195
VDRL test with, 192–193
Anticancer drugs, 28
Anticonvulsant drugs, 71, 98
Antidepressant drugs, 288, 289
Antidiuretic hormone (ADH), 290–291
adrenocorticotropic hormone (ACTH) and, 284
dehydration test (Miller-Moses test) for, 291
radioimmunoassays of, 290
serum and urine osmolarity of, 290
syndrome of inappropriate secretion of (SIADH), 290, 291
water loading test for, 291
Antigens, 168–169, 185–187
antibodies to tissue, 187–195
Anti-intrinsic factor antibodies, 188, 189
Antimicrobial removal devices (ARDs), 150
Antimicrobial sensitivity testing, 151–154
Antimicrosomal antibodies, 188, 189
Antimitochondrial antibodies, 188–189, 234
Antinuclear antibodies (ANAs), 187, 188, 189–191, 192
Antinuclear factors
rheumatic diseases with, 205–206
synovial fluid, 203
Anti-parietal cell antibodies, 187, 188, 189
Anti-smooth muscle antibodies, 187, 188, 189
Antistreptolysin O (ASLO) test, 168, 169–170
Antithrombin III (AT III), 55–56
Antithyroglobulin, 188, 189
Antithyroid preparations, 239
Antitreponemal antibody tests, 192
Anti-trichinella antibodies, 267
Antitrypsin deficiency, 234
Aplastic anemia, 36, 50
L-arginine hydrochloride, 287
Arias syndrome, 238, 240
Arterial blood gases, 132–135
Arteriovenous (A-V) malformation, 122
Arthritis, 192, 202, 203, 204, 207; see also Rheumatoid arthritis and other specific types of arthritis
Arthropies, on synovial fluid, 199, 201
Ascorbic acid, 226
Aspartate aminotransferase (AST), 232; see also Serum glutamic-oxaloacetic transaminase (SGOT)
Aspergillus species, 147
Aspirin, 55, 74, 203, 208
Asthma, 40, 123, 178, 179
Atherosclerosis, 111
Atopic eczema, 177
Autoimmune diseases, 177
antibodies to tissue antigens in, 187
hypoadrenergic states with, 334
T lymphocytes in, 175
Autoimmune hemolytic anemia, 183
Axotemia, 97, 102, 104

Bacillus species, 147–148
Bacteremia, 150, 152
Bacteria
antibiotic combinations and, 156–159
antimicrobial sensitivity testing of, 151–154
blood cultures for, 149–151
C3 and C4 in, 182
disk diffusion test for, 151–152
immunoglobulins and, 176
indirect immunofluorescence assay (IFA) for antigen to, 167
leukocytosis with, 37
minimal bactericidal concentration (MBC) of antibiotics for, 151, 153–154
minimal inhibitory concentration (MIC) of antibiotics for, 151, 153–154
quantitation of, 148–149
serum bactericidal concentration (SBC) assay (Schlichter Test) of, 154–155
small bowel and malabsorption, 223, 225
T cells in immune response to, 175
tolerance of, 155–156
tube dilution assay of, 152–154
Bacterial endocarditis, 154, 155
Bacterial meningitis, 155, 266
Bacterial pneumonia, 140
Bacteriuria, 149
Bacteroides species, 150
Barium studies
esophagram, 122
gastrointestinal, 29
Barr bodies, 336, 337
Basopenia, 34
Basophilic stippling, 43
Bayes' formula, 12
B cells, 175, 176
Benadryl, 211
Bence-Jones protein, 94, 185
Benzidine, 226
Benzyl alcohol, 318
Berylliosis, 308
Beta-hydroxybutyric acid, 273–274
6-betahydroxycortisol, 323
3-betahydroxydehydrogenase deficiency, 331
11-beta-hydroxylase blockade, 284
Beta thalassemia minor, 29
Bicarbonate
anion gap and, 78
hyperkalemia and, 88
pregnancy and, 365
renal tubular acidosis (RTA) with, 98
Bile acids
deficiency of, 225
diarrhea and, 228
liver function and, 236–238, 245
malabsorption of, 222, 223
pregnancy and, 374
Bile salts, 243
diarrhea and, 227, 228
malabsorption of, 222, 223
Biliary atresia, 243, 246
Biliary cirrhosis, 188, 189
antimitochondrial antibody in, 234
bilirubin in, 239
copper storage in, 246
Biliary tract stones, 240
Bilirubin, amniotic fluid, 357–359, 381–382
Bilirubin, serum
hemolysis with, 30
jaundice with, 263
liver function with, 238–239, 240, 243, 245, 249
pregnancy and, 373
Bilirubin, urine
hypertension with, 115
liver function with, 239–240, 245
Bilirubinuria, 238, 239
Blacks

hematuria in, 109
  white cell count normal range in, 34
Blastomycosis, 142
Bleeding time test, 51, 55
Blood component antibodies, 187, 191–192
Blood cultures, 149–151
  antimicrobial removal devices (ARDs) in, 150
  drawing blood in, 149–150
  infective endocarditis on, 149–150
  sputum examination and, 138
Blood gases, 77–83
  arterial, 132–135
Blood loss, 26, 29; see also Occult blood loss
Blood urea nitrogen (BUN)
  acute glomerulonephritis with, 107, 108
  acute interstitial nephritis with, 108, 109
  glomerular filtration rate (GFR) and, 97
  hematuria with, 109
  hyperkalemia with, 88
  hypertension with, 115
  nephrotic syndrome with, 106, 107
  pregnancy and, 376
  renal failure and, 102, 104, 105, 267
B lymphocytes, 175, 176
Bone alkaline phosphatase measurements, 304
Bone disease, 241, 242, 302–303
Bone marrow aspiration
  anemia on, 25, 28
  iron and, 29–30, 356
  leukocytosis and, 38
  lymphocytosis and, 39
  pancytopenia and, 50
  Pappenheimer bodies in, 43
Bone metastases, 308
Breast cancer
  alpha feto protein in, 349
  carcinoembryonic antigen (CEA) in, 347
  receptors in, 350–352
"Breast-milk jaundice," 239, 240
Breath tests, in malabsorption, 221, 222, 223, 224, 225
Bromocriptine, 290
Bromosulphthalein (BSP)
  liver function and, 240–241, 245
  pregnancy and, 367–373
Bronchogenic carcinoma, 142
Bronchography, 122, 139
Broth dilution assays, 152–154
Brucella, 166
Bruton's congenital, sex-linked agammaglobulin-
    emia, 176
BSP, see Bromosulphthalein (BSP)
Buccal smear, in gonadal disease, 336
BUN, see Blood urea nitrogen (BUN)
Burr cells, 44, 46, 47

CAH, see Congenital adrenal hyperplasia (CAH)
Calcitonin (CT)
  acute pancreatitis with, 217
  carcinoid tumors with, 342
  multiple endocrine neoplasia syndromes (MENs)
    with, 340
  serum levels of, 298
Calcium, fasting fractional excretion of (FECa),
    303–304
  hypercalcemia with, 308–310
  kidney stone disease with, 320–321
  osteoporosis with, 312
Calcium, serum, 302, 303
  acute pancreatitis with, 217

hypercalcemia with, 308–310
hyperphosphatemia with, 317
hypocalcemia with, 314–315
hypoglycemia with, 277
hypophosphatemia with, 316
kidney stone disease with, 320–321
malabsorption with, 220
osteomalacia with, 319
Paget's disease with, 313
pregnancy and, 364
pulmonary disease with, 142
Calcium, urine, 303–304
  hypocalcemia with, 308–310
  hyperphosphatemia with, 317
  hypophosphatemia with, 316
  kidney stone disease with, 320–321
  osteomalacia with, 319
  osteoporosis with, 312
  Paget's disease with, 313
Calcium gluconate, 340
Calcium infusion test, 213
Calcium metabolism, 302–318
Calcium oxalate kidney stone disease, 307, 311,
    313, 320–321
Calcium pyrophosphate arthropathy, 199
Campylobacter infection, 146, 227
Cancer
  Cushing's disease and, 325
  eosinophilia with, 40, 41
  hypercalcemia differential diagnosis and, 308
  monocytosis in, 41
  neutropenia with chemotherapy in, 35
  see also Oncology and specific sites and types
    of cancer
Candida albicans, 148, 150
Candida species, 147, 175, 180
Carbamazepine, 68, 70, 318
Carbenicillin, 156
Carbohydrate malabsorption, 220–221, 227
Carbohydrate metabolism, in pregnancy, 362–
    363
Carbon dioxide production (VCO$_2$), 135–136
Carcinoembryonic antigen (CEA), 8–9, 347
Carcinoid syndrome, 342
Cardiac enzymes, 112–113
  Cardiomyopathy, 117–118
Cardiovascular disease, 111–118
  cardiac enzymes and, 112–113
  cardiomyopathy in, 117–118
  cholesterol and triglycerides in, 111–112
  hypertension and, 113–116
  renovascular hypertension in, 116–117
Carotene, 220
Casts, urinary sediment with, 92; see also Red
    cell casts
CAT, see Computerized axial tomography
    (CAT)
Catecholamines
  hypoadrenergic states and, 334
  pheochromocytoma and, 330, 332, 333
  renovascular hypertension with, 117
Cations, 78
C-cell hyperplasia (CCH), 339, 340
CEA, see Carcinoembryonic antigen (CEA)
Cellular immune system, 175, 177; see also
    Immunology
Celsius temperature, 22
Cephalosporins, 150
Cerebrospinal fluid (CSF), 263–267
  cell count and differential in, 264

countercurrent immunoelectrophoresis (CIE) of, 266
cytomorphological studies of, 264
fungi in, 266–267
gamma globulin in, 265
glucose level of, 264
Gram stain for, 145
handling of specimen of, 263
IgG-albumin index of, 265
lactic acid levels in, 264
microbial tests with, 266
myelin basic protein in, 265
oligoclonal bands in, 265
protein in, 264–265
serological examination of, 165–166
syphilis tests with, 266
Ceruloplasmin, 193, 246, 247, 367
Charcot-Leyden crystals, 138
Chemstrips, 274
Chenodeoxycholic acid, 236, 237
Chest roentgenography, 119–121, 122–123
computerized axial tomography (CT) in, 123–124
portable, 120
pulmonary disease on, 119–124
tomography in, 121
ultrasound in, 123
CH50, 183, 203, 206
Chlamydial infection, 163
Chloramphenicol, 67, 68
Chlordiazepoxide, 330
Chloride
hypokalemia with, 88
phosphorus ratio with, 307
pregnancy and, 365
Chlorpromazine, 289, 330
Cholangiolytic hepatitis, 240
Cholangitis, 242
Cholecystokinin-pancreozymin (CCK-PZ), 219
Cholestasis, 237, 239, 240, 241, 243, 244, 246
of pregnancy, 373, 374
Cholestatic alcoholic hepatitis, 236
Cholesterol, 111–112
cardiovascular disease and, 111–112
liver function and, 236, 239
nephrotic syndrome with, 106
normal values by age for, 112, 113
pregnancy and, 367, 373
synovial fluid, 199
Cholic acid, 236, 237
[¹⁴C] Cholyl glycine breath test, 222, 225
Chondrocalcinosis, 199
Choriocarcinoma, 338, 354
Chromosome abnormalities, 38, 359–360
Chronic disease, anemia of, 25, 26, 29
Chronic lymphocytic leukemia, 39–40, 45, 187, 191
Chronic obstructive lung disease, 123
Chylomicrons, 112, 222
Chylothorax, 141
Chymotrypsin, 218
Cimetidine, 75, 289, 338
Cirrhosis, 9, 205
alpha feto protein in, 349
antibodies in, 188, 189, 191
bilirubin in, 238
cholesterol in, 236
cryptogenic, 189
globulins in, 234
growth hormone in, 288
hyperaldosteronism with, 326

prolactin and, 289
Clinistix, 272
Clinitest tablets, 272, 273
Clofibrate, 111
Clonidine, 332, 333
Clostridium difficile toxin, 227
Clotting disorders, 51–53
Clotting factor assays, 58–59; see also Factor headings
Coagglutination, 169
Coagulation studies, in pregnancy, 363–364
Coccidioidomycosis, 179, 308
Colchicine, 208
Colorectal carcinoma, 8–9, 347
Column temperature measurements, 22
Coma, hyperglycemic non-ketonic (HNKC), 275
Complement fixation (CT) assay, 167, 170, 171
histoplasmosis with, 141–142
rubella infection with, 366
Complement system
acute glomerulonephritis with, 108
acute-phase reactants with, 193
hematuria and, 109
hemolytic assays of, 183
nephrotic syndrome with, 106
pleural fluid, 141
quantitative assessment of, 180, 182–184
rheumatic diseases with, 206–207
synovial fluid, 203
Complement C1, 207
Complement C1 esterase inhibitor (C1 E1), 182, 183–184
Complement C1q
quantitation of, 182, 185, 186
rheumatic diseases with, 207
Complement C2, 207
Complement C3
hemolytic anemia with, 192
quantitation of, 180, 181, 182–183
rheumatic diseases with, 206, 207
Complement C4, 184
quantitation of, 180, 182–183
rheumatic diseases with, 207
synovial fluid, 203
Complement C5 through 9, 183
Computerized axial tomography (CT)
pituitary abnormalities on, 292
pulmonary disease on, 123–124
renovascular hypertension on, 117
Concentration, SI unit for, 20–21
Confirmation tests, 13, 14–15
Confounding variables, 4–5
Congenital adrenal hyperplasia (CAH), 322
17 ketosteroids (17 KS) in, 338
laboratory tests in, 330, 331
pregnancy and, 378
Congenital rubella syndrome, 366
Congestive heart failure, 242, 326
Connective tissue disorders, 180, 193, 194
Contrast studies of chest, 122
Coombs positive hemolytic anemia, 45, 114
Coombs test, 30
Copper, and liver function, 244–247
Copper sulfate tests, in diabetes mellitus, 272–273
Coproporphyria, 257, 258, 259, 260
Coronary artery disease
cholesterol and triglycerides and, 111
exercise tolerance test (ETT) in, 1, 12, 15
Corticosteroid-binding globulin (CBG), 322
Corticosteroids

leukocytosis with, 37
renovascular hypertension and, 117
Corticosterone, 322, 331
Cortisol, 322
  antidiuretic hormone (ADH) and, 284, 290, 291
  congenital adrenal hyperplasia (CAH) and, 331
  dexamethasone suppression test (DST) for, 324, 325
  hypercortisolism with, 323, 324
  hyporeninemic hypoaldosteronism with, 329
  insulin hypoglycemia and, 283
  osteoporosis with, 313
  pituitary function and, 281–282
  plasma-free, 322
Cortisol, urine-free (UFC), 323
  dexamethasone suppression test (DST) and, 325
Cortisone, 322
Cosyntropin injection tests, with adrenocortico-tropic hormone (ACTH), 282–283, 323
Coulter counters, 56–57
Counterimmunoelectrophoresis (CIE), 169, 170, 266, 349
Coxsackievirus B, 256
C-peptide, and insulin, 277
CPK, see Creatine phosphokinase (CPK)
Craniopharyngioma, 290
C-reactive protein (CRP), 193–194
Creatine phosphokinase (CPK), 112–113, 267
  cardiac, 112–113
  muscle diseases with, 267
Creatinine, serum
  acute glomerulonephritis with, 107, 108
  anemia and, 30
  carcinoid syndrome with, 342
  hematuria with, 109
  hyperkalemia and, 88
  hypertension with, 115
  kidney stone disease and, 313–318
  nephrotic syndrome with, 106, 107
  pancreatitis and, 361–362
  pregnancy and, 376
  renal failure and, 102, 104, 105, 267
  rheumatic diseases with, 208
  urine phosphorus measurements with, 304
Creatinine clearance
  acute glomerulonephritis with, 107, 108
  acute interstitial nephritis with, 109
  acute pancreatitis with, 216
  anemia and, 30
  glomerular filtration rate (GFR) with, 96–97
  hematuria with, 109, 110
  nephrotic syndrome with, 107
  pregnancy and, 376
  renal failure and, 102, 104, 105
Crenated cells, 46, 47
Crigler-Najjar syndrome, 238, 240
Crohn's disease, 177, 207
Cryoglobulinemia, 100, 183, 186–187
Cryoglobulins, 108, 185, 186–187, 207
Cryoproteins, 186–187
Cryptococcal antigen, 169, 267
Cryptococcus neoformans, 142, 147, 171, 266
Cryptogenic cirrhosis, 189
Crystals, synovial fluid, 198–199
Cultures
  blood, see Blood cultures
  diarrhea on, 227
  synovial fluid, 203–204
Cushing's disease (CD), 114, 324

Cushing's syndrome (CS), 312
  adrenocorticotropic hormone (ACTH) in, 281, 282, 283
  cortisol in, 282, 322, 323
  dexamethasone suppression tests (DST) in, 323, 324–326
  forms of, 324
  hirsutism in, 338
  laboratory tests in, 323–324
  pregnancy and, 377
Cyclic AMP (cAMP), and parathyroid hormone (PTH), 306–307
Cyclic AMP, urine (UcAMP), 306–307
  hypercalcemia and, 308–310
  hypocalcemia and, 314–315
  hypophosphatemia and, 316
  kidney stone disease and, 320–321
  osteomalacia with, 319
Cyclic neutropenia, 36
Cytomegalovirus, 256, 365
  lymphocytosis with, 38, 39
  serological data on, 171
Cyclophosphamide, 28, 50, 352
Cystic fibrosis, 214, 217
Cystine, 98, 311
  kidney stone disease and, 313, 320–321
Cystinuria, 98, 311, 321
Cystitis, 109
Cytosine arabinoside, 28

Dane particle, 250
Dead space (V_D), lung, 136
Decubitus ulcers, 149
Dehydration test, with antidiuretic hormone (ADH), 291
Dehydroepiandrosterone (DHEA), 330, 331
Dehydroepiandrosterone sulfate (DHEAS), 334–335
  congenital adrenal hyperplasia (CAH) with, 330, 331
  hirsutism and, 338
Delayed-type hypersensitivity (DTH) skin test, 175, 176, 177, 180
Deoxycholic acid, 236, 237
11-deoxycortisol, 284, 322
21-deoxycortisol, 322
Deoxycorticosterone, 328
Depression
  cortisol and, 322
  growth hormone in, 288
Dermatitis, 179
Dermatomyositis, 191
Desmolase, 331
Dexamethasone, 322
Dexamethasone-suppressible adrenal hyperplasia (DSAH), 326, 329
Dexamethasone suppression test (DST)
  adrenal hyperplasia and, 329
  Cushing's syndrome (CS) with, 323, 324–326
  high-dose, 325–326
  low-dose two-day, 324–325
  overnight single-dose, 324
  pregnancy and, 377
Dextrostix, 274
Diabetes insipidus, 86
  antidiuretic hormone (ADH) and, 290, 291
  nephrogenic, 291
  pregnancy and, 375
  urinary concentrating ability in, 98, 100
Diabetes mellitus (DM), 242, 269–275, 312, 338

antibodies in, 188
blood glucose monitoring in, 274
complications of, 274–275
diagnosis of, 269–272
etiology of, 271
fasting plasma glucose (FPG) and oral glucose
  tolerance test (OGTT) in, 269–270
glomerulosclerosis and, 104
glucose level testing in, 15
growth hormone in, 286
hyperglycemic non-ketonic coma (HNKC) in, 275
hypertension in, 115, 116
monitoring, 272–275
pregnancy and, 271–272
primary (idiopathic) versus secondary, 270–271
urine glucose in, 272–273
urine ketones in, 273–274
Diabetic ketoacidosis (DKA), 80, 100, 216, 274–
  275, 316
Diarrhea, 226–228
  infantile, 177
  stool tests in, 227–228
Diazepoxides, 239
Diazoxide, 332
Diethylstilbestrol, 338
Diffusion tests, lung, 132
Digitalis, 116, 338
DiGeorge's syndrome, 175
Digoxin, 61, 62, 65, 68, 73–74
1,25-dihydroxyvitamin D (1,25 OH2 D), 307,
  308–310
Dilantin, see Phenytoin (Dilantin)
Dimorphic anemia, 31
Diphenhydramine hydrochloride, 211
Diphtheroids, 149
Diphylobotrium latum, 222
Dipstick tests
  hematuria with, 109
  hypertension with, 115
  nephrotic syndrome with, 105, 107
  urinary proteins on, 94
Direct Coomb's test, 191–192, 193
Direct fluorescent antibody test, 168, 170
Disaccharidases, and malabsorption, 223, 224
Discoid lupus, 191
Disk diffusion test, 151–152, 155
Disopyramide, 68, 72–73
Disseminated intravascular coagulation (DIC),
  47, 54
Dithiotreitol, 166
Diuretics
  diabetes mellitus and, 270, 271
  hyperaldosteronism with, 327, 328, 329
  hypokalemia with, 88
  hypomagnesemia with, 318
  metabolic alkalosis with, 81
  stress polycythemia with, 33
Diverticulitis, 347
DNase B, 168, 169–170
Döhle bodies, 37
Down's syndrome, 359
Drugs and drug levels, 61–76
  anemia and, 28
  compartment model in, 63
  eosinophilia from, 40
  errors in use of, 65–66
  glucose tolerance tests and, 270
  half-life determinations in, 65
  minimal inhibitory concentration (MIC) with, 61

neutropenia induced by, 35
peak concentrations in, 64
pharmacokinetics of, 62–64
pheochromocytoma tests and, 332, 333
plasma protein binding and, 63–64
prolactin and, 289
rate of elimination of drug and, 62–63
recommendations for obtaining, 64–65
steady state in, 63
therapeutic range of, 61–62
toxicity of drugs and, 62, 64, 65
trough levels in, 64–65
see also specific drugs and classes of drugs
DST, see Dexamethasone suppression test (DST)
Dubin-Johnson syndrome, 239, 240
Duchenne's muscular dystrophy, 267, 360
Duodenal ulcer, 31, 212, 213
Dyphylline, 75

Echinocytes, 46, 47
Eclampsia, 312
Ectopic ACTH syndrome, 322, 324, 325, 326
Ectopic pregnancy, 354
Eczema, 177, 179
Edema, hereditary angioneurotic (HAE), 183–184
EDTA, 37, 47
Ehrlich's reagent, 258–260
Electrocardiogram (EKG), and potassium levels,
  87, 88–89
Electrolytes, 78–79
  diarrhea and, 227–228
  hypertension and, 115–116
  kidney stone disease and, 313
  pregnancy and, 364–365
Electrophoresis
  cardiomyopathy and, 117
  cerebrospinal fluid (CSF), 265, 266
  hemoglobin, 357
  kidney stone disease and, 318
  lipoprotein, 112
  urine protein, 94, 105
Elimination rate of drugs, 62–63
Elliptocytes, 44, 45
Embolism, pulmonary, 122, 123
Emphysema, 136, 142
Encephalitis, 166, 171, 264
Encephalomyelitis, acute disseminated, 265
Endogenous unipolar depression, 322, 323, 324
Energy, in SI measurement, 22
Entamoeba histolytica, 227
Enteric hyperoxaluria, 311
Enterococcal endocarditis, 154, 156, 158–159
Enterococcal infection, 149, 158–159
Enzyme-linked immunosorbent assay (ELISA), 179
Enzyme-linked immunospecific assay (EIA), 167–
  168, 171
Enzymes
  cardiac, 112–113
  SI units for activity of, 22–23
Eosinophilia, 40–41, 267
  pulmonary disease with, 137
Eosinophilic gastroenteritis, 223
Eosinophils, in sputum examination, 137–138
Ephedrine, 332, 333
Epinephrine, 55
  leukocytosis with, 37
  multiple endocrine neoplasia syndrome (MENs)
    with, 341
  pheochromocytoma and, 330, 332, 333

Epithelial cells, in urinary sediment examination, 92
Epstein-Barr virus, 172
E rosettes, 175
Error in laboratory tests, 4–5
Erythroblastosis fetalis, 380–382
Erythrocyte casts, 92
Erythrocytes
  antibodies to, 187, 191–192
  pleural field, 140
Erythrocyte sedimentation rate (ESR), 44, 194–195
Erythrocytosis, 33–34
Erythrohepatic protoporphyria, 257
Erythropoietic porphyria, 257, 258, 259
Erythropoietin, 34
Esbach's picric acid-citric acid reagent, 94
Escherichia coli, 151, 152, 227
Esophagram, barium, 122
Esophagus diseases, 211
Essential cryoglobulinemia, 187
Essential hypertension, 113, 116
Estradiol, 334, 335
  amenorrhea with, 337, 338
  female infertility and, 339
  gynecomastia with, 338
  hypogonadism screening with, 285–286
  indications for use of, 291, 292
Estrogens, 323, 335
  breast cancer receptors and, 350–351, 352
  cholestasis with, 239
  cortisol and, 322
  dexamethasone suppression test (DST) and, 324
  growth hormone tests with, 287
  osteoporosis with, 313
  prolactin and, 289
  testosterone levels and, 334
  thyroid hormone binding capacity and, 293, 296
  vaginal smear for, 337
Estrone, 335
Ethosuximide, 68, 70
Ethylenediaminetetraacetic acid (EDTA), 37, 47
Ethylene glycol, 80
Eunuchoid habitus, 337
Exclusion tests, 13–14
Exercise, and growth hormone, 286, 288
Exercise tolerance tests (ETT)
  coronary artery disease with, 1, 12, 15
  pulmonary function and, 136–137
Expiratory reserve volume (ERV), lung, 125, 126

Factitious hypoglycemia, 277
Factitious hyponatremia, 84
Factor B, 182
Factor D, 183
Factors, I, II, V, VII, X, 235, 363
Factor VIII, 53, 59, 363
Factor IX, 53, 235
Factor Xa, 55–56
Factors XI, XII, 53–54, 363
Falciparum, 44
Familial hypocalciuric hypercalcemia, 310
Fanconi syndrome, 97–98
Fasting fractional excretion of calcium, see
  Calcium, fasting fractional excretion of (FECa)
Fasting hypoglycemia, 275–276, 277
Fasting plasma glucose (FPG), 269–270
Fat breath test, 222

Fat malabsorption, 221–222
Fat tests, 211, 218, 222
Fc portion of IgG, 185–186
FECa, see Calcium, fasting fractional excretion of (FECa)
Fecal tests, see Stool tests
Fecatest, 223
Felty's syndrome, 191, 205
Female infertility, 339
Ferricyanide, 267
Ferritin
  anemia and, 29, 30
  iron deficiency with target cells on, 44
  liver function and, 247–248
  malabsorption and, 220
  Pappenheimer bodies and, 43
  pregnancy and, 356
  thrombocytosis and, 49
Fiberoptic bronchoscopy, 122
Fibrin degradation products, and pregnancy, 363–364
Fibrinogen, 193, 194
Fibrinolysis, and pregnancy, 363–364
Fibrosis, pulmonary, 126
First-order elimination of drugs, 62–63
Flocculation tests, 233
Florinef, 328
Flow-volume curve, lung, 128
Fluorescence microscopy, 160
Fluorescent treponemal antibody absorption test, 192–193, 266
Fluoroscopy of chest, 122
5-fluorouracil, 351, 352
Foam stability index (FSI), in amniotic fluid, 383
Folate deficiency, 28–29, 31, 357
Folic acid, and malabsorption, 220
Follicle-stimulating hormone (FSH), 335, 336, 348
  amenorrhea with, 337
  female infertility and, 339
  hypogonadism with, 286
  impotence and, 338
  indications for use of, 291, 292
  male infertility and, 339
  pregnancy and, 374
  virilization disorders and, 337
Food allergy, 179, 224
Forced expired volumes (FEVs), lung, 127–129
Forced midexpiratory flow rate (FEF_{25-75}), lung, 127–128
Forced vital capacity (FVC), lung, 127–129
Free erythrocyte protoporphyrin (FEP), 29
Free thyroxine (FT_4), 292–293
  by dialysis, 296, 300
  pregnancy and, 380
  by radioimmunoassay (RIA), 296
  thyroid-stimulating hormone (TSH) and, 297
Free thyroxine index (FT_4I), 294, 296, 300
  hyperthyroidism and, 301
  hypothyroidism and, 297–298, 301
  pregnancy and, 380
  stress and, 300, 302
  thyroiditis and, 300, 302
Free triiodothyronine (FT_3), 293
Free triiodothyronine index (FT_3I), 293, 294, 297
Frequency, in SI measurement, 21
Froin's syndrome, 265
FSH, see Follicle-stimulating hormone (FSH)
Functional hypoprolactinemia, 289

Functional residual capacity (FRC), lung, 124–125, 126
Fungi, 148
  cerebrospinal fluid (CSF), 266–267
  immune response to, 175, 178
  indirect immunofluorescence assay (IFA) with, 167
  intestinal contents in malabsorption and, 223
  sputum examination of, 139
Furosemide, 108
Fusidic acid, 318

Galactorrhea, 281
Gamma globulin, 182, 265
Gamma glutamyl transpeptidase, 304
  liver function with, 244, 245, 249
  pregnancy and, 374
Gas exchange tests, 132–137
Gastric acid tests, 211–212
Gastric carcinoma, 212
Gastric washings, with mycobacteria, 160
Gastrin, 211, 213, 228
Gastrinoma, 212, 213, 214, 228, 340
Gastritis, 188, 189, 212, 213
Gastroenteritis, 223
Gastroenteropathy, 226
Gastrointestinal neoplasms, 9, 347, 349
Gastrointestinal tract diseases, 211–228
  barium studies of, 29
  diagnosis of, 213
  diarrhea in, 226–228
  malabsorption in, 219–223
  occult blood losses in, 223–226
  protein loss quantitation in, 226
  serum amylase in, 215
Gaussian distribution model, 5
Genetic analysis, in gonadal disease, 336–337
Gentamicin, 66–67, 68, 151, 152, 318
Germ cell tumors, 348, 349
Giant cell arteritis, 194
Giardia lamblia, 177, 223, 224, 227
Gilbert's syndrome, 237, 239, 240
Globulins, and liver function, 233–234, 249
Glomerular filtration rate (GFR), 95–97
  acute glomerulonephritis with, 107
  blood urea nitrogen (BUN) with, 97
  creatinine clearance and, 96–97
  inulin clearance in, 96
  pregnancy and, 376
  renal failure with, 101, 104
  sodium conservation and, 101
  urinary concentrating ability with, 98, 99
  urine phosphorus with, 304, 305
Glomerulonephritis, 92, 107–108
  chronic renal failure with, 104
  follow-up tests in, 108
  hematuria with, 109
  immunoglobulins in, 182, 183, 187
  proteinuria with, 93
  red blood cell casts in, 92
Glomerulosclerosis, diabetic, 104
Glucagon
  acute pancreatitis with, 217
  growth hormone tests with, 288
  hypoglycemia with, 277
  pheochromocytoma and, 332
Glucocorticoid production disorders, 318–326
Glucocorticoids, 297
  glucose tolerance and, 270

  osteoporosis and, 312
  pituitary function with, 282
  pregnancy and, 377
  radioimmunoassay (RIA) of, 318–322
  stimulation tests for, 323
  urine tests for, 322–323
Glucose, cerebrospinal fluid (CSF), 264
Glucose, serum
  acute pancreatitis with, 217
  diabetes mellitus monitoring with, 274
  fasting plasma (FPG), 269–270
  hypertension with, 116
  hypoglycemia with, 278
  osteoporosis with, 313
  pregnancy and, 362
Glucose, urine
  diabetes mellitus monitoring with, 272–273, 274
  Fanconi syndrome with, 97
  home capillary monitoring of, 274
Glucose oxidase, in diabetes mellitus, 267, 273, 274, 275, 362
Glucose tolerance tests, 15, 269–270
  oral (OGTT), 269–270, 272, 276, 278
  pregnancy and, 362–363
Gluten enteropathy, 223, 224
Glycosuria, 98, 115
Glycosylated hemoglobin, 274
Goiter, 188, 298, 300, 301
Gold standard tests, 1
Gonadal disease, 334–339
Gonadal function tests, 334–337
  diagnosis of gonadal disease with, 337–339
  genetic analysis in, 336–337
  gonadotropins and, 335–336
  semen analysis in, 337
  sex steroids in, 334–335
  vaginal smear in, 337
Gonadotropin-releasing hormone (GnRH), 286, 336
Gonadotropins, 335–336
  female infertility and, 339
Gonacoccal arthritis, 203, 204
Gonacoccal sepsis, 207
Goodpasture's syndrome, 188
Gout
  synovial fluid examination in, 197, 198, 199, 200, 202
  uric acid and, 208
Gram-negative sepsis, 207
Gram-negative septicemia, 183
Gram stains, 145–146
Granulocytopenia, 34, 155
Granulomas, 267
Grave's hyperthyroidism, 188, 189
  iodine scan in, 299
  laboratory tests in, 301
  thyroid-stimulating immunoglobulins (TSI) in, 299
Growth hormone (GH), 334
  acromegaly and hypersecretion of, 281
  arginine infusion test with, 287
  carcinoid syndromes with, 342
  deficiency of, 286, 287
  exercise and, 288
  glucagon-propranolol test for, 288
  hypoglycemia with, 276, 287
  insulin tolerance test (ITT) for, 284, 287
  L-dopa and, 287

oral glucose tolerance test (OGTT) in, 288
serum levels of, 286
somatomedin levels and, 286–287
stimulation tests of, 287–288
thyrotropin-releasing hormone (TRH) and, 285, 288
G6PD deficiency, 28, 43
G6PD enzymes, and platelet counts, 49
Guaiac tests, 223
Guillain-Barré syndrome, 264
Gynecologic conditions, 215
Gynecomastia, 336, 338

Haemophilus influenzae type b, 169
Half-life of drugs, 65
Hamartoma, 121
Haptoglobin, 193
hemolysis with, 30
pregnancy and, 367
Hashimoto's thyroiditis, 188, 189
Hay fever, 179
hCG, *see* Human chorionic gonadotropin (hCG)
Heart disease, 1, 12; *see also* Cardiovascular disease
Heavy chain disease, 185
Heavy metals, and liver function, 244–249
Heinz bodies, 30, 43
Helper T cells, 176
Hemagglutination inhibition (HIA) antibody, in rubella, 365–366
Hematest, 223
Hematochezia, 26
Hematocrit
anemia and, 27, 31
hypertension and, 113
lymphocytosis with, 39
normal values for, 26
polycythemia and, 31, 32
pregnancy and, 355–356
pulmonary disease with, 137
Hematological diseases, 25–59
normal values for tests in, 25, 26
red cell morphology in, 41–44
see also specific diseases and syndromes
Hematologic neoplasms, 35
Hematology, in pregnancy, 354–357
Hematuria, 109–110
nephrosis with, 106, 108
Heme deficiency, in porphyrias, 257–258
Heme pigment, 103, 109
Hemoagglutination assay, 166, 172
Hemoccult, 223
Hemochromatosis, 118, 199, 204
HLA typing in, 248–249
liver function and, 247, 248, 249
Hemodialysis, 146
Hemoglobin
glycosylated, in diabetes mellitus, 274
hypertension and, 113
neonatal, 382
normal values for, 26
polycythemia and, 32
pregnancy and, 355–356
Hemoglobin A_2, and F (fetal) anemia, 29
Hemoglobinopathies, 43, 44
anemia and, 28
pregnancy and, 357
tests for, 30
Hemoglobinuria, 267

Hemolysis
anemia and, 29–30
fetal, 357, 359
neonatal, 380–382
Hemolytic anemia, 29–30, 103
antibodies in, 189, 192
autoimmune, 183
diseases or drugs associated with, 192, 193
red cell morphology in, 43, 44, 45, 48
Hemolytic disease of newborn, 380–382
Hemolytic uremic syndrome, 103
Hemophilia, 53, 360
hepatitis non-A, non-B diagnosis and, 256
posttransfusion, 254
surface antigen (HB$_s$Ag) in, 107, 108, 251–253, 254, 255, 349
surface antigen antibody (anti-HB$_s$) in, 251, 254–256
virus in, 187
Hepatocellular disease
alkaline phosphatase in, 241
alpha feto protein in, 349
bilirubin in, 239
ceruloplasmin in, 246
gamma glutamyl transpeptidase in, 244
iron storage in, 248
5′ nucleotidase (5′N) in, 243
Hepatoma, 233, 236, 249
Hereditary angioneurotic edema (HAE), 183–184
Hereditary spherocytosis (HS), 45–46
Heroin, 193
Herpes simplex, 171, 256
Herpetic encephalitis, 266
High density lipoprotein cholesterol, 367
Hirsutism, 338
Histamine, 178, 332
Histoplasmosis, 141–142, 308
HLA typing
hemochromatosis with, 248–249
rheumatic diseases with, 207–208
Hemorrhage, subarachnoid, 263
Hemosiderin, 30
Hemosiderosis, 179
Heparin, 56, 58, 312, 322
Hepatitis, 232, 233
alpha feto protein in, 349
bile acids in, 237
cholangiolytic, 240
chronic active, 189, 233, 237
globulins, in, 233
5′ nucleotidase (5′N) in, 243
serum glutamic-oxaloacetic transaminase (SGOT) in, 232, 233
serum glutamic-pyruvate transaminase (SGPT) in, 233
serum transaminase levels for, 1
synovial fluid examination and, 203
viral, *see* Viral hepatitis
Hepatitis A, 249–250
hepatitis non-A, non-B diagnosis and, 256
virus antibody (anti-HAV) in, 250
Hepatitis B, 249, 250–256
antigen systems in, 250–251
core antigen antibody (anti-HB$_c$) in, 251, 252, 254, 255, 256
"e" antigen (HB$_e$AG) in, 251, 253, 255
"e" antigen antibody (anti-HB$_e$) in, 251, 252, 253–254, 255
Hodgkins' disease, 242

Hoesch test, 260
Hoffman ferricyanide procedure, 267
Hollander test, 211–212
Hormonal diarrhea, 228
Hormone tests, gastrointestinal, 211
Howell-Jolly bodies, 43, 44, 58
  leukocytosis with, 38
  sickle cell anemia with, 47
Human chorionic gonadotropin (hCG), 335–336
  beta subunit of (β-hCG), 348, 353–354
  gynecomastia and, 338
  as oncology marker, 348
  pregnancy and, 276, 335–336, 353
Human chorionic somatomammotropin, 362
Human placental lactogen (hPL), 353, 362, 374
Humoral immune system, 175, 177; see also
  Immunology
Hungry bone syndrome, 313
Hyaline casts, 92
Hyaluronidase, 168, 169
Hydatidiform mole, 348, 354
Hydralazine, 332
Hydrocortisone suppression test, 307
Hydrogen breath test, 221, 223
Hydrogen (H⁺) ion concentration, 77
17-hydroxycorticosteroids (17 OHCS), 322–323
  adrenal insufficiency with, 327
  Cushing's syndrome (CS) with, 324, 326
  dexamethasone suppression test (DST) and,
    324–325
  pregnancy and, 377
5-hydroxyindoleacetic acid (5HIAA)
  carcinoid syndrome with, 342
  diarrhea and, 228
11-hydroxylase deficiency, 284, 331, 378
17-hydroxylase deficiency, 330, 331
18-hydroxylase deficiency, 331
21-hydroxylase deficiency, 330, 331, 378
Hydroxyapatite crystals, in synovial fluid, 199
17-hydroxyprogesterone, 378
27-hydroxyprogesterone, 330
Hydroxyproline, 307, 313
17-hydroxysteroids (17-OHS), 282, 284
5 hydroxytryptamine (5HT), 342
5 hydroxytryptophan (5HTP), 342
Hydroxyurea, 28
25-hydroxyvitamin D (25 OH D), 307, 319
Hyperadrenergic disorders, 330–333
Hyperalbuminemia, 303
Hyperaldosteronism, 318
  hypertension and, 114, 115
  metabolic alkalosis with, 81
  peripheral renal activity (PRA) values in, 326,
    327, 328
  plasma aldosterone in, 327–328
  primary (PH), 326
Hyperaminoacidemia, 287
Hyperbilirubinemia, 238, 239
Hypercalcemia, 98, 104, 142
  differential diagnosis of, 308–310
  familial hypocalciuric, 310
  hydrocortisone suppression test in, 307
  kidney stone disease and, 321
  parathyroid hormone (PTH) and, 306
Hypercalciuria
  kidney stone disease and, 313, 318, 320
  urine calcium in, 303, 304
Hypercarotenemia, 263
Hyperchloremia, 100

Hyperchloremic acidosis, 79–80
Hypercorticoidism, and metabolic acidosis, 81
Hypercortisolism, 323–324
  adrenocorticotrophic hormone (ACTH) and,
    322
Hypercoagulable states, 55–56
Hypereosinophiliac syndrome, 40, 41
Hypergammaglobulinemia, 234
Hyperglobulinemia, 44, 142, 303
Hyperglycemia
  acute pancreatitis with, 217
  cerebrospinal fluid (CSF) glucose levels in, 264
  hyponatremia with, 84, 85
  urine glucose in, 272
Hyperglycemic non-ketonic coma (HNKC), 275
Hyperinsulinemia, 276, 277
Hyperkalemia, 87–88, 101, 108
  acidosis with, 82
  adrenal insufficiency and, 282
  aldosterone and, 326, 328
  causes and treatment of, 88, 89
  congenital adrenal hyperplasia (CAH) and,
    330
  mineralocorticoid deficiency in, 329
Hyperlipidemia, 105
  acute pancreatitis with, 217
  hyponatremia with, 84
Hyperlipiduria, 105
Hyperlipoproteinemia, 217
Hypermagnesemia, 312
Hypernatremia, 83, 85–86, 87
Hyperosmolality, with hypernatremia, 85
Hyperoxaluria, 311, 321
Hyperparathyroidism, 100, 199, 217
  hypercalcemia and, 308
  hypophosphatemia and, 316
  kidney stone disease and, 320
  multiple endocrine neoplasia syndromes
    (MENs) with, 339, 340
  parathyroid hormone (PTH) in, 306
  urine cyclic AMP (UcAMP) in, 307
  urine pH in, 312
Hyperphosphatemia, 317
Hyperpigmentation, 282
Hyperprolactinemia, 285, 289, 336
Hyperproteinemia, 84
Hyperprothrombinemia, 235
Hyperreninemia, with hyperaldosteronism, 327
Hypersensitivity, in immunology, 178–180
Hypersplenism, 50
Hypertension, 113–116
  electrolytes in, 115–116
  glucose in, 116
  hematologic testing in, 113–115
  minimum laboratory evaluation in, 114
  portal, 238
  pregnancy and, 354, 376–377
  renal status in, 115
  renovascular, 116–117
Hyperthyroidism, 100
  cortisol and, 322
  gynecomastia with, 338
  17-hydroxycorticosteroid (17 OHCS) in, 323
  hyperphosphatemia and, 317
  iodine scan in, 299
  laboratory tests in, 300, 301–302
  osteoporosis with, 312
  testosterone in, 334
  thyroglobulin in, 298

thyroid function tests in, 296
thyroid-stimulating hormone (TSH) in, 298
triiodothyronine (T$_3$) in, 297
Hypertonicity
hypernatremia with, 84, 85
serum potassium and, 87
Hyperuricemia, 311
Hyperuricosuria, 313, 321
Hyperventilation
metabolic acidosis with, 80
progesterone-induced, in pregnancy, 365
Hypoadrenalism, 323
Hypoadrenergic states, 334
Hypoalbuminemia, 105, 303
Hypoaldosteronism, 329
Hypocalcemia, 314–315
acute pancreatitis with, 217
cardiomyopathy with, 118
magnesium in, 304
Hypochromia, 43
Hypocortisolism, 291, 326, 327
Hypogammaglobulinemia, 36, 176, 178
Hypoglobulinemia, 303
Hypoglycemia, 275–279
alcoholic, 276
alcoholic ketoacidosis (AKA) with, 274
alimentary, 278
factitious, 277
fasting, 275–276, 277
growth hormone and, 287
hyperinsulinemic, 277
idiopathic or functional, 277
insulin-induced, 211–212, 283, 323
reactive, 270, 278
urine glucose in, 272
Hypoglycorrhachia, 264, 266
Hypogonadism, 285–286, 312, 336
follicle-stimulating hormone (FSH) in, 286
gonadotropin-releasing hormone (GnRH) in, 286
gynecomastia with, 338
laboratory tests in, 337
luteinizing hormone (LH) in, 286
male infertility in, 339
pituitary function tests in, 291
testosterone and estradiol in screening for, 285–286
Hypokalemia, 87, 88–89
aldosterone and, 326, 328, 329
alkalosis with, 81, 82
cardiomyopathy with, 118
congenital adrenal hyperplasia (CAH) and, 330
hypertension with, 115–116
renal diseases with, 100, 101
Hypomagnesemia, 217
causes of, 312, 318
hypocalcemia and, 314
laboratory tests in, 312
Hyponatremia, 83–85, 116, 291
acute and chronic determination in, 85
factitious, 84
serum sodium in, 83
Hypoosmolality, with hyponatremia, 83, 84, 85
Hypoparathyroidism
hypocalcemia and, 314
hypophosphatemia with, 317
parathyroid hormone (PTH) in, 306
Hypophosphatasia, 319
Hypophosphatemia, 316
cardiomyopathy with, 118

osteomalacia with, 319
phosphorus measurement and, 304
Hypopituitarism, 282
Hypoprolactinemia, 289
Hypoproteinemia, 247
Hyporeninemic hypoaldosteronism, 329
Hypothalamus
free thyroxine (FT$_4$) and triiodothyronine (FT$_3$) levels and, 293
hypogonadism and, 286
Hypothyroidism, 100
cortisol metabolism in, 282
17-hydroxycorticosteroids (17-OHCS) in, 323
hyponatremia in, 291
laboratory tests in, 300, 301
pituitary function tests in, 291
pregnancy and, 380
primary versus secondary, 297–298
prolactin and, 288
reverse triiodothyroxine (rT$_3$) in, 298
sex hormone-binding globulin (SHBG) in, 334
thyroid-stimulating hormone (TSH) in, 297–298, 380
triiodothyronine (T$_3$) in, 297, 380
Hypovolemia, 377
Hypoxemia, 134–135

Idiopathic adrenocortical hyperplasia (IAH), 326, 328–329
Idiopathic membranoproliferative glomerulo-nephritis, 207
Idiopathic thrombocytopenic purpura (ITP), 48–49
Ig, see Immunoglobulin *headings*
Immune complex diseases, 182
complement system in, 207
synovial fluid examination in, 203
Immune complexes, detection of, 185–187
Immunodeficiency, 175–178
B lymphocytes in, 176
immunoglobulins in, 176–177
T lymphocytes in, 175–176
Immunoelectrophoresis (IEP)
cardiomyopathy with, 117
cerebrospinal fluid (CSF) with, 266
countercurrent (CIE), 169, 170, 266, 349
immunoglobulin analysis with, 184–185
urine protein, 94
Immunodiagnosis, 163–172
Immunoglobulin A (IgA), 177
immunoelectrophoresis (IEP) of, 184
liver function with, 234
quantitative assessment of, 180, 181
serum levels with age of, 177
Immunoglobulin D (IgD), 177
Immunoglobulin deposition disease, 185
Immunoglobulin E (IgE), 177
quantitative assessment of, 180
RAST (radioallergosorbent tests) of, 179–180
serum measurement of, 179
wheal and flare skin tests with, 178–179
Immunoglobulin G (IgG), 176, 177
agglutination tests with, 166, 169
antibody to, 163
cerebrospinal fluid (CSF), 265
complement cascade and, 183
Fc portion of, 185–186
hemolytic anemia and, 192, 193
hepatitis A and, 250
hypogammaglobulinemia with, 178

idiopathic thrombocytopenic purpura (ITP)
with, 49
IgM antibody differences with, and diagnosis,
164–165
immunoelectrophoresis (IEP) of, 184, 185
quantitative assessment of, 180, 182
serum levels with age of, 177
Immunoglobulin M (IgM), 177
agglutination tests with, 166
complement cascade and, 183
hemolytic anemia and, 193
hepatitis A and, 250, 256
hypogammaglobulinemia with, 178
IgG antibody differences with, and diagnosis,
164–165
immunoelectrophoresis (IEP) of, 184, 185
immunofluorescence with, 171
liver function with, 234
quantitative assessment of, 180
rubella and, 171, 366
serum levels with age of, 177
Toxoplasma gondii with, 172
Immunoglobulins, 176–177
B lymphocytes and, 176
cerebrospinal fluid (CSF), 165–166, 265
cryoproteins and cryoglobulins and, 186–187
immunoelectrophoresis (IEP) of, 184–185
proteinuria with, 93
quantitative assessment of, 180–185
serum levels with age of, 177
thyroid-stimulating (TSI), 299
Immunology, 175–195
B lymphocytes in, 176
cryoproteins/cryoglobulins in, 186–187
delayed-type hypersensitivity (DTH) skin
testing in, 175, 176, 177, 180
IgE serum measurements in, 179
immediate versus delayed hypersensitivity in
tests in, 178–180
immune complexes detection in, 185–187
immunodeficiency testing in, 175–178
immunoelectrophoresis (IEP) in, 184–185
immunoglobulins in, 176–177
quantitation of immunoglobulins and complement in, 180–185
RAST (radioallergosorbent tests) in, 179–180
synovial fluid examination in, 203
syphilis with, 266
T lymphocytes in, 175–176
wheal and flare skin tests in, 178–179
Impotence, 338
Inappropriate antidiuretic hormone secretion,
syndrome of (SIADH), 290, 291
Inclusions, red cell, 38, 41, 43, 58
Indexes
accuracy for positive and negative prediction
with, 9–13
distribution of test values in, 6–7
sensitivity and specificity in, 7–9
Indian childhood cirrhosis, 246
Indirect Coomb's test, 192, 193
Indirect fluorescence tests, 167, 170
Indirect immunofluorescence assays (IFA), 167–
168, 170, 171, 190
Indocyanine green, in liver function tests, 241,
245
Indomethacin, 108, 329
Infantile eczema, 179
Infections and infectious diseases, 145–161

acute glomerulonephritis with, 107
antibiotic combinations in, 156–159
antimicrobial sensitivity testing of, 151–154
bacterial tolerance in, 155–156
blood cultures in, 149–151
ceruloplasmin in, 246
C-reactive protein in, 194
disk diffusion test in, 151–152
Gram-stained specimen in, 145–146
immunodiagnosis of, 163–172
immunoglobulins and, 177, 187
interpretation of quantitation of organisms in,
148–149
iron storage in, 248
leukocytosis in, 37
leukopenia and, 36
lymphocytosis with, 38–39
mixed saprophytic flora in, 149
mycobacteria in, 159–161
neutropenia with, 35
nucleated red cells in, 43
polymorphonuclear leukocytes (PMNs) and,
145–146
pregnancy and, 365–367
serum bactericidal concentration (SBC) assay
(Schlichter Test) in, 154–155
T cell tests in, 180
thrombocytopenia with, 48
tissue stains used with, 146–148
tube dilution assay in, 152–154
see also Bacteria; Viral infections; *and specific
infections*
Infectious arthritis, 197
Infectious endocarditis, 152
blood cultures of, 150–151
staining of samples in, 147–148
Infectious hepatitis, 38, 39
Infectious mononucleosis
antibodies in, 189, 190
lymphocytosis with, 38, 39
serological data on, 171–172
Infertility
female, 339
male, 334, 337, 339
Inflammatory bowel diseases, 9, 311, 347
Insect sensitivity, 178
Inspiratory capacity (IC), 124, 125
Inspiratory reserve volume (IRV), 124
Insulin
gastric secretion tests with, 211–212
hypoglycemia with, 211–212, 275–276,
283, 323, 324
pregnancy and, 362
Insulinoma, 276–277, 278, 340
Insulin tolerance test (ITT)
adrenocorticotropic hormone (ACTH) with,
283–284, 323
growth hormone and, 284, 287
prolactin on, 284, 289
Intermittent proteinuria, 95
International System of Units (SI), 17–23
advantages and disadvantages of, 23
compound prefixes used in, 19
development of, 17–18
units and presentation in, 18–23
Interstitial diseases, 93, 95, 98
Interstitial nephritis, 92, 104
acute, 108–109
hypocalcemia diagnosis and, 314

hypomagnesemia with, 318
Intestinal lymphangiectasia, 223, 225
Intestinal lymphoma, 223, 225
Intrinsic factor (IF)
    anemia and, 28
    antibodies to, 188, 189
    stomach diseases with, 211, 212
    vitamin B$_{12}$ absorption and, 222
Inulin clearance, 96
Iodine
    radioactive uptake (RAIU) test with, 299–301
    thyroiditis with, 300, 302
Iopanoic acid (Telepaque), 297
Iron
    anemia and, 29
    bone marrow evaluation of, 29–30
    liver function and storage of, 244, 247–249
    malabsorption and, 220
    pregnancy and, 356
Iron deficiency
    anemia and, 27–28, 29–30, 31, 223, 356
    ovalocytes in, 45
    target cells in, 44
Islet cell antibodies, 188
Isoamylases, 216
Iso-hemagglutinins, 178
Isoproterenol, 332

Jaundice
    cerebrospinal fluid (CSF) examination in, 263
    liver function tests in, 234, 235, 237, 239, 240, 241

Kanamycin, 66, 68
Karyotype
    amniotic fluid and, 359–360
    gonadal disease and, 336–337
Kernicterus, 382
Ketoacidosis, diabetic, 80, 100, 216, 274–275, 316
Ketones, urine, in diabetes mellitus, 273–274, 275
Ketonuria, 276
17-ketosteroids (17KS), 323
    congenital adrenal hyperplasia (CAH) and, 330, 331
    hirsutism with, 338
    pregnancy and, 378, 379
Kidney disease, see Renal headings
Kidney stone disease, 303
    calcium oxalate, 307, 311, 313, 320–321
    crystallographic analysis of, 311, 313
    cystine, 98
    hematuria with, 109, 110
    hyperoxaluric, 311
    laboratory evaluation of, 313–318, 320–321
    magnesium ammonium phosphate, 311, 313, 320–321
    radiographic studies in, 313
    uric acid, 311
    urine uric acid in, 307
Kinky hair syndrome, 247
Kirby-Bauer test, 151–152, 155
Klinefelter's syndrome, 336, 337, 339
Kolmer test, 266
Kwashiorkor, 246, 247

Laboratory tests, 1–16
    accuracy for positive and negative prediction

on, 9–13
    aggregate of positive results in, 15
    clinician evaluation of results of, 161
    confounding variables on, 4–5
    evaluation of, 13–15
    as gold standard tests, 1
    indexes of proficiency of, 6–13
    interpretation of, 1
    laboratory error in, 4–5
    range of normal on, 1–6
    sensitivity and specificity of, 7–9
    as "surrogate tests," 1
    tandem use of, 14–15
Lactation, and prolactin, 289
Lactic acid
    cerebrospinal fluid (CSF), 266
    hyperglycemic non-ketonic coma with, 275
Lactic acidosis, 80, 82
Lactic dehydrogenase (LDH)
    cardiac, 112–113
    hemolysis with, 30
    muscle diseases with, 267
    pleural fluid, 140, 141
    pregnancy and, 373
Lactose tolerance test, 220–221
Lactulose, 227
Lange colloidal gold test, 265
Lasix, 329
Latex agglutination, 166, 168, 169, 170, 171
Latex rheumatoid factor test, 205
Laurell electrophoresis, 181
Laxatives, 227
LDH, see Lactid dehydrogenase (LDH)
L-dopa
    growth hormone and, 287
    pheochromocytoma and, 332, 333
    prolactin and, 290
Lead poisoning, 29
LE cell, 202
    factor, 189–190
    test, 205, 206
Lecithin/sphingomyelin (L/S) ratio, 382–383
Legionella species, 138, 146, 147, 170
Legionellosis, 146, 170
Leprosy, 193, 205
Leucine, 277
Leucine aminopeptidase, 244, 245
Leukemia
    ceruloplasmin in, 246
    eosinophiliac, 40
    iron storage in, 248
    leukocytosis and, 38, 39
    monocytosis with, 41
    neutrophiliac, 38
    nucleated red cells in, 43
    osteoporosis diagnosis and, 312, 313
    see also specific types of leukemia
Leukemic arthritis, 202
Leukocyte alkaline phosphatase (LAP), 31
Leukocyte casts, 92
Leukocyte mobilization study, 36
Leukocytes
    diarrhea tests with, 227
    pregnancy and, 357, 358
Leukocytosis, 37–38
    blood smear review in, 38
    lymphopenia with, 36
    monocytosis with, 41
    splenectomy and, 37–38

Leukopenia, 34–37
LH, *see* Luteinizing hormone (LH)
Lidocaine, 68, 73
Light chains, 94
  immunoelectrophoresis (IEP) with, 184, 185
  nephrotic syndrome with, 105
  proteinuria with, 93, 94
Lipase, 216–217
Lipids
  acute pancreatitis with, 217
  fat absorption and, 222
  pleural fluid, 41
  pregnancy and, 367, 373
Lipoprotein electrophoresis, 112
Lithium, 98, 100
Lithocholic acid, 236
Liver biopsy, 246
Liver cancer, 234
Liver disease, 44, 100, 231–260
  alcohol-induced, 233
  alpha feto protein in, 349
  cortisol in, 322
  17-hydroxycorticosteroids (17-OHCS) in, 323
  neutropenia with, 36
  osteoporosis and, 312, 313
  prothrombin time (PT) with, 54
  spiky red cells in, 47
  target cells in, 44
Liver failure, with hypoglycemia, 276
Liver function tests, 231–249
  albumin in, 234–235
  alkaline phosphatase in, 241–242, 304
  bile acids in, 236–238
  bilirubin (serum) in, 238–239, 240
  bilirubin (urine) in, 239–240
  BSP in, 240–241
  cholesterol in, 236
  clearance function and bile formation in, 236–244
  flocculation tests in, 233
  gamma glutamyl transpeptidase in, 244
  globulins in, 233–234
  heavy metals in, 244–249
  indocyanine green in, 241
  inflammatory activity tests in, 231–234
  leucine aminopeptidase in, 244
  5′ nucleotidase (5′N) in, 242–243
  pregnancy and, 367–374
  prothrombin time in, 235–236
  selection of, 249
  serum glutamic-oxaloacetic transaminase (SGOT) in, 231–233
  serum glutamic pyruvate transaminase (SGPT) in, 233
  synthetic function tests in, 234–236
  urobilinogen in, 239–240
Löffler's pneumonia, 40
Low density lipoprotein triglyceride, 367
Lucey-Driscoll syndrome, 238–239, 240
Lundh test, 219
Lung
  compliance test of, 130
  fetal maturity of, 382–383
  volume tests of, 124–126
Lung cancer, 123–124, 338
  alpha feto protein in, 349
  carcinoembryonic antigen (CEA) in, 347
Lung disease, *see* Pulmonary disease
Lung scans, 122–123

Lupus erythematosis, 100, 106, 108
  LE cell in, 202, 205, 206
Lupus nephritis, 108
Luteinizing hormone (LH), 348
  amenorrhea with, 337
  female infertility and, 339
  hypogonadism with, 286
  impotence and, 338
  indications for use of, 291, 292
  male infertility and, 339
  measurement of, 335, 336
  pregnancy and, 353, 354, 374
  virilization disorders and, 337
Lymphangiectasia, intestinal, 223, 225
Lymph node B cells, 176
Lymphocytes
  immunodeficiency testing with, 177
  pleural fluid, 140
Lymphocytic leukemia, chronic (CLL), 39–40, 45, 191
Lymphocytic thyroiditis, 302
Lymphocytosis, 38–40, 172
  chronic lymphocytic leukemia (CLL) with, 39–40
Lymphoma
  eosinophilia with, 41
  hyperphosphatemia with, 317
  hypocalcemia and, 315
  immunoglobulins in, 187
  intestinal, 223, 225
  osteoporosis and, 312, 313
Lymphopenia, 36–37
Lymphosarcoma cell leukemia, 39, 40
Lymphotic leukemia, chronic, 39–40, 43, 187, 191
Lysozyme, with proteinuria, 93

McArdle's myophosphorylase deficiency, 267
Macroamylasemia, 216
Macrocytic anemia, 28
Macrocytosis, 28–29, 41, 42
Macrolide antibiotics, 75
Macrophages, alveolar, 137, 146
Macrophages, urinary, in nephrotic syndrome, 106
Magnesium, serum, 302
  acute pancreatitis with, 217
  diarrhea and, 227
  hypocalcemia with, 304
  pregnancy and, 364
Magnesium, urine
  hypocalcemia with, 304
  hypomagnesemia with, 312, 318
Magnesium ammonium phosphate (MAP) stones, 311, 313, 320–321
Magnesium metabolism, 312
Malabsorption, 219–223
  absorption tests in, 223
  bacterial overgrowth in small bowel in, 223
  bile acid, 222
  carbohydrate, 220–221, 227
  carcinoid syndrome and, 342
  cause of, 224–225
  diarrhea in, 227
  fat, 221–222
  hydrogen breath test in, 221
  hypomagnesemia with, 318
  indicators of, 220
  lactose tolerance test in, 220–221
  protein, 222
  stool fat tests in, 221–222
  tests for diagnosis of, 220–222

vitamin B$_{12}$, 222
D-xylose tolerance test in, 220
Malaria parasites, 44, 58
Male infertility, 334, 337, 339
Malignancy, see Cancer; Oncology
Malignant hypertension, 104
Malignant melanoma, 189
Malnutrition, 312
    cortisol metabolism in, 282
    growth hormone in, 288
Mandelamine, 342
Marihuana, 338
Marrow panhypoplasia, 36
Mass, in SI units, 20
Maximal breathing capacity (MBC), 130
Maximal voluntary ventilation (MVV), 130
M-component, in cardiomyopathy, 117
MCV, see Mean corpuscular volume (MCV)
Mean corpuscular hemoglobin (MCH), 56, 57
Mean corpuscular hemoglobin concentration
    (MCHC), 56, 57
Mean corpuscular volume (MCV), 56
    anemia, 28, 29, 30, 31
    normal values for, 26
    red cell abnormalities on, 42
    thrombocytosis on, 49
Mean platelet volume (MPV), 57
Mediastinum lesions, 121
Medroxyprogesterone acetate, 339
Medullary carcinoma of thyroid (MCT), 298, 339,
    340, 341
Medullary cystic disease of kidney, 100
Medullary sponge kidney, 313, 320
Megakaryocytopenia, 49
Megaloblastic anemia, 45, 356
Melanocyte antibodies, 188
Melanoma, 189
Melena, and anemia, 26
Men, infertility in, 334, 337, 339
Menetrier's disease, 212, 213
Meningitides, 264
Meningitis
    bacterial, 155, 266
    cerebrospinal fluid (CSF) in, 264, 266
    immunoglobulins in, 166
    streptococcal, 170
    tuberculous, 266
    viral, 264, 266
Menke's X-linked copper deficiency, 247
MENs, see Multiple endocrine neoplasia syndromes
    (MENs)
Menstruation
    anemia and, 26, 27
    female infertility and, 339
Meprobamate, 323, 330
2-mercapthoethanol, 166
Mesangiocapillary glomerulonephritis, 106, 108
Metabolic acidosis, 79–80, 82, 100
    blood gasses in, 77, 78
    diabetic ketoacidosis with, 274
    elevated anion gap in, 79
    hyperventilation in, 80
    mixed acid-base disturbances with, 82–83
Metabolic alkalemia, and blood gases, 78
Metabolic alkalosis, 81, 106
    hypokalemia with, 88
    mixed acid-base disturbances with, 82–83
Metabolic disease, 302–303
Metabolic inhibition test, 170

Metamethasone, 322
Metanephrine, 330, 332, 333
Metastatic carcinoma, 142, 202, 204
Methanol, 80
Methotrexate, 352
Methyldopa, 289, 338, 342
Methylxanthines, 332, 333
Metyrapone
    adrenal stimulation with, 323
    adrenocorticotropic hormone (ACTH) and,
        284, 323
    Cushing's syndrome (CS) with, 324, 326
    pregnancy and, 377
Microangiopathic hemolytic anemia, 47, 103
Microbial tests, with cerebrospinal fluid (CSF), 266
Micrococcus species, 149
Microcytosis, 29, 41, 194
Micromyeloblasts, 39
Miliary tuberculosis, 142
Milk-alkali syndrome, 308, 311, 312, 321
Miller-Moses test, 291
Mineralocorticoid production disorders, 326–329
    deficiency in, 282, 329
    excess states in, 326–329
Minimal bactericidal concentration (MBC) of anti-
    biotics, 151, 153–154, 155
Minimal inhibitory concentration (MIC) of anti-
    biotics, 151, 153–154, 155, 156
Mithramycin, 315
Mixed acid-base disturbances, 77, 78, 82
    clinical approach to, 81, 82–83
    normal pH in, 83
Mixed connective tissue disease, 191, 192, 206
Mixed saprophytic flora, 149
Mole concentrations, 20–21
Molecular weight, 17
Monarticular arthritis, 204
Monilial esophagus, 211
Monoclonal gammopathies, 93, 182, 265
Monocytes, in pregnancy, 357
Monocytic leukemia, 41
Monocytopenia, 34
Monocytosis, 41
Mononucleosis, 179, 256
Mucin clot test, 198
Mucus tests, 212
Multiple endocrine neoplasia syndromes (MENs),
    339–341
    MEN 1, 340
    MEN 2 (2a), 339, 340–341
    MEN 3 (2b), 341
Multiple myeloma, 44, 105, 117, 312
    cortisol in, 322
    immunoglobulins in, 182, 187
    urinary proteins in, 93, 94
Multiple sclerosis, 265
Mumps meningoencephalitis, 264
Muscle diseases
    creatine phosphokinase (CPK) in, 267
    myoglobinuria in, 267
Muscle enzyme, in rheumatic diseases, 208
Myasthenia gravis, 130, 188, 189, 267
Mycobacteria
    cerebrospinal fluid (CSF) examination of, 266
    T cells in immune response to, 175
Mycobacterium species, 146, 147
Mycobacterium tuberculosis, 159–161
Mycoplasma pneumoniae, 170
Mycoplasma species, 138, 170

Myelin basic protein, in cerebrospinal fluid (CSF), 265
Myeloblastic leukemia, 39
Myelocytic leukemia, 38
Myelogenous leukemia, 279
Myeloid metaplasia, 48
Myeloma, 179
  hypercalcemia and, 308
  immunoglobulins in, 185
  osteoporosis and, 312, 313
Myelomonocytic leukemia, 41
Myocardial infarction, 112, 195, 244
Myoglobinuria, 267
Myxedema, 188

Nalidixic acid, 330
Neisseria species, 149
Neoplasms, see Cancer; Oncology; and specific sites and types of cancer
Nephelometry, 181, 182
Nephrocalcinosis, 109, 313
Nephrogenic diabetes insipidus, 100, 291
Nephrotic syndrome (nephrosis), 93, 105–107
  copper storage in, 246, 247
  cortisol in, 322
  hyperaldosteronism with, 326
  leucine aminopeptidase in, 244
Nephrotomogram, 101
Neural tube defects, 379
Neuroblastoma, 347
Neurological diseases, 263–267
Neuromuscular diseases, 267
Neurosyphilis, 265, 266
Neutropenia, 34–36, 156
  antibodies in, 191
  chronic idiopathic, 35–36
  cyclic, 36
  drug-induced, 35
  monocytosis with, 41
  normal ranges for, 34–35
  pancytopenia with, 50
  sputum examination and, 138
Neutrophilia, 37
"Neutrophilic leukemia," 38
Neutrophils
  antibodies to, 191
  pleural fluid, 140
  pregnancy and, 357, 358
Newborns
  hemolytic disease of, 380–382
  hyperbilirubinemia in, 238–239
  IgG antibody in, 165
  respiratory distress syndrome in, 382
Niacin, 318
Nitrogen
  blood urea, see Blood urea nitrogen (BUN)
  lung washout tests with, 125, 131–132
  stool, in chronic pancreatitis, 218
Nitroglycerine, 332
Nitroprusside tests, in diabetes mellitus, 273–274, 275
Nocardia species, 147
Norepinephrine
  hypoadrenergic states with, 334
  pheochromocytoma and, 330, 332, 333
Normal range of values on laboratory tests, 1–6
  confounding variables and, 4–5
  Gaussian distribution model in, 5
  indexes of test proficiency and, 6–7

laboratory error and, 4–5
  problems with use of, 2–6
Nucleated red cells, 43
5′ nucleotidase (5′N), in liver function, 242–243, 245, 249, 304

Oat cell carcinoma of lung, 338
Obstructive jaundice, 241
Obstructive lung disease, 123, 126
Occult blood loss, 223–226
Ochronosis, 204
Oligomenorrhea, 339
Oncology, 347–352
  acid phosphatase in, 349–350
  alpha feto protein in, 348–349
  breast cancer receptors in, 350–352
  carcinoembryonic antigen (CEA) in, 347
  human chorionic gonadotropin (hCG) in, 348
  T cell tests in, 180
  see also Cancer
Opiates, 289
Oral contraceptives, 270, 322, 323
Oral glucose tolerance test (OGTT), 269–270, 272, 276, 278, 288
Orogratin, 297
Orthostatic hypotension, 330
Osmolality
  antidiuretic hormone (ADH) and, 290
  diarrhea with, 227–228
  hypernatremia with, 85–86
  hyponatremia with, 83–84
  pregnancy and, 365
  serum sodium and, 83
  urine, 99
Osmotic fragility test, 45, 46
Osmotic gap, in hyponatremia, 84
Osteoarthritis, 195
Osteogenic sarcoma, 313
Osteomalacia, 312
  hypocalcemia and, 315
  laboratory evaluation of, 319
Osteomyelitis, 155, 205
Osteopenia, 312–313
Osteoporosis, 312–313
Otitis media, 177
Oval fat bodies, 92, 93, 106
Ovalocytes, 44, 45
Ovarian failure, 337
Ovarian tumors, 189, 338
Oxylate, 311
  hypertension with, 115
  kidney stone disease with, 320–321
Ox cell hemolysin test, 171
Oxtriphylline, 75
Oxygenation, arterial measurement of, 132–135
Oxytocin, 375

Paget's disease, 313
Pancreatic cancer, 214, 215, 217, 219, 349
Pancreatic diseases, 214–219
Pancreatic insufficiency, 214, 217, 225
Pancreatitis, 9
  alcoholic, 217
  amylase/creatine clearance ratio (Cam/Cer) in, 361–362
  carcinoembryonic antigen (CEA) in, 347
  hypocalcemia and, 314
Pancreatitis, actue, 214–217
  amylase in, 361

amylase/creatine clearance ratio (Cam/Cer) in, 216
calcium in, 217
hyperglycemia nonketonic coma with, 275
immunoreactive trypsin in, 217
isoamylases in, 216
leucine aminopeptidase in, 244
lipase tests in, 216–217
lipids in, 217
macroamylasemia in, 216
Pancreatitis, chronic, 217–219
amylase in, 216, 275
chymotrypsin output in, 218
duodenal content tests in, 219
stool tests in, 218
urine tests in, 218
Pancytopenia, 49–50
Pandy's test, 265
Papillary necrosis, and hematuria, 109
Pappenheimer bodies, 43, 47
Paraaminobenzoic acid (PABA), 218
Paracoccidioidomycosis, 142
Paraldehyde, 80
Parasitism, 40, 163, 179, 223
Parathyroid disease, 302–318
Parathyroid gland hyperplasia, 339
Parathyroid hormone (PTH)
hypercalcemia with, 308–310
hyperphosphatemia with, 317
hypocalcemia with, 314–315
hypophosphatemia with, 316
kidney stone disease with, 320–321
osteomalacia with, 319
osteoporosis with, 313
radioimmunoassay (RIA) of, 305–306
Parietal cell antibodies, 187, 188, 189
Paroxysmal nocturnal hemoglobinuria, 30
Partial thromboplastin time (PTT), 51–55, 58
Particle counts, in SI units, 21
Peak concentration of drugs, 64
Pellagra, 247
Pemphigus, 188
Pencil forms, 44, 45
Penicillamine, 267
Penicillinase (β-lactamase), 150
Penicillins, 61, 108, 150, 159, 330
Pentagastrin, 340
Pentazocine, 330
Pepsin tests, 211, 212
Perfusion scanning, 122, 123
Pernicious anemia, 28, 212, 213, 356
antibodies in, 188, 189
pH
mixed acid-base disturbances and, 83
urine, see Urine pH
Pharmacokinetics, 62–64
of commonly used drugs, 66–76
compartment model in, 63
Phenobarbital, 67, 68, 70, 323, 324
Phenothiazines, 342
cholestasis with, 239
neutropenia with, 35
prolactin and, 288, 289
Phentolamine, 332
L-phenylalanine mustard, 351
Phenylbutazone, 323
Phenylephrine, 332
Phenytoin (Dilantin)
cortisol metabolism and, 282

dexamethasone suppression test (DST) and, 324
diabetes mellitus and, 270, 271
17-hydroxycorticosteroids (17-OHCS) and, 323
metyrapone in 11-hydroxylase block and, 284
pharmacokinetics of, 68, 70–71
rate of elimination of, 63
Pheochromocytoma, 114, 326, 330–333
multiple endocrine neoplasia syndromes (MENs) with, 339, 340, 341
Phlebotomy, 31
Phosphate, 78
Fanconi syndrome with, 97
hypocalcemia and, 314–315
Phosphatidyl glycerol (PG), in amniotic fluid, 382, 383
Phosphorus, serum, 304
chloride ratio with, 307
hypercalcemia and, 308–310
kidney stone disease and, 313
malabsorption and, 220
osteomalacia with, 319
pregnancy and, 365
Phosphorus, urine, 304
chronic renal failure with, 104
hyperphosphatemia with, 316, 317
Phosphorus, urine, tubular maximum for reabsorption (TmP/GFR), 304, 305, 306
hypercalcemia with, 308
hyperphosphatemia with, 317
hypocalcemia with, 314–315
hypophosphatemia with, 316
kidney stone disease with, 320–321
osteomalacia with, 319
osteoporosis with, 312
Phytohemagglutinin (PHA), T-cell mitogen, 176, 177
Pituitary adenomas, 288, 289, 336
Pituitary disease, 291
antidiuretic hormone (ADH) in, 290
gynecomastia with, 338
pituitary function tests in, 291–318
presentation in, 281
Pituitary function tests, 281–291
antidiuretic hormone (ADH) in, 290–291
growth hormone (GH) in, 286–288
hypogonadism and, 285–286
objectives of, 281, 283
pituitary-adrenal axis in, 281–284
pituitary disease diagnosis with, 291–318
pituitary-gonadal axis in, 285–286
pituitary-thyroid axis in, 285, 293
pregnancy and, 374–375
prolactin in, 288–290
screening and confirmatory tests with, 291, 292
Pituitary mass effect, 281, 292
Pituitary tumors
antidiuretic hormone (ADH) in, 290
growth hormone (GH) deficiency in, 287
multiple endocrine neoplasia syndrome (MENs) with, 339, 340
prolactin in, 288, 289, 336
Plasma cells, 176
Plasmodium vivax, 44
Platelets, 49, 51, 57
antibodies to, 187, 191
lymphocytosis with, 39
normal values for, 26
pregnancy and, 357

thrombocythemia with, 49
thrombocytosis with, 49
Pleural fluid examination, 140–141
Pleuritis, uremic, 140
Pneumococcal meningitis, 266
Pneumococcal pneumonia, 138, 170
Pneumonia, 138, 140, 146, 170
Poikilocytosis, 43, 44–48
Polyarteritis nodosa, 191, 243
Polychromatophilia, 29, 31, 43, 46
Polycystic kidney disease, 104
Polycystic ovarian syndrome, 338, 339
Polycythemia, 31–34, 194
  erythrocytosis with, 33–34
  hypertension and, 114
  red cell volume in, 32–33
  stress, 33
Polycythemia vera, 31–32, 33, 34
  thrombocytopenia in, 49
Polymorphonuclear leukocytes (PMNs)
  inflammatory response to infection with,
    145–146
  pleural fluid, 140
  sputum, 137
  synovial fluid, 202
Polymyalgia rheumatica, 194
Polymyositis, 192, 206, 267
Polyvinyl pyrrolidone (PVP), 226
Porphobilin, 260
Porphobilinogen (PBG), 257, 258, 260
Porphyrias, 256–260
  enzyme deficiencies causing, 256, 257
  erythropoietic, 257, 258, 259
  heme-deficient, 257–258
  variegate, 257, 258, 259, 260
Porphyrinogins, 260
Portal cirrhosis, 237
Portal hypertension, 238
Postural proteinuria, 95
Potassium, serum, 86–89
  hyperaldosteronism with, 326, 327, 329
  hyperkalemia with, 87–88
  hypertension with, 115
  hypokalemia with, 88–89
  pregnancy and, 364
Potassium, stool, in diarrhea, 227, 228
Potassium, urine
  hyperaldosteronism with, 326
  hyperkalemia with, 88
  renal disease and, 101
Prealbumin, thyroxine (T_4) binding, 295
Prednisolone, 322
Prednisone, 322
Preeclampsia, 47
Pregnancy, 353–383
  adrenal function in, 377–378
  alpha feto protein (AFP) in, 349, 378–379
  amniotic fluid bilirubin in, 357–359
  amylase in, 360–362
  anemia evaluation in, 356–357
  carbohydrate metabolism in, 362–363
  coagulation studies in, 363–364
  cortisol in, 322, 323
  diabetes mellitus and, 271–272
  electrolytes in, 364–365
  erythroblastosis fetalis and hemolytic disease
    of newborn and, 380–382
  fetal lung maturity in, 382–383
  glucose tolerance tests and, 270, 271

hematology in, 354–357
hemoglobin and hematocrit in, 355–356
human chorionic gonadotropin (hCG) in, 276,
  335–336, 353
17-hydroxycorticosteroids (17-OHCS) in, 323
hypoglycemia in, 276
infectious diseases and, 365–367
intrauterine, 354
leukocytes in, 357
lipids in serum in, 367
liver function tests in, 243, 244, 246, 247,
  367–374
pituitary hormones in, 374–375
plasma volume changes in, 354, 355
platelets in, 357
red cell mass in, 355
renal function in, 376–377
rubella in, 365–367
testing for, 353–354
testosterone values and, 334
thyroid function in, 380
Preleukemia, 36
Prerenal azotemia, 102, 104
Pretest disease likelihood, 12–13, 14
Prevalence of disease, 12–13
Primidone, 67, 69, 323
Probenecid, 208
Procainamide, 62, 69, 71–72
Progesterone, 322
  breast cancer receptors and, 350, 351
  congenital adrenal hyperplasia (CAH) and,
    331
  hyperventilation in pregnancy and, 365
  measurement of, 335
  pregnancy and, 377
Progestins, 330, 350, 351
Proinsulin, 277
Prolactin, 288–290, 334
  amenorrhea with, 281, 337
  chlorpromazine and, 289
  dopaminergic agonist in suppression of, 290
  female infertility and, 339
  gynecomastia and, 338
  impotence and, 338
  insulin tolerance test (ITT) for, 284, 289
  male infertility and, 339
  measurement of, 336
  pituitary tumors with, 287
  pregnancy and, 374
  serum levels of, 288–289
  stimulation tests for, 289
  thyrotropin-releasing hormone (TRH) and, 289
Properdin, 182, 183
Propoxyphene, 70, 330
Propranolol, 288, 297
Propylthiouracil, 35, 297
Prostatic cancer, 349–350
Protein
  cerebrospinal fluid (CSF), 264–265
  chronic renal failure with, 104
  ^{51}C-labeled, in stool tests, 226
  drug binding to, 63–64
  hematuria with, 109
  malabsorption of, 222, 247
  pleural field, 140
  pregnancy and, 367
  proteinuria and, 94
  quantitation of loss of, 226
  SI measurements of, 20–21

tests for urinary, 94
thyroid-binding, 293, 295
Protein A, 169
Protein immunoelectrophoresis (IEP), 184–185
cardiomyopathy with, 117
kidney stone disease with, 318
Proteinuria, 93–95
acute glomerulonephritis with, 107
hematuria with, 109
oval fat bodies with, 92
postural, 95
urinary protein tests in, 94
Prothrombin, in malabsorption, 220
Prothrombin time (PT), 51–55, 58
clotting cascade in, 51, 52–53
liver function with, 235
pregnancy and, 363
Protoporphyria, 257, 258, 259
Pseudogout, 197, 198, 199, 200
Pseudohyperkalemia, 87–88
Pseudohyponatremia, 84
Pseudohypoparathyroidism, 314, 317
Pseudomonas aeruginosa, 150, 156
Pseudotumor cerebri, 207
Psoriatic arthritis, 207
Psychotropic drugs, 40
Pulmonary disease, 119–142
clinical laboratory tests in, 137–142
computerized axial tomography (CT) in, 123–124
contrast studies in, 122
eosinophilia in, 40, 41
fluoroscopy in, 122
lung scans in, 122–123
pleural fluid examination in, 140–141
pulmonary function tests in, 124–137
roentgenographic examination of chest in, 119–124
serological tests in, 141–142
sputum examination in, 137–139
tomography in, 121
ultrasound of thorax in, 123
Pulmonary embolism, 122, 123
Pulmonary fibrosis, 126, 205
Pulmonary function tests, 124–137
airflow in, 126–130
arterial blood gases in, 132–135
diffusion in, 132
exercise testing in, 136–137
gas exchange tests in, 132–137
lung compliance in, 130
lung volumes in, 124–126
single breath nitrogen washout test in, 131–132
Pulmonary infiltration with eosinophilia (PIE) syndrome, 40
Pyelonephritis, 92, 149
Pyrogen stimulation test, 323
Pyrophosphate arthropathy, 199
Pyruvate kinase deficiency, 47
Pyuria, 108

Quinacrine, 318
Quinidine, 48, 318
Quinidine gluconate, 71
Quinidine sulfate, 69, 71

RA cells, synovial fluid, 198
Radial immunodiffusion, 181, 182, 186
Radioallergosorbent tests (RAST), 179–180
RAIU, see Iodine, radioactive uptake (RAIU) test

Raji cell binding assay, 185–186, 207
Range of normal, see Normal range of values on laboratory tests
RAST (radioallergosorbent tests), 179–180
Raynaud's phenomenon, 187
RBC, see Red blood cells (RBC)
Reactive hypoglycemia, 270, 278
Reagin test, 266
Red blood cells (RBC)
antibodies against, 191–192
cerebrospinal fluid (CSF), 263, 264
color abnormalities in, 43
complement fixation (CF) assay with, 167
hypertension with, 115
microorganisms in, 44
morphology of, 41–44
pleural fluid, 140
polycythemia and, 32–33
pregnancy and, 355, 356
range of abnormalities in, 41–42
T. gondii agglutination assay with, 166
variants of, 42
Red cell casts
acute glomerulonephritis with, 107
hematuria with, 109
nephrosis with, 106
renal failure with, 103, 104
Red cell distribution width (RCDW), 57
Regan isoenzyme, 242
Reiter's cells, 202
Reiter's syndrome, 207
Renal disease, 91–110
assessment of renal integrity in, 91–95
laboratory tests in, 101–110
potassium secretion in, 101
proteinuria in, 93–95
renal function tests in, 95–101
sodium conservation and, 100–101
urinary sediment examination in, 91–93
Renal failure, acute, 101–103
acute interstitial nephritis with, 108
dexamethasone suppression test (DST) and, 324
growth hormone in, 286, 288
17-hydroxycorticosteroids (17-OHCS) in, 323
hypercalcemia and, 309
hyperkalemia and, 88
hypermagnesemia with, 312
hyperphosphatemia with, 317
hypertension and, 115
osteomalacia with, 319
oxalate in, 311
pregnancy and, 376–377
prolactin and, 288–289
Renal failure, chronic, 103–105
hypocalcemia and, 314
Renal function tests, 95–101
anemia and, 30–31
cystinuria with, 98
distal tubular acidification in, 100
distal tubular function on, 98–101
Fanconi syndrome with, 97–98
glomerular filtration rate (GFR) in, 96–97
potassium concentration in, 101
proximal tubular function on, 97–98
sodium conservation in, 100–101
urinary concentrating ability in, 98–99
Renal insufficiency, 96, 98
Renal stones, see Kidney stone disease
Renal tubular acidosis (RTA)

distal, 100
hypomagnesemia with, 318
hypophosphatemia and, 316
kidney stone disease and, 320
osteomalacia with, 319
proximal, 98
urine pH in, 311, 312
Renin
adrenal tumors with, 115
renovascular hypertension with, 116–117
Renovascular hypertension, 116–117
Reserpine, 289, 330, 338
Residual volume (RV), lung, 125
Resin uptake test, *see* Triiodothyronine resin
uptake test (T₃RU)
Respiratory acidosis, 80–81
blood gases in, 78
mixed acid-base disturbances with, 82–83
Respiratory alkalosis, 81
blood gases in, 78
hypophosphatemia and, 316
mixed acid-base disturbances with, 82
pregnancy and, 365
Respiratory distress syndrome in newborn, 382
Respiratory tract infections, 138, 177
Reticulocytes, 26, 28
Reticulocytosis, 29, 30
Reverse triiodothyroxine (rT₃), 298, 300
Rhabdomyolysis, 267
Rheumatic diseases, 197–209
antinuclear factor in, 205–206
biopsy of tissue in, 209
complement levels in, 206–207
HLA typing in, 207–208
sedimentation rate studies in, 204–209
synovial biopsy in, 204
synovial fluid examination in, 197–204
Rheumatic fever, 201
Rheumatoid arthritis, 35, 141, 195, 246, 247
antibodies in, 188, 191, 192
antinuclear factor in, 206
immunoglobulins with, 179, 183
sheep cell agglutination test (SCAT) in, 205
synovial fluid examination in, 200, 202, 203
Rheumatoid factor, 36, 169, 185, 203, 204, 205
Rh group, 192
Rh hemolytic disease, 381
Rhinitis, 178, 179
Ribonucleoprotein antigen, 191, 192
Rickets, 163, 319
Ring chromosome, 359
Ro antigen, 190
Rocket electrophoresis, 181
Roentgenography, chest, *see* Chest roentgenog-
raphy
Ropes test, 198
Rotor syndrome, 239, 240
Rouleaux, 41, 43–44
Rubella, 256, 365–367
evaluation timing in, 367, 368–372
serological data on, 171

Salicylic acid, 63, 69, 74–75, 80
Salivary gland disease, 215, 216
Salmonella, 227
Sarcoidosis, 142, 179, 180, 265
hypercalcemia and, 308
kidney stone disease and, 321
Schilling test, 212, 213

chronic pancreatitis with, 218
macrocytosis in anemia and, 28
malabsorption on, 222, 223, 225
Schistocytes, 46, 47
Schlichter test, 154–155
Scleroderma, 190, 191, 192, 206
Sclerosing cholangitis, 239
Scratch tests, 179
Screening tests, 13, 14–15
Secretin test, 213, 219
Sella tomography, 292
Semen analysis, 334, 337, 339
Seminoma, 348
Sensitivity of laboratory tests, 1, 6, 7–9
accuracy for positive and negative prediction
and, 10
aggregate of positive results with, 15
calculation of, 8, 9–10
exclusion test and, 14
screening test and, 14
spectrum of disease in tested population and,
8–9
tandem use of other tests with, 14–15
Sepsis
gonococcal, 207
gram-negative, 151–152, 207
Septicemia, 183
Serology, 163–172
agglutination tests in, 166
antibody measurement in, 166–168
antigen detection in, 168–169
basic principles of, 163–164
cerebrospinal fluid (CSF) in, 165–166
complement fixation (CF) assays in, 167
diarrhea with, 227
enzyme-linked immunospecific assay (EIA) in,
167–168
IgM antibody-IgG antibody differences in, 164–
165
indirect immunofluorescence assays (IFA) in,
167–168
pulmonary disease with, 141–142
saving sera in, 163–164
specific infections in, 169–172
Serotonin, 342
Serum glutamic-oxaloacetic transaminase (SGOT)
cardiac, 112
liver function with, 231–233, 249
muscle disease with, 267
pregnancy and, 373
Serum glutamic pyruvate transaminase (SGPT)
liver function with, 233, 249
muscle disease with, 267
pregnancy and, 373
Serum sickness, 203, 207
Sex hormone-binding globulin (SHBG), 335, 378
Sex hormone deficiency, and pituitary disease, 281
SGOT, *see* Serum glutamic-oxaloacetic trans-
aminase (SGOT)
SGPT, *see* Serum glutamic pyruvate transaminase
(SGPT)
Sheep cell agglutination test (SCAT), in rheumatoid
arthritis, 205
Sheep red blood cells (SRBC), 175, 183
Shigella, 227
Short bowel syndrome, 213, 225
Shunts, venous admixture, 135
SI, *see* International System of Units (SI)
Sickle cell, 44, 47–48

Sickle cell anemia, 47, 100
Sickle cell disease, 44, 194
Sickle cell trait, 109
Sickle-hemoglobin C hemoglobinopathy, 47
Sickle thalassemia, 44, 47–48
Sideroblastic anemia, 43
Single breath nitrogen washout test, 131–132
Sjögren's syndrome, 100, 188, 189, 190, 191,
    192, 205, 206
Skin disorders, 40, 41
Skin tests
    allergen, 180
    delayed-type hypersensitivity (DTH), 175, 176,
        177, 180
    scratch tests in, 179
    wheal and flare, 178–179
SLE, *see* Systemic lupus erythematosis (SLE)
Small bowel
    malabsorption and bacterial overgrowth in, 223,
        225
    obstruction of, 342
Small intestine diseases, 219–223; *see also*
    Malabsorption
Sm antigen, 191, 206
Smoking, and carcinoembryonic antigen (CEA), 347
Smooth muscle antibodies, 187, 188, 189
Sodium, dietary, in hyperaldosteronism, 327
Sodium, serum, 83–86
    hypernatremia with, 85–86
    hypertension with, 116
    hyponatremia with, 83–85
    pregnancy and, 364
Sodium, stool, and diarrhea, 227, 228
Sodium, urinary, 102
    fractional excretion of (FE_{Na}), 102
    renal disease and, 100–101
Sodium ipodate, 297
Sodium nitroprusside test, in cystinuria, 98
Sodium urate crystals, synovial fluid, 199
Somatomedins, 286–287
Somogyi unit, 22
Specificity of laboratory tests, 1, 6, 7–9
    accuracy for positive and negative prediction
        and, 10
    aggregate of negative results in, 15
    calculation of, 8, 9–10
    confirmation test and, 14
    screening test and, 14
    spectrum of disease in tested population and,
        8–9
    tandem use of other tests with, 14–15
Spherocytes, 28, 44, 45–46
Spherocytosis, 194
Sphingomyelin, 382–383
Sphygmomanometers, 22
Spiky red cells, 44, 46–47
Spirometry, 137
Spironolactone, 318, 329, 330, 338
Splenectomy
    idiopathic thrombocytopenic purpura (ITP)
        after, 49
    leukocytosis with, 37–38
    lymphocytosis and, 38
    spiky red cells after, 47
    target cells after, 44
Splenomegaly
    neutropenia with, 35, 36
    pancytopenia with, 49, 50
    polycythemia and, 31, 32, 33, 34

    thrombocytopenia with, 55
Sporotrichosis, 142
Sprue, 224, 246, 342
Spur cells, 46
Sputum examination, 137–139
    cytological examination in, 139
    Gram stain in, 138, 145
    legionellosis in, 170
    Mycobacterium tuberculosis with, 159–160
    transtracheal aspiration in, 139
Stains
    Gram, 145–146
    tissue, 146–148
Staphylococcal enteritis, 146
Staphylococci infections, 148
Staphylococcus aureus, 155, 169
Staphylococcus epidermis, 149
Steady state in drug therapy, 63, 65
Steatorrhea, 218, 235
Steroid crystals, synovial fluid, 199
Steroids
    calcium in hypercalcemia diagnosis with, 308–
        310
    cholestasis with, 239, 241
    lymphopenia with, 36
    ovarian pathology and, 379
    pituitary function with, 282
Stomach cancer, 212
Stomach diseases, 211–213
    gastric secretion tests in, 211–212
    gastrin tests in, 213
    intrinsic factor (IF) secretion tests in, 212
    pepsin and mucus secretion tests in, 212
Stomatocytes, 44, 48
Stones
    biliary tract, 240
    kidney, *see* Kidney stone disease
Stool tests
    anemia and, 30
    ^{51}C-labeled proteins in, 226
    diarrhea with, 227–228
    fat malabsorption on, 221–222, 224, 225
    gastrointestinal diseases on, 211
    Gram stain of, 146
    pancreatitis with, 218
Storage pool disease (SPD), 55
Streptococcal glomerulonephritis, 183
Streptococcal infections, 149
    acute glomerulonephritis with, 107, 108
    antibody to, 168
    antigen tests for, 169, 170
    serological data on, 168, 169–170
Streptococcal meningitis, 170
Streptococcus faecalis, 159
Streptococcus faecium, 159
Streptococcus pneumoniae, 170
Streptokinase/streptodornase, 175, 180
Streptolysin, 168
Streptomycin, 159
Stress
    cortisol and, 322
    growth hormone and, 286
    prolactin and, 289
    thyroid function tests and, 300, 302
Stress polycythemia, 33
Subacute bacterial endocarditis (SBE), 151, 183,
    186, 203, 205
Subacute sclerosing panencephalitis, 265
Subarachnoid hemorrhage, 263

Substance, SI unit for amount of, 17, 20
Sucrose tolerance test, 221
Sulfa drugs, 108
Sulfasalicylic acid test, 94, 105
Sulfonylureas, 239
Surrogate tests, 1, 12–13
Synovial fluid biopsy, 204
Synovial fluid examination, 183, 197–204
    classification of sample fluid in, 198, 200–201
    crystals seen in, 198–199
    cultures in, 203–204
    differential analysis by stained smear of, 202–203
    handling sample in, 197–198
    immunologic measurements on, 203
    white cell count in, 199–202
Syphilis, 192, 266, 365
Systeme International d'Units (SI), *see* International System of Units (SI)
Systemic lupus erythematosis (SLE), 141
    antibodies in, 189–190, 191, 192, 193, 195
    C3 and C4 in, 182, 183, 186
    LE cell factor in, 189–190
    nephrotic syndrome with, 106
    neutropenia in, 35
    synovial fluid examination in, 201, 202, 203

T_3, *see* Triiodothyronine (T_3)
T_4, *see* Thyroxine (T_4)
Tamm-Horsfall protein, 92
Tamoxifen, 351, 352
Tapeworm, 222
Target cells, 44, 45
T cells, 175–176
    delayed-type hypersensitivity (DTH) skin testing of, 175, 180
    mitogen phytohemagglutinin (PHA), 176, 177
Teardrop-shaped red cells, 44, 48
Technetium scans, with thyroid function, 299, 300, 302
Telepaque, 297
Temperature, in SI measurement, 22
Temporal arteritis, 243
Terbutaline, 332
Testape, 272, 273
Testicular cancer
    alpha feto protein in, 349
    gynecomastia in, 338
    human chorionic gonadotropin (hCG) in, 348
Testosterone, 334, 335
    congenital adrenal hyperplasia (CAH) with, 330
    free concentration of, 334
    gynecomastia and, 338
    hypogonadism screening with, 285–286
    indications for use of, 291, 292
    male infertility and, 339
    osteoporosis with, 313
    pregnancy and, 377–378, 379
    virilization disorders and, 337
Tetanus toxoid, 175, 180
Tetracycline, 98
Tetrahydroaldosterone, 328
Thalessemia, 29, 31, 44, 357
Theophylline, 69, 75–76
Thiazides
    acute interstitial nephritis with, 108
    calcium measurements and, 303
    hypercalcemia and, 310
    hypertension with, 116
    thrombocytopenia with, 48

Thrombocytopenia, 48–49, 54, 55
    antibodies in, 191
    chronic lymphocytic leukemia with, 39
    pancytopenia with, 50
Thrombocythemia, 49
Thrombocytosis, 49
Thromboembolism, 56
Thrombotic thrombocytopenic purpura (TTP), 47
Thymoma, 267
Thyroglobulin, 298
Thyroid, medullary carcinoma of (MCT), 298, 339, 340, 341
Thyroid antibodies, 187, 188
Thyroid-binding proteins, 293, 295, 380
Thyroid carcinoma, 188, 298, 299, 326
Thyroid disease, 292–302
Thyroid function tests, 294–299
    calcitonin (CT) levels in, 298
    free thyroxine (FT_4) and free thyroxine index (FT_4I) in, 296
    free thyroxine (FT_4) by dialysis in, 296, 300
    free thyroxine (FT_4) by radioimmunoassay (RIA) in, 296
    free thyroxine concept in, 292–293
    free triiodothyronine index (FT_3I) in, 294
    ^{123}iodine (^{123}I) scans in, 299–301
    osteoporosis and, 312
    pregnancy and, 380
    reverse thyroxine (rT_3) in, 298
    technetium pertechnetate ($^{99m}TcO_4^-$) scans in, 299
    thyroglobulin levels in, 298
    thyroid hormone binding proteins in, 293
    thyroid-stimulating immunoglobulins (TSI) in, 299
    total thyroxine (TT_4) in, 294–295
    triiodothyronine radioimmunoassay (T_3RIA) in, 296–297
    triiodothyronine resin uptake test (T_3RU) in, 293–294
    ultrasound of thyroid in, 301
Thyroid hormone deficiency, and pituitary disease, 281
Thyroiditis, 189, 301
    iodine scan in, 299
    laboratory tests in, 300, 302
Thyroid nodule, 340
    calcitonin levels in, 298
    laboratory tests in, 300, 302
Thyroid-stimulating hormone (TSH)
    hyperthyroidism with, 298
    hypothyroidism with, 297–298, 301, 380
    pregnancy and, 353, 354, 374, 375, 380
    thyroid function and, 291, 292, 297–298, 300
Thyroid-stimulating immunoglobulins (TSI), 299
Thyrotropin-releasing hormone (TRH)
    growth hormone and, 288
    hyperthyroidism with, 297, 301
    prolactin and, 289
    stress and, 300, 302
Thyrotoxicosis, 242, 310
Thyroxine-binding globulin (TBG), 295
Thyroxine (T_4), 293
    free, *see* Free thyroxine (FT_4); Free thyroxine index (FT_4I)
    pregnancy and, 380
    kidney stone disease and, 318
    osteoporosis with, 313
    total, *see* Total thyroxine (TT_4)

triiodothyronine (T₃) production and, 297
Tidal volume (V_T), lung, 124
Time, in SI units, 21
T lymphocytes, *see* T cells
Tobramycin
  combination therapy with, 158, 159
  pharmacokinetics of, 66–67, 69
Tolbutamide, 277
Tolerance, bacterial, 155–156
Tomography
  of chest, in pulmonary disease, 121
  see also Computerized axial tomography (CT)
Total lung capacity (TLC), 125, 126, 128
Total parenteral nutrition, 318
Total thyroxine (TT₄), 292, 293, 294–295, 300
  hyperthyroidism with, 301, 302
  hypothyroidism with, 301
  stress and, 300, 302
  thyroiditis with, 300, 302
Total triiodothyronine (TT₃), 293, 296, 300
Toxemia of pregnancy, 362, 377
Toxin ingestion, 80
Toxoplasma gondii, 163, 166, 172
Toxoplasmosis, 38, 39, 365
Tracheomalacia, 130
Transaminase, 1
  hepatitis B with, 254
  liver function and, 248, 249
Transcortin, 322
Transferrin
  liver function and, 247, 248
  pregnancy and, 356, 367
Transtracheal aspiration, in sputum examination,
    139
Treponema pallidum immobilization (TPI) test,
    193
TRH, *see* Thyrotropin-releasing hormone (TRH)
Triamcinolone, 322
Triamterene, 329
Trichinosis, 267
Trichophyton, 175
Trichopoliodystrophy, 247
Tricyclic antidepressant drugs, 288, 289
Triglycerides, 111–112
  cardiovascular disease and, 111–112
  fat malabsorption and, 222
  normal values by age for, 112, 113
  pregnancy and, 367, 373
Triiodothyronine (T₃), 285, 293
  free (FT₃), 293
  free index (FT₃I), 293, 294, 297
  kidney stone disease and, 318
  osteoporosis and, 313
  physiology of production of, 297
  pregnancy and, 380
  total (TT₃), 293, 296, 300
Triiodothyronine (T₃) by radioimmunoassay (RIA),
    296–297
  hyperparathyroidism with, 301, 302
  stress and, 302
Triiodothyronine resin uptake test (T₃RU), 292,
    293–294, 295, 300
  hyperthyroidism with, 301
  stress and, 300, 302
  thyroiditis with, 300, 302
Trophoblastic disease, 348
Trough levels of drugs, 64–65
Trypsin, 217
Tryptophan, 342

TSH, *see* Thyroid-stimulating hormone (TSH)
Tube dilution assay, 152–154
Tuberculin test, 1, 15, 175
Tuberculosis, 1, 15, 140, 142, 159–161, 201, 205
  hypercalcemia and, 308
  T cell tests in, 180
Tuberculous meningitis, 266
Tubular necrosis, acute, 101–102
Turner's syndrome, 337
Tyramine, 332

UcAMP, *see* Cyclic AMP, urine (UcAMP)
UDP glucuronyl transferase, 238–239
Ulcerative colitis, 191
Ultrasound
  of thorax, 123
  thyroid function with, 301
Unipolar depression, 322, 323, 324
Upper respiratory tract infections, 177
Urea nitrogen, blood, *see* Blood urea nitrogen
    (BUN)
Uremia, 80, 82
Uremic pleuritis, 140
Uric acid, serum
  drugs affecting, 203, 208
  kidney stone disease with, 320–321
  rheumatic diseases with, 203, 208
Uric acid, urine, 307–311
  hypertension with, 115
  kidney stone disease with, 320–321
  pregnancy and, 376–377
  rheumatic diseases with, 208, 209
Uric acid stones, 307–311, 320–321
Urinary concentrating ability, 98–99, 99–100
Urinary sediment examination, 91–93
  abnormal values in, 92–93
  acute glomerulonephritis with, 107
  acute renal failure with, 103
  normal values in, 91–92
Urinary tract infections, 115, 148, 152
Urine colony count, 148–149
Urine culture and sensitivity (C&S), 311, 320–321
Urine pH, 311–312
  kidney stone disease with, 320–321
  osteomalacia with, 319
Urine tests
  chronic pancreatitis with, 218–219
  Gram stain in, 145
  osmolality of, 99, 103
  refractive index of, 99
  specific gravity of, 99
Urobilinogen, 239–240, 245
Uroporphyrin, 257, 258
Uroporphyrinogen, 260
Urticaria, 179, 184, 195

Vaccine, polyvalent pneumococcal, 170
Vaginal smear, in gonadal disease, 337
Vagotomy, 212
Valproic acid, 69, 70
Vanillylmandelic acid (VMA)
  diet with, 332
  multiple endocrine neoplasia syndromes
    (MENs) with, 341
  pheochromocytoma and, 330–332, 333
Van den Bergh reaction, 238
Variegate porphyria, 257, 258, 259, 260
Vasculitis
  acute glomerulonephritis with, 107, 108

C3 and C4 in, 182
erythrocyte sedimentation rate (ESR) in, 194, 195
immunoglobulins in, 187
rheumatoid factor tests in, 205
Vasoactive intestinal polypeptides (VIP)-secreting tumor, 228
Vasopressin
  adrenocorticotropic hormone (ACTH) and, 284, 323
  hypoadrenalism with, 323
  pregnancy and, 375
Venereal Disease Research Laboratory (VDRL), 107, 192–193, 266
Venous admixture, 135
Ventilation/perfusion (V/Q) ratios, 133
Ventilation scans, 122, 123
Ventilatory failure, 81
Very low density lipoprotein cholesterol, 367
Vibrio cholera, 227
Viral arthritis, 203
Viral hepatitis, 183, 189, 249–256
  bilirubin in, 239
  "e" antigen (HB$_e$Ag) in, 253
  "e" antigen antibody (anti-HB$_e$) in, 253–254
  hepatitis A diagnosis in, 249–250
  hepatitis B diagnosis in, 250–252
  hepatitis non-A, non-B diagnosis in, 256
  serology of, 249–256
  serum glutamic-oxaloacetic transaminase (SGOT) in, 233
  surface antigen (HB$_s$Ag) in, 252–253
  surface antigen antibody (anti-HB$_s$) in, 254–256
Viral infections
  antibody response in, 165
  C3 and C4 in, 182
  complement fixation (CF) assay with, 167
  immunoglobulins and, 176, 177
  serological tests with, 163
  sputum examination with, 138–139
  stains and techniques for, 146, 147
  T cells in, 175, 180
  thrombocytopenia with, 48
Viral meningitis, 264, 266
Viridans streptococci, 149, 150
Virilization disorders, 337, 379
Vital capacity (VC), lung, 125
Vitamin A, 220, 309
Vitamin B$_6$, 342
Vitamin B$_{12}$, 42
  anemia and, 28, 29
  intrinsic factor (IF) and, 212
  malabsorption and, 220, 222, 223
  pancreatitis and, 218
Vitamin C, 226
Vitamin D, 307, 319
  kidney stone disease and, 321
  osteomalacia and, 319
  toxicity of, 308, 321
Vitamin K
  factors II, VII, IX, and X in liver and, 235
  prothrombin time (PT) with, 54
Vitiligo, 188
Von Willebrand's disease, 53

Waldenstrom's macroglobulinemia, 185, 187, 191
Wasserman test, 266
Water
  hypernatremia and excretion of, 86
  sodium excess and, 83

Water loading test, and antidiuretic hormone (ADH), 291
Watson-Schwartz test, 258, 260
Wegner's granulomatosis, 108, 194
Westergren erythrocyte sedimentation rate (ESR), 194
Wheal and flare skin tests, 178–179
Whipple's disease, 223, 225
Wilson's disease, 246, 247, 267
Wintrobe erythrocyte sedimentation rate (ESR), 194
White blood cells (WBC)
  acute glomerulonephritis with, 107
  cerebrospinal fluid (CSF), 263, 264
  hypertension and, 113–114
  leukopenia and, 34–37
  neutropenia and, 34–35, 36
  new technology for counts of, 57–58
  normal ranges for, 26, 34–35
  synovial fluid, 199–202
  urinary sediment examination with, 91–92
  variations in, with repeats, 34
White cell casts, in chronic renal failure, 104
Women, infertility in, 339

Y chromosome, 337, 338
Year, 21
Yeast cells, cerebrospinal fluid (CSF), 267
Yersinia, 227

X-rays, *see* Chest roentgenography
D-xylose tolerance test, 220, 223, 224

Zero-order elimination of drugs, 62–63
Zollinger-Ellixon syndrome, 213